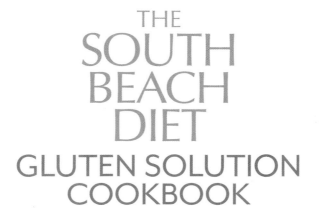

THE
SOUTH
BEACH
DIET

GLUTEN SOLUTION
COOKBOOK

THE
SOUTH
BEACH
DIET
GLUTEN SOLUTION
COOKBOOK

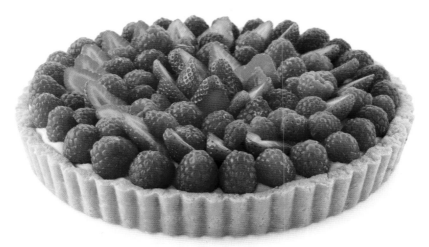

ARTHUR AGATSTON, MD

© 2013 by Arthur Agatston, MD

The South Beach Diet® is a Registered Trademark of the SBD Holdings Group Corp.

All rights reserved. No part of this publication may be reproduced or transmitted in any form
or by any means, electronic or mechanical, including photocopying, recording, or any other information
storage and retrieval system, without the written permission of the publisher.

Rodale books may be purchased for business or promotional use or for special sales.
For information, please write to:
Special Markets Department, Rodale Inc., 733 Third Avenue, New York, NY 10017.

Printed in the United States of America

Rodale Inc. makes every effort to use acid-free ♾, recycled paper ♲.

Book design by Carol Angstadt

Photographs by Mitch Mandel/Rodale Images

Food styling by Adrienne Anderson

Prop styling by Paige Hicks

On the front cover: Green and White Pasta, page 204; Summer Berry Tart, page 260;
and Oat Cake Quesadillas, page 90

On the back cover: Lemon Zucchini Bread, page 44

On the title page: Summer Berry Tart, page 260

Library of Congress Cataloging-in-Publication Data is on file with the publisher.

ISBN-13: 978–1–62336–047–4   hardcover

Distributed to the trade by Macmillan

2   4   6   8   10   9   7   5   3   1   hardcover

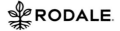

We inspire and enable people to improve their lives and the world around them.
rodalebooks.com

TO MY WIFE, SARI,
AND SONS, EVAN AND ADAM

CONTENTS

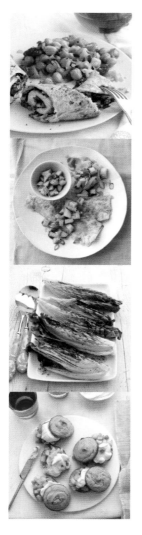

ACKNOWLEDGMENTS

THERE ARE MANY PEOPLE who deserve credit for the time and energy they devoted to this book.

At Rodale, I would like to thank executive editor Trisha Calvo for her editorial expertise; art director Carol Angstadt for the striking design; photographer Mitch Mandel for his creative vision; food stylist Adrienne Anderson for making the recipes look so good; and prop stylist Paige Hicks for the beautiful backgrounds. I would also like to thank senior project editor Nancy N. Bailey for shepherding the book to completion and Beth Lamb, Brent Gallenberger, and Kristin Kiser for their marketing expertise.

For creating all of the original gluten-free recipes in this book, my special thanks go to Kate Slate, Sandra Rose Gluck, and Vanessa Maltin Weisbrod.

My appreciation as well to my agent, Mel Berger, of William Morris Endeavor, and publicists Sandi Mendelson and Cathy Gruhn of Hilsinger-Mendelson East in New York City.

I would also like to thank South Beach Diet nutrition director, Marie Almon, for the considerable time she spent planning and reviewing the book, and editorial director, Marya Dalrymple, for overseeing the project while also helping me to remain gluten aware.

Finally, this book, and *The South Beach Diet Gluten Solution* book that inspired it, would not have happened without the insights and support of my wife and partner, Sari Agatston.

FOREWORD

ON THE SOUTH BEACH DIET, we have always recommended eating a wide variety of healthy whole foods, including whole grains like wheat, barley, and rye that contain the protein gluten. And that hasn't changed. So how does a gluten-free cookbook fit in with our long-standing South Beach Diet eating principles?

To answer that, let me go back in time for a moment. The ironic thing is, just as I never intended to write a best-selling diet book when I created the South Beach Diet back in the early 1990s, I never expected to be writing about gluten today. But then, a few years ago, I had an epiphany when I realized I had new information to share that could potentially affect the lives of millions of people. I decided to write *The South Beach Diet Gluten Solution*, and now this companion cookbook.

The South Beach Diet Gluten Solution came about because for years I had noticed that many individuals on Phase 1 of the South Beach Diet, which was *intentionally* grain free but *unintentionally* gluten free, not only lost weight but often felt so great that they hesitated to progress to Phase 2. When they reintroduced gluten-containing grains on Phase 2, they often stopped feeling great. I eventually realized that gluten was the culprit explaining these observations. So I created the South Beach Diet Gluten Solution Program (see page 2) to help people figure out whether gluten could be at the root of their health problems.

There's no question that for some people—about 1 percent of the population—gluten can be a matter of life or death. These people have a condition known as celiac disease. True celiacs, as they are called, are so sensitive to gluten that even a small amount can make them very sick. Gluten damages the lining of the small intestine in those with celiac disease, preventing the absorption of certain nutrients. This can lead to a host of health problems ranging from chronic diarrhea and abdominal cramping to osteoporosis and even the risk of some cancers.

Unless you are part of that 1 percent (and only special tests will let you know if you are), it's unlikely that you will need to live a completely gluten-free lifestyle.

But I have found that many of my patients are nevertheless gluten sensitive—they don't have celiac disease, but consuming gluten still leads to problematic symptoms. What's interesting is that the level of gluten sensitivity varies from person to person. It's not a black or white condition.

That said, the only way that you can find out just how gluten sensitive you are, if at all, is to give up gluten for a few weeks. When people who are gluten sensitive eliminate foods containing gluten, they start to feel much better, often within a few days. They have better digestion, fewer headaches, sounder sleep, sharper mental focus, more energy, clearer skin and are generally in a better mood. They may even feel relief from more serious chronic conditions, like fibromyalgia, psoriasis, and thyroiditis. It's when they slowly begin to reintroduce gluten-containing foods in small quantities, after being off them for a while, that they learn which of these foods—or how much of them—can be consumed without triggering symptoms. It's the process of eliminating then gradually reintroducing gluten-containing foods that allows you to become what I call gluten aware.

I firmly believe that each individual needs to determine his or her own level of gluten sensitivity and awareness while enjoying the widest range of nutrient-rich foods possible: high-fiber vegetables, fruits, and whole grains, as well as lean protein and good fats. Remember, gluten free doesn't mean grain free (there are plenty of gluten-free whole grains such as brown rice, wild rice, and quinoa that are good for you), and it certainly doesn't mean sacrificing essential nutrients like vitamins, minerals, and fiber. It also doesn't mean giving up all bread, pasta, and those occasional decadent desserts, as you'll see by paging through this book.

In working with our nutritionist and recipe developers to create this cookbook, I knew I wanted to give people healthy gluten-free recipes that they could draw upon as they were embarking on my Gluten Solution Program, and well beyond. I wanted recipes that, like all of the healthy South Beach Diet dishes in all of our cookbooks, were free of refined starches, sugar, and artery-clogging saturated fats, and packed with plenty of wholesome nutrients. I wanted recipes that were so delicious that no one would ever realize they were gluten free.

I got what I wanted: 175 mouthwatering recipes that will help you achieve better health whether you turn out to be gluten sensitive or not. And yes, the recipes in this book will help you lose weight if you want to. As the creator of the South Beach Diet, I wouldn't have it any other way.

—Arthur Agatston, MD

*Batter-Baked Cod with
Homemade Mango Chutney
(see page 126)*

COOKING THE GLUTEN SOLUTION WAY

WELCOME to the world of healthy and delicious gluten-free cooking, South Beach Diet style. We've applied the same proven principles that have helped millions of South Beach dieters lose weight and achieve better health to a flavor-packed cookbook for those concerned about gluten. Yes, you will lose weight if you enjoy our gluten-free recipes as part of an overall healthy eating plan. And by eating gluten free for a few weeks, you're likely to see common symptoms of gluten sensitivity such as bloating, abdominal pain, headaches, stiff joints, fatigue, sinus problems, brain fog, depression, and skin rashes disappear too.

Many people are under the misconception that gluten free is synonymous with inferior taste. That certainly does not have to be the case, as the recipes in this book will prove. What is true, though, is that unless carefully planned, a gluten-free diet can be *nutritionally inferior* to one that contains wheat, barley, and rye, particularly if a person relies on gluten-free packaged products as staples. While gluten-free foods may not contain the troublesome protein, they're often packed with saturated fat, sugar, and sodium. Many also include high-glycemic refined ingredients like white rice flour and potato starch that can cause swings in your blood sugar and trigger cravings.

These are concerns you won't have to worry about when you cook from this book. Each recipe was developed with good nutrition and flavor in mind. In fact, these dishes do more for your health than subtract gluten from your diet. They protect against heart disease, cancer, and diabetes. And they have been designed to help you lose weight if you want to—something that not every gluten-free diet program or cookbook can deliver. In other words, they are good for your overall

1

health, even if gluten doesn't turn out to be a problem for you. And they're also recipes you'll want to make time and again for your family and friends (who may or may not be gluten sensitive) because they're easy to make and they taste so good.

ABOUT THE SOUTH BEACH DIET GLUTEN SOLUTION PROGRAM

You certainly don't have to be gluten free to enjoy the recipes in this book, but having an overview of the South Beach Diet Gluten Solution Program's basic tenets may help you better understand how gluten could be affecting your life.

As with the original South Beach Diet, the Gluten Solution Program has three phases, which are designed to help you lose weight and ultimately achieve better health. Which phase you start on depends on how much weight you have to lose and whether you have cravings for sugary and starchy carbohydrates. You'll learn whether you are gluten sensitive—and to what degree—by giving up gluten for 4 weeks, then gradually reintroducing foods containing gluten to see if they trigger symptoms.

Note: While the Gluten Solution Program itself is not specifically designed for people with celiac disease, who must remain totally gluten free for life, the recipes in this book can be enjoyed by anyone with this condition (be sure to check labels on all ingredients carefully).

One important difference between the South Beach Diet Gluten Solution Program and some other gluten-free plans is the inclusion of non-gluten-containing whole grains. We do eliminate all grains on Phase 1 of the Gluten Solution Program, just as we do on Phase 1 of the original South Beach Diet, in order to stabilize your blood sugar and help you get a grip on cravings. But beginning on Gluten Solution Phase 2, we reintroduce healthy whole grains that don't contain gluten—amaranth and buckwheat and brown rice, to name a few—but do contain fiber, as well as vitamins and minerals that are hard to get in other foods. In addition, as always, our emphasis is on getting plenty of other good carbohydrates as well, such as vegetables, beans, and whole fruits.

Take a look at the glossary of ingredients that are used in this book, which begins on page 270. It will give you an overview of just how many naturally gluten-free foods you can choose from when planning meals from breakfasts to desserts. As you page through the recipes and look at all the taste-tempting photos, you'll quickly realize that gluten free doesn't mean giving up the foods you love, or sacrificing flavor or satisfaction.

What follows is a description of the Gluten Solution phases in a nutshell. For complete information on the program, you may want to read *The South Beach Diet Gluten Solution*, which offers complete food lists for each phase as well as additional recipes and meal plan ideas. You can also visit southbeachdiet.com/glutensolution for more information and support.

GLUTEN SOLUTION (GS) PHASE 1

If you have more than 10 pounds to lose and have cravings for sugar and starchy foods as well as symptoms of gluten sensitivity, you should start on GS Phase 1. During the 2 weeks on GS Phase 1, you won't be eating any wheat, barley, or rye, or products made from these grains, and you'll do your best to avoid products with gluten additives, such as certain types of soy products, imitation crabmeat, and blue cheese. In fact, as with the original South Beach Diet plan, you won't be eating any grains at all, or fruits for that matter, because we want you to get the blood sugar swings that cause your cravings under control. If that sounds difficult, don't worry. We have plenty of tasty, satisfying Phase 1–appropriate recipes in this book. You'll be losing weight fairly rapidly—up to 10 pounds in 2 weeks—and your gluten-sensitivity symptoms will begin to diminish and perhaps disappear. After 2 weeks you will move on to GS Phase 2 (see "If you are entering GS Phase 2 from GS Phase 1," below).

GLUTEN SOLUTION (GS) PHASE 2

If you have fewer than 10 pounds to lose and no cravings but do have gluten-sensitivity symptoms, you can begin the Gluten Solution Program on Phase 2 and stay gluten free—but not grain free—for 4 weeks. Your weight will drop steadily, although more slowly than if you were to have started on GS Phase 1, about 1 to 2 pounds a week. Since you don't have a lot of weight to lose, you can have three gluten-free starches and three servings of fruits per day the first week, utilizing the recipes in this book. If you aren't dropping 1 to 2 pounds a week, cut back on the number of starches and fruit servings. You will experiment with adding gluten back into your diet after being gluten free for 4 weeks, but you'll remain on GS Phase 2 until you reach a healthy weight.

If you are entering GS Phase 2 from GS Phase 1, you'll continue to stay gluten free for 2 more weeks, but you should *gradually* introduce gluten-free grains and fruits, working up to three servings of each per day over the 2-week period (if your weight loss stalls, cut back). You will experiment with adding gluten back into your diet after being gluten free for a total of 4 weeks, but you'll remain on GS Phase 2 until you reach a healthy weight.

If you have no weight to lose and no cravings, but are experiencing gluten-sensitivity symptoms, you can do a modified GS Phase 2. This means you won't have to limit yourself to three gluten-free starches and three fruits a day, as is required for those with cravings or those who want to drop pounds. After 4 weeks of being gluten free, you move on to GS Phase 3.

No matter where you begin the Gluten Solution Program, at the end of 4 weeks on the program, gradually reintroduce some healthy, gluten-containing starches, swapping them for the gluten-free starches. (If you have been diagnosed with celiac disease, do not reintroduce gluten into your diet.) We recommend adding one gluten-containing food to your diet each day during the first week and carefully monitoring your reaction to it. If you're fine with one serving of gluten each day, you can add a second daily serving of a gluten-containing food the second week, working up to a maximum of three a day as the week progresses. You will know quickly if a food triggers symptoms (and/or cravings); if so, stop eating it. It may take a few weeks of trial and error to find your level of gluten tolerance, and you may discover that you aren't gluten sensitive at all.

GLUTEN SOLUTION (GS) PHASE 3

This is the maintenance phase of the Gluten Solution Program. You have achieved your healthy goal weight on GS Phase 2, you know what triggers your cravings and/or your gluten-sensitivity symptoms, and you know how to make the right food choices for you. You have become gluten aware, not gluten phobic, and you know that no food is absolutely off-limits, unless you say it is.

All of the recipes in this book have been marked with the appropriate phase, depending on the ingredients a recipe contains. Remember, Phase 1 recipes can be included on Phase 2, and all can be enjoyed on Phase 3, whether you are on the Gluten Solution Program or the traditional South Beach Diet.

HOW TO USE THIS BOOK

For ease of use, we've organized this book the way most people like to cook, beginning with a variety of breakfast dishes, moving on to appetizers and snacks, then main dishes, and finally tantalizing desserts. For those who like lighter meals, there are chapters on soups and sandwiches, as well as salads, and for those who prefer not to eat meat, a chapter of meatless main dishes. The chapter on side dishes will prove very useful as you plan meals for the week.

As you look at the specific recipes, do so with an eye to what phase of the diet you're on. If you're on Gluten Solution Phase 1, for example, you'll be avoiding starches (bread, pasta, rice) and sugars (including fruits and fruit juice), just as you would on the traditional South Beach Diet program, but you'll still find plenty of satisfying recipes to choose from, including some Phase 2 recipes where we've simply swapped out an ingredient to make the recipe GS Phase 1 friendly (you'll see these marked Phase Switch). Once you're on GS Phase 2 or GS Phase 3, you can of course enjoy all the recipes in the book.

Every recipe features Hands-On Time (the active time you spend in the kitchen chopping, stirring, seasoning, and so on) and Total Time (how long it takes to make a dish from start to finish), including a notation if a dish needs to marinate or chill for any length of time. In addition, if a recipe can be made in 30 minutes or less, and more than half of the recipes in this book can, you'll see the icon, below, to indicate this.

Where pertinent, you'll find tips for making the dishes ahead, along with suggestions on how to refrigerate or freeze finished dishes for future use. We have also provided ideas for turning one recipe into another (called Variations). For example, our Slow-Cooker Pulled Beef (page 186) could serve 12 for a party, or you can make it ahead, freeze it, and turn it into a variety of dishes like Beef Tostadas, Quick Beef Soup, Beefy Pasta, or Sloppy Joes. Our Green Lentil Salad (page 114) can easily become a main dish by adding whatever type of lean protein you prefer (we suggest pork). Also keep in mind that you always can alter a recipe to use what's seasonal or freshest at the market. If the cod or halibut looks better than the grouper, for example, use it in the California Fish Tacos (page 128). In summer, when peaches or strawberries are at their best, use one of them instead of apples in the Caramelized Apple Mini-Shortcakes (page 256).

Whichever recipes appeal to you, we suggest that you read through them in advance, plan a week's worth of menus, then make sure you have all the ingredients and equipment on hand (see page 13 for kitchen gear essentials). This will save you time and money too.

SURVEYING YOUR KITCHEN

The key to a healthy kitchen often lies in what's not in it rather than what is, and this is particularly true when you're embarking on a gluten-aware lifestyle. The first step is to take a good look at the contents of your cupboards, fridge, and freezer, and remove problem foods, particularly the highly processed sugary and starchy carbs—

GLUTEN-FREE PHASE 1 DESSERTS

You'll be giving up all starches and fruits on Phase 1 of the Gluten Solution Program, but that doesn't mean you can't have dessert. Here are two of our South Beach Diet Phase 1 favorites. After 2 weeks on GS Phase 1, you'll be able to sample all the delicious gluten-free desserts found in this book, beginning on page 249. For more GS Phase 1 desserts, go to southbeachdiet.com/glutensolution.

CHILLED ESPRESSO CUSTARD
HANDS-ON TIME: 10 MINUTES · TOTAL TIME: 25 MINUTES PLUS CHILLING TIME

1½ cups 1% milk

2 large eggs, beaten

3 tablespoons monk fruit natural no-calorie sweetener (baking formula)

2 teaspoons espresso powder

1 teaspoon vanilla extract

Ground cinnamon, for topping

In a medium bowl, whisk together the milk, eggs, monk fruit sweetener, espresso powder, and vanilla until well blended. Pour into four 6-ounce custard cups and place the cups in a deep skillet.

Fill the skillet with water to come halfway up the custard cups. Bring the water to a simmer over high heat. Reduce the heat to low, cover the pan with foil, and continue to simmer for 10 minutes. Carefully remove the cups from the pan, cover the custards with plastic wrap (it can touch), and refrigerate for at least 3 hours or overnight. When ready to serve, sprinkle with cinnamon.

MAKES 4 (6-ounce) SERVINGS ▶ Per serving: 81 calories, 3.5 g fat, 1.5 g saturated fat, 6 g protein, 6 g carbohydrate, 0 g fiber, 86 mg sodium

the full-fat ice cream, the candy bars, the chips, the pretzels—that shouldn't be in any healthy eater's kitchen in the first place. The next step is to remove or put away *all foods that contain gluten* for 4 weeks if you're following the Gluten Solution Program. You won't need these foods for the recipes in this book anyway.

You should also check your fridge and freezer for anything that has exceeded its expiration date, looks less than savory, or has freezer burn. Also open up containers of

CREAMY LEMON-VANILLA RICOTTA SOUFFLÉS
HANDS-ON TIME: 15 MINUTES · TOTAL TIME: 30 MINUTES

Olive oil cooking spray

1 cup part-skim ricotta cheese

2 large eggs, separated

3 tablespoons monk fruit natural no-calorie sweetener (baking formula)

2 teaspoons grated lemon zest

½ teaspoon lemon extract

½ teaspoon vanilla extract

Pinch of salt

Preheat the oven to 375°F. Lightly coat four 4-ounce ramekins with cooking spray.

In a large bowl, whisk together the ricotta, egg yolks, 1 tablespoon of the monk fruit sweetener, lemon zest, and lemon and vanilla extracts until well combined.

In another large bowl, with an electric mixer at high speed, beat the egg whites and salt until soft peaks form, 2 to 3 minutes. Add the remaining 2 tablespoons of monk fruit sweetener and continue beating until stiff peaks form.

Gently fold one-third of the egg whites into the ricotta mixture just until combined. Repeat with the remaining egg whites.

Spoon the ricotta mixture into the ramekins. Bake until the soufflés have risen and are set and lightly browned, about 15 minutes. Serve immediately.

MAKES 4 (½-cup) SERVINGS ▶ **Per serving:** 130 calories, 7 g fat, 4 g saturated fat, 10 g protein, 5 g carbohydrate, 0 g fiber, 180 mg sodium

herbs and spices and put them to the "smell test." If any smell musty or have no smell at all, they are too old and should be thrown out and replaced. Also taste all your salad and cooking oils to make sure that they haven't become rancid. If they smell or taste acrid, throw them out.

Here's a quick guide to clearing out your pantry for those who are interested in following the Gluten Solution Program. You'll be getting rid of foods containing gluten and also those that are simply bad for you, period. Some of these foods only need to be removed from your kitchen during GS Phase 1 and can be gradually reintroduced on GS Phase 2. Those that contain gluten must be eliminated for 4 weeks.

BAKED GOODS: Breads, bagels, rolls, cakes, cookies, crackers, cupcakes, muffins, waffles, and all other baked goods if you are on GS Phase 1. You can gradually reintroduce gluten-free baked goods on GS Phase 2 and then those containing gluten (in moderation, of course) after you've been gluten free for 4 weeks.

BEVERAGES: Fruit juices, sugary sodas, wine, beer, spirits, and any other sugary drink particularly with high-fructose corn syrup. Red and white wine and certain other gluten-free spirits can be reintroduced on GS Phase 2.

CANDY: All candies, except those that are gluten free and sugar free. Gluten-free dark chocolate can be reintroduced in moderation on GS Phase 2.

CEREALS: All cereals on GS Phase 1. Low-sugar, high-fiber, gluten-free cereals can be enjoyed on GS Phase 2, with additional cereals added after 4 weeks of being gluten free.

CONDIMENTS, DRESSINGS, AND SEASONINGS: All condiments that are not gluten free, particularly soy sauce (check labels) and teriyaki sauce. Also barbecue sauce, honey mustard, ketchup, and any other condiment or sauce made with corn syrup, molasses, or sugar.

DAIRY AND CHEESE: Whole and 2% milk, full-fat soy milk, full-fat and frozen yogurt, and ice cream; cheeses made with anything but 1%, part-skim, or fat-free milk; full-fat cheeses.

FATS/OILS: All solid vegetable shortening or lard, butter, and hydrogenated or partially hydrogenated oils.

FLOUR: All flours and packaged products made with flour (such as pancake and waffle mixes) as well as gluten-free flours and cornmeal on GS Phase 1. Gluten-free flours and cornmeal can be reintroduced on GS Phase 2, as can flours with gluten once you've been gluten free for 4 weeks.

FRUIT: Fresh fruits, dried fruits, frozen fruits, and canned fruits. As explained earlier, you give up these foods for only 2 weeks in order to get control of swings in blood sugar and cravings. Even nutritious fruit has sugar. Fresh, frozen, and canned fruits (not in heavy syrup) and dried fruits can be part of your diet on GS Phase 2.

MEAT AND POULTRY: Anything processed with sugar (honey-baked or maple-cured ham, for instance); fatty fowl such as goose and duck legs; pâté; dark-meat chicken and turkey (legs and wings); processed fowl such as packaged chicken nuggets or patties; beef brisket, liver, rib steaks, skirt steak, bacon (except Canadian and turkey), bologna, pepperoni (except turkey), salami, and other fatty meats.

PASTA: All pasta. Gluten-free pasta is permitted on GS Phase 2, and pasta containing gluten can be gradually introduced once you've been gluten free for 4 weeks.

POTATOES AND OTHER STARCHY VEGETABLES: You can have carrots, corn, sweet potatoes, winter squash, and other starchy vegetables again on GS Phase 2. However, white and instant potatoes and beets should be on the menu only occasionally and only once you've lost the weight you need to.

RICE: All rice, including white rice, jasmine rice, and sticky rice. You can introduce white and brown basmati rice, black rice, regular brown rice, and wild rice on GS Phase 2.

SNACK FOODS: All unhealthy packaged snacks such as cheese puffs, chips, pretzels, and cookies, even if they're gluten free. You can enjoy high-fiber, high-protein, low-sugar, gluten-free snack bars on GS Phase 2 and gradually reintroduce some that contain gluten once you've been gluten free for 4 weeks.

SOUP: All powdered soup mixes (many are full of trans fat and sodium) and any canned soups containing cream, hydrogenated oils, or gluten additives, such as modified food starch.

SWEETENERS: Ditch white sugar, brown sugar, honey, molasses, and corn syrup as stand-alone products permanently. You can use agave nectar in moderation on GS Phase 1 and stevia, monk fruit natural no-calorie sweetener, and other sugar substitutes if you so choose. In this book we use only all-natural agave nectar and monk fruit sweetener in our recipes.

VEGETARIAN MEAT SUBSTITUTES: Seitan, soy bacon, soy burgers, soy chicken, soy crumbles, soy hot dogs, soy sausage, and tofu with seasonings that might contain gluten. You may be able to introduce some of these products, once you determine your level of gluten sensitivity.

BECOME A SAVVY FOOD SHOPPER

Now that you've cleaned out your kitchen, it's time to fill it up again. Gluten-aware shopping requires the same "skills" you'd normally bring to buying healthy foods for yourself and your family. It's just that you'll have to get into the habit of not putting anything with gluten into your basket for a while, including the whole-wheat breads and pastas that may have become a staple at your house. You may also find that you'll have to go further afield to locate some ingredients like amaranth, black soybeans, and masa harina, which may not be in your local supermarket but are often available at health-food stores or online (see page 295).

PLAN MEALS IN ADVANCE

To save time, and money, it's best to plan your meals a week ahead, make a list of all the ingredients you'll need for each recipe (ideally organized by the way the store is laid out to save shopping time), and then shop as few times as possible. Plan for a visit to the farmers' market or food co-op too, and don't forget about the food you may have signed up to get from a Community Supported Agriculture (CSA) group. By making a complete shopping list, you'll be better able to knock off foods from the list that you may already have. The list will also help you figure out your grocery expenses ahead of time and prevent unhealthy impulse buys from creeping into your cart.

As you're making the list, consider who in your family will be home when and whether you'll need to make take-along breakfasts, snacks, and lunches during the week. Also plan for some meals using leftovers. For example, the chilled Baked Salmon with Spinach and Couscous (page 135) is delicious for lunch the next day; the Turkey Moussaka (page 162) can easily be frozen and reheated; and leftover Orange-Maple Pork Tenderloin (page 191) can be used more than once in stir-fries and salads or for sandwiches on gluten-free johnnycakes (see page 87).

In many families, there may only be only one person who is trying to avoid gluten (including a child at the suggestion of a pediatrician), but there's really no point in cooking multiple meals. All of the recipes in this book are so tasty that you won't get any complaints, even from the kids, when you make recipes like Crispy-Topped Mac and Cheese (page 214), "Sesame" Noodles (page 225), and Pork Meatballs with Broken Spaghetti (page 196). And for those who are avoiding meat as well as gluten, there's an entire chapter of meatless gluten-free dishes that can be enjoyed on more than just "Meatless Mondays."

Remember, healthy gluten-aware cooking doesn't mean that everything at every meal has to be made from scratch. Many supermarkets offer a wide variety of prepared foods, like rotisserie chicken and turkey breast, baked salmon, and steamed shrimp, as well as prechopped and shredded vegetables, bagged lettuce mixes, sliced and chopped fruits, shredded reduced-fat cheeses, and chopped garlic and onions, that are gluten free and great time-savers. Just read labels carefully (see "Be a Gluten Sleuth," below) and ask how a precooked dish has been prepared.

BE A GLUTEN SLEUTH

Once you've compiled your shopping list and are actually in the store, it's not quite as simple as grabbing the first can of chicken broth you see or choosing any soy sauce or deli meat. Learning how to read product labels is essential if you really want to avoid gluten in your diet. If you've been on the traditional South Beach Diet plan, you already know that we strongly recommend looking at both the Nutrition Facts panel *and* the ingredient list to ensure you're buying nutritious foods that aren't highly refined and that don't have high levels of saturated fats, trans fats, sugars, or sodium. You'll also have to search the label for gluten in its obvious and hidden forms.

Fortunately, the FDA now requires that any product labeled "gluten free" must contain less than 20 parts per million (ppm) of gluten—the amount most people with celiac disease can safely tolerate. Food manufacturers under FDA jurisdiction also have to identify, *in plain English,* any ingredient from a list of eight major food allergens. This means that if a food contains milk, eggs, fish, crustacean shellfish, tree nuts, peanuts, *wheat*, or soybeans, the label is required to say so. This identification can be done in one of two ways: 1) by listing the allergen in the ingredient list in parentheses after a food, or 2) by adding a "Contains" statement at the end of the ingredient list.

In the first instance, enriched flour in the ingredient list would have a parenthetical next to it that clearly states *(wheat);* lecithin would have *(soy);* whey would have *(milk);* and so on. With the second option, you'd simply see Contains: Wheat, Soy, and Milk. Some manufacturers choose to do both. But because gluten is not only found in wheat—and barley, rye, and oats are not covered by the labeling law—you will still have to read the ingredient list carefully if the "Contains" option is all that's used. Most careful gluten-aware buyers use the "Contains" statement only as a quick way to eliminate a product, not as a quick way to determine if it is safe. Luckily, rye is not used in that many foods, and the label usually lists it simply as "rye" when it is there. Barley may be listed as barley malt or as malt, malt syrup, malt extract, malt flavoring, or simply as "flavoring." As for oats, you can assume that if they are listed without the words "gluten free" next to them, they may be contaminated with wheat.

Some manufacturers also voluntarily add a line to the food label that reads something like this: "Manufactured in a facility that also produces products made with wheat" or "Manufactured on equipment that also produces products that contain wheat." Note that our South Beach Diet gluten-free products and the equipment they are produced on are routinely tested and guaranteed to meet or exceed the FDA standard for "gluten free." Our products are also certified by the Gluten-Free Certification Organization.

So these are the basics. But gluten can still hide in the ingredient list under various other guises. Some of the words to watch out for include *binder* or *binding, thickening* or *thickener, emulsifier, edible starch, gum base, filler, modified food starch* (this is usually made from corn, but if it contains wheat, it must say so) or *modified starch, special edible starch, triticale, rusk, wheat alternative,* and *maltodextrin* (even though this word begins with *malt,* it is gluten free and is usually made from corn, potato, or rice; if wheat is used, the label would have to say *wheat maltodextrin* or *maltodextrin [wheat]*). Another potential gluten-containing ingredient, hydrolyzed vegetable protein (HVP), must specify the vegetable or grain it's made from, such as hydrolyzed wheat protein, which is not gluten free, or hydrolyzed soy protein, which is.

The bottom line here is: If in doubt, call the manufacturer. Many products list the phone number right on the package.

START COOKING

Now that you've planned and shopped, it's time to have some fun in the kitchen. Knowing that you've got most of your ingredients on hand before you start to cook makes food preparation a lot easier.

Whether you're cooking for yourself, your family, or a group of friends, making gluten-free dishes relies on the same healthy cooking techniques you're probably already familiar with—steaming, grilling, stir-frying, and sautéing (in olive oil, not butter!), as well as roasting and baking. You'll find that most recipes in this book will allow you to get an entire meal on the table in well under an hour, even if you're a novice cook. But there are a few, like the Tofu-Mushroom Lasagna (page 216),

Asparagus, Portobello, and Tuna Bake (page 142), Golden Chicken Cottage Pie (page 164), and Italian Tamales (page 176), that do require more time and effort. It will be worth it.

COOK AHEAD

If you work long hours or are busy with kids, consider cooking ahead, since you may not always have time to whip something up from scratch for every meal. Knowing there's a meal already prepared in the fridge or freezer to simply reheat is certainly a major stress-reliever. On weekends, when possible, cook a few dishes in big batches. By preparing more food than you need at one time, you'll be able to turn one meal into two (or more!). Soups and stews like our Chicken, Butternut, and Quinoa Soup (page 66), Hearty Tomato and Meatball Soup (page 69), Chunky Turkey and Black-Eyed Pea Stew (page 172), and Chickpea-Fennel Stew with Greens (page 208) are good examples of dishes that can be made in larger batches, then frozen for future meals. You can also make and freeze extra meatballs from the Pork Meatballs with Broken Spaghetti recipe (page 196); extra loaves of "Everything" Oat Bread (page 86); or almost any of the other baked goods in this book. See the Make Ahead tips included in many recipes for ideas of what can be prepared in advance.

If weekend cooking is impossible, try to do some prepping in the evenings when you can. Cut up veggies, chop herbs, and precook ground beef, turkey, and chicken, for example. Then refrigerate them so you can put a meal together faster when you get home from work or your day's activities.

HAVE THE RIGHT GEAR

The best cooks rely on quality kitchen tools, which can be huge time-savers. The good news is that unless you have celiac disease, or are living with someone who does, or you are extremely gluten sensitive, you won't need to buy a dedicated toaster, colander, sifter, baking pans, cutting boards, and other utensils to prevent cross contamination in your kitchen.

What you will need is some essential equipment that can save you time slicing, dicing, beating, whipping, and blending. If you're familiar with the South Beach Diet, you already know that cooking with nonstick skillets, saucepans, griddles, and grill pans is essential if you want to use less fat. But there are a

(continued on page 16)

DOES IT OR DOESN'T IT? A GLUTEN CRIB SHEET

Here's a short list of the most common foods that contain gluten, and some you wouldn't have expected, along with a list of safe grains for those who are going gluten free.

FOODS TO WATCH OUT FOR

Keep an eye out for wheat, barley, and rye under many guises.

Barley

Barley enzymes

Barley extract

Barley grass

Barley malt

Barley pearls

Bran

Bread flour

Bulgur

Bulgur wheat

Couscous

Croutons

Dextrin

Dinkel (also known as spelt)

Durum wheat

Einkorn wheat

Emmer wheat

Farina

Farro or faro (also known as spelt)

Flour containing wheat, barley, rye, or any of their derivatives, including bleached flour and enriched bleached flour

Fu (dried wheat gluten sold as sheets or cakes; used in Asian dishes)

Graham flour

Hordeum vulgare (a type of barley)

Hydrolyzed wheat gluten

Hydrolyzed wheat protein

Kamut (a fine whole-meal flour made from low-gluten, soft-textured wheat; also known as chapati flour)

Macha (spelt wheat)

Malt

Malt extract

Malt flavoring

Malt syrup

Malt vinegar

Matzo and matzo meal

Meat, poultry, seafood, or vegetables that are breaded, floured, served with a sauce made from wheat, or marinated in a wheat-based sauce such as soy or teriyaki

Mir wheat

Rice malt

Rice syrup, brown (it may contain barley)

Rye

Seitan (a meatlike food derived from wheat gluten used in many vegetarian dishes)

Semolina

Spelt

Sprouted wheat or barley

Tabbouleh

Triticale

Udon

Vital wheat gluten

Wheat

Wheat berries

Wheat bran

Wheat bread

Wheat flour

Wheat germ

Wheat oil

Wheat protein

Wheat starch

SNEAKY GLUTEN

Many of these foods may be made with or without gluten, so you need to read labels carefully. Most people don't have to worry about the gluten in lipstick, nutritional supplements, or medicine, but if you're highly gluten sensitive, you might.

Bacon, imitation (may contain wheat)

Baking powder

Beer (all forms except those labeled gluten free)

Breading, coating mixes, and panko

Brewer's yeast (if a by-product of beer)

Chocolates and candies (may contain fillers, wheat flour, or barley malt)

Communion wafers (may contain wheat)

Cooking spray for baking (may contain wheat flour)

Croutons

Fillers (could be wheat)

Flour or cereal products

Lipstick/lip gloss (may contain gluten fillers)

Marinades/dressings (may contain malt/fillers)

Medications/vitamins/ herbal supplements (may contain wheat/ gluten fillers)

Miso (may contain barley)

Mustard, yellow (may contain wheat)

Mustard powder (may contain wheat)

Nondairy creamer

Oats, oatmeal, and other oat products (may be cross-contaminated)

Pastas made with wheat, including couscous, orzo

Poultry, self-basting

Processed deli meats, reduced-fat sausages, hot dogs, or other smoked, cured, or processed meats that have modified food starches used as a binder

Sauces, gravies with modified food starch or other gluten additives

Seafood, imitation (may contain wheat)

Soy sauce or soy sauce solids (may contain wheat)

Spice blends (may contain wheat)

Stock, broth, or bouillon (may contain gluten additives like modified food starch)

Stuffings/dressings

Surimi (artificial crab)

Teriyaki sauce

Thickeners (roux)

Toothpaste (dental products)

Yogurt (flavored) and other flavored dairy products

SAFE GRAINS

Many people get confused when it comes to grains. Here are some gluten-free grains that can be enjoyed.

Amaranth

Buckwheat, 100% (despite its name, it's not wheat)

Corn

Cornmeal

Millet

Oats (if certified gluten free by the manufacturer)

Quinoa

Rice, basmati (brown and white)

Rice, black

Rice, brown

Rice, wild

Teff

number of other tools that will make preparing the recipes in this book so much quicker and easier:

SHARP KNIVES: Good sharp knives can really speed up food preparation. And you don't have to spend a fortune buying a matching 12-piece set, since all you really need are four: a 3- or 4-inch paring knife for peeling, mincing, and slicing small items; an 8- or 10-inch chef's knife for chopping, dicing, mincing, and julienning, and for slicing meat, fish and poultry; a long, serrated bread knife (which you can also use for slicing tomatoes or tofu); and an 8- or 10-inch carving knife with a slender blade.

A good knife can be made of carbon steel, stainless steel, or high-carbon stainless, but most people prefer knives made from high-carbon stainless because they hold their edge and shiny appearance longer and are easier to sharpen. To hold maximum sharpness, always keep your knives in a free-standing rack or attach them to a magnetic strip. Never store them in a kitchen drawer where their delicate edges will be abraded by other gadgets kept there. To clean your knives, always wash by hand (never in the dishwasher). Too much water and harsh detergents can dull and distort both handles and blades.

FOOD PROCESSOR: A food processor is ideal for chopping, slicing, and shredding vegetables as well as for grinding beef, poultry, and pork for burgers and meatballs. It will come in handy for grinding the meat for the Sirloin Burgers with Grilled Scallions (page 188) and Pork Meatballs with Broken Spaghetti (page 196). A food processor is also a quick way to make the dough for a pie crust like Citrus Yogurt Pie (page 254). For some recipes, we've indicated that a standard blender may work just as well.

MINI FOOD PROCESSOR: This indispensable gadget is available with a bowl capacity of 1½ to 3 cups. It doesn't take up much space on your counter and comes in handy for speedily chopping herbs and garlic. It is also ideal for making your own nut flours for dishes like Coconut-Almond Chicken Strips (page 56) and grinding nuts to add to a salad dressing as we do for Artichoke, Edamame, and Walnut Salad (page 106). Make sure the mini processor you buy has a good-size feed tube.

SPICE GRINDER OR COFFEE GRINDER: You can use this instead of a mini food processor for grinding nuts and seeds (buy one and dedicate it to this purpose). You can also grind your own espresso beans to make "instant" espresso powder for the Chocolate Walnut Espresso Cake (page 253).

ELECTRIC HAND MIXER OR STAND MIXER: You'll need either a hand or stand mixer for quickly beating egg whites and for preparing batter for a number of baked goods in this book. As its name suggests, a hand mixer is a convenient handheld mixing device with one or two beaters. Stand mixers are larger and have more powerful motors than hand mixers. They generally have a special bowl that is locked in place while the mixer is operating. A typical home stand mixer will include a wire whip for beating egg whites; a flat beater for mixing batters; and a dough hook for kneading. Either type of mixer is fine for the recipes in this book.

IMMERSION/STICK BLENDER: This handheld tool makes easy work of puréeing soups, sauces, dips, and smoothies. It has a long, narrow stem with rotary blades at the end so you can immerse it right in the pot, bowl, or glass (and avoid dirtying the food processor or blender). Look for one with a powerful motor that is lightweight enough to hold comfortably. Cordless models offer the greatest convenience. We use an immersion blender for a wide variety of tasks, from puréeing sweet potatoes for the Golden Chicken Cottage Pie (page 164) and strawberries for Strawberry-Apple Breakfast Fool (page 34) to thickening the broth for Chickpea-Fennel Stew with Greens (page 208).

LARGE SAUCEPAN/DUTCH OVEN: Many of the soups and stews in this book, like Butternut and Black Bean Stew (page 206) and Green Curry with Scallops and Peppers (page 138), call for a large saucepan or Dutch oven (4 to 7 quarts is ideal) with a tight-fitting cover. A Dutch oven, which is basically a large pot with "ear" handles, is particularly convenient because it can be used on the stovetop and in the oven. Look for a nonstick Dutch oven, which is easier to clean than the enameled cast-iron models.

SLOW COOKER: With a slow cooker you can get a dinner going early in the day and forget about it until it's time to eat. Or, in a reverse move, you can use the slow cooker overnight to make big soups, chilis, and stews to freeze for later use. We simmer the beef for Slow-Cooker Pulled Beef (page 186) for 7 hours in a slow cooker.

TART PAN: You will need a 9-inch tart pan with a removable bottom to make the Summer Berry Tart (page 260). Though it's not essential, a pan with a nonstick coating makes for easier removal and cleaning.

MUFFIN TIN: We use a standard 12-cup muffin tin for our Coconut-Apple Muffins (page 25), Gingerbread Muffins (page 26), and Caramelized Apple

Mini-Shortcakes (page 256). A jumbo muffin tin is ideal for the Mini Salmon Loaves (page 136), but you can also use a regular muffin tin and produce smaller loaves.

BELGIAN WAFFLE IRON/MAKER: You'll need a waffle iron for our Belgian Waffles (page 24). Even if it's nonstick, spraying it with a little olive oil cooking spray before pouring in the batter will make it easier to get the waffles out.

GRILL PAN: A ridged grill pan is ideal for grilling meat, fish, and vegetables on the stovetop and for making grilled cheese sandwiches. Though it can't replace the flavor of open-flame grilling, it does make nice char-grill marks. Some grill pans even come with hinged tops for making panini. We call for a grill pan for Spice-Rubbed Grilled Duck Breasts with Fresh Plum Salsa (page 168), Pan-Grilled Turkey Cutlets with Thai Relish (page 171), and Sirloin Burgers with Grilled Scallions (page 188), among other recipes. If you don't have a grill pan, you can use a cast-iron skillet instead.

TOASTER OVEN: This appliance is ideal for many tasks, including toasting nuts and reheating dishes you've made ahead and frozen.

STEAMER: You can use a steamer basket or collapsible steamer insert for steaming the vegetables in this book. We steam asparagus for our Asparagus in a Blanket (page 51) and sweet potatoes for the Chicken and Sweet Potato Salad with Spicy Peanut Dressing (page 96). A bamboo steamer basket works well for the Ginger-Garlic Eggplant Skewers (page 61).

MEAT MALLET: Having a meat mallet on hand makes flattening meat or even crushing peppercorns easier than using a heavy skillet. We flatten pork chops for the Braised Pork Rolls (page 193).

MICROPLANE ZESTER/GRATER AND BOX GRATER: These tools are ideal for grating or shredding fresh Parmesan and other hard cheeses, and for grating citrus zest, whole nutmeg, fresh ginger, and chocolate. You can also use the Microplane zester or box grater for quickly grating garlic and for grating apple and onion, as we do for the Piggy Burgers (page194).

Y-SHAPED PEELER: With so many fancy peelers on the market, this old-fashioned gadget (with just one moving part) often gets overlooked. Because it easily follows the shape of any fruit or vegetable, it's the fastest way to peel apples for our Strawberry-Apple Breakfast Fool (page 34), squash for Butternut and Black Bean Stew (page 206), and jícama for Jícama Cheese Toasties (page 83). Look for a peeler with a comfortable handle.

KITCHEN SCISSORS: If you're always using your household shears for kitchen tasks, now is the time to buy a dedicated pair. You'll find endless uses for them, from trimming the excess fat from poultry and beef to snipping out the tough stems from kale for Sautéed Kale, Bacon, and Sun-Dried Tomatoes (page 245) and chard for Rainbow Chard Salad with Sesame-Carrot Dressing (page 115).

SKEWERS: You'll need eight 10- or 12-inch skewers (or 16 smaller skewers if your steamer won't accommodate the longer ones) for the Ginger-Garlic Eggplant Skewers (page 61) and 6-inch or larger skewers for Chicken Kebabs with Minted Feta Sauce (page 152).

INSTANT-READ THERMOMETER: A good instant-read thermometer is the best way to test the temperature of roasted meats and poultry. Use one to ensure that the pork tenderloin is cooked perfectly to 145°F for Garlicky Roast Pork and Tomato Salad (page 102) and Mustard-Roasted Pork and Apple Salad (page 101).

NOW ENJOY

Cooking and eating as many meals as possible at home is healthier and far more satisfying than resorting to take-out food as so many families now do in this rush-rush world. Nationally, it is estimated that one in three meals is eaten out of the home, mainly at fast-food restaurants, and there's no question that the drive-thru is where America's problems with gluten overload begin.

If you know you've got health problems related to gluten, or someone in your family does, or you simply want to see if eliminating gluten for a while makes you feel better, cooking at home with the recipes from this book will help.

On the South Beach Diet, we have always recommended eating three wholesome meals a day as well as a midmorning and midafternoon snack to prevent the drop in blood sugar that typically results when you don't eat often enough. Skipping meals of course leads to fatigue and then cravings—often for those gluten-laden doughnuts, snack cakes, and pretzels that have caused you to feel bad enough to buy this book in the first place.

Those days of missed meals (and gluten overload) are over. With *The South Beach Diet Gluten Solution Cookbook* you'll nearly 200 healthy gluten-free solutions for breakfasts, lunches, dinners, snacks, and, yes, desserts, at your fingertips and you'll be well on your way to better health for life.

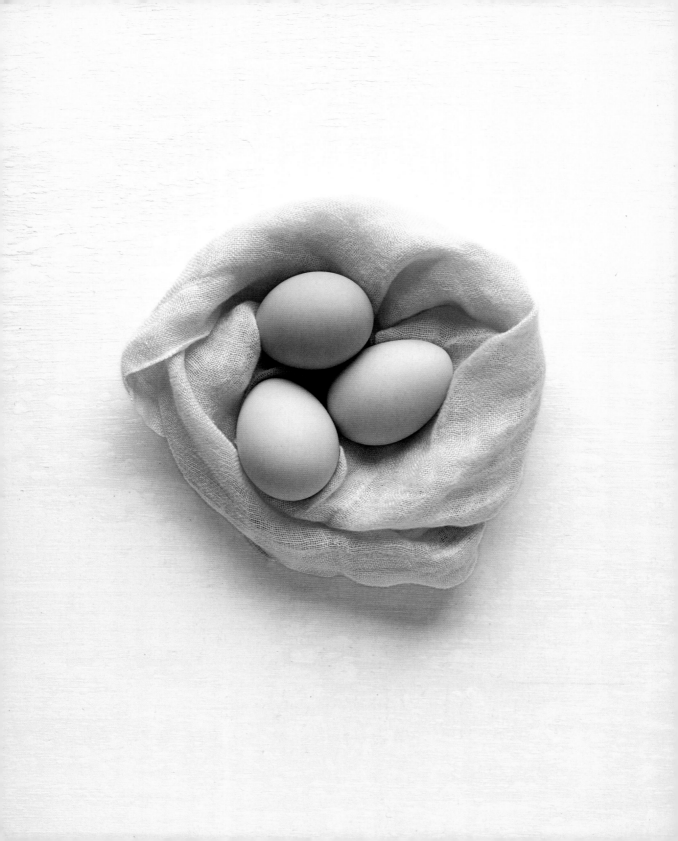

BREAKFAST

Gluten-aware or not, Rule Number One for a healthy diet (and weight loss): Never skip breakfast, even on the busiest of days. In this chapter you'll find plenty of easy-to-make, energizing egg dishes (eggs don't raise blood cholesterol in most people), as well as fiber-rich pancakes, waffles, biscuits, scones, muffins, and cereal made with gluten-free flours and grains. On hectic mornings, take along our protein-rich Banana Cream Pie Breakfast Shake or Strawberry-Apple Breakfast Fool.

BACON-PECAN BREAKFAST BISCUITS

HANDS-ON TIME: 10 MINUTES   TOTAL TIME: 40 MINUTES

PHASE 2

For a complete breakfast, split and toast these savory drop biscuits and top with a soft-boiled or poached egg, or with ¼ cup nonfat (0%) plain Greek yogurt or part-skim ricotta. Sprinkle with chopped chives, if desired.

⅓ cup pecans

1¼ cups brown rice flour

¼ cup nonfat dry milk powder

3 tablespoons flaxseed meal or ground chia seeds

¾ teaspoon gluten-free baking powder

¼ teaspoon salt

½ cup liquid egg whites

2 tablespoons extra-virgin olive oil

1 cup grated yellow squash (1 small squash, 5 ounces)

2 ounces gluten-free all-natural uncured Canadian bacon, finely diced

Preheat the oven to 350°F. Line a baking sheet with parchment paper.

In a mini food processor, grind the pecans with ¼ cup of the flour until the nuts are finely ground. Transfer to a medium bowl. Add the remaining 1 cup flour, the milk powder, flaxseed meal, baking powder, and salt. Blend well.

Make a well in the center of the dry ingredients and add the egg whites, oil, and ⅓ cup water. Stir until the dry ingredients are evenly moistened. Add the squash and Canadian bacon and use your hands to blend into the dough (as though you were making a meatloaf).

Using a ¼-cup measure, scoop out generous ¼ cups of dough and place on the baking sheet 2 inches apart (for a total of 8). With moistened hands, pat the dough into discs about ½ inch high and 2½ inches across.

Bake until lightly browned and a toothpick inserted in the center comes out clean, about 30 minutes. Transfer to a rack to cool.

MAKES 8 BISCUITS (1 per serving) ❭ **Per biscuit:** 185 calories, 8 g fat, 1 g saturated fat, 6 g protein, 22 g carbohydrate, 2.5 g fiber, 215 mg sodium

❬MAKE AHEAD❭ **The baked biscuits can be refrigerated for up to 1 week or frozen for up to 3 months. To freeze, arrange on a baking sheet and freeze solid, then transfer to a freezer container. Split and reheat in a toaster oven (thaw first if frozen).**

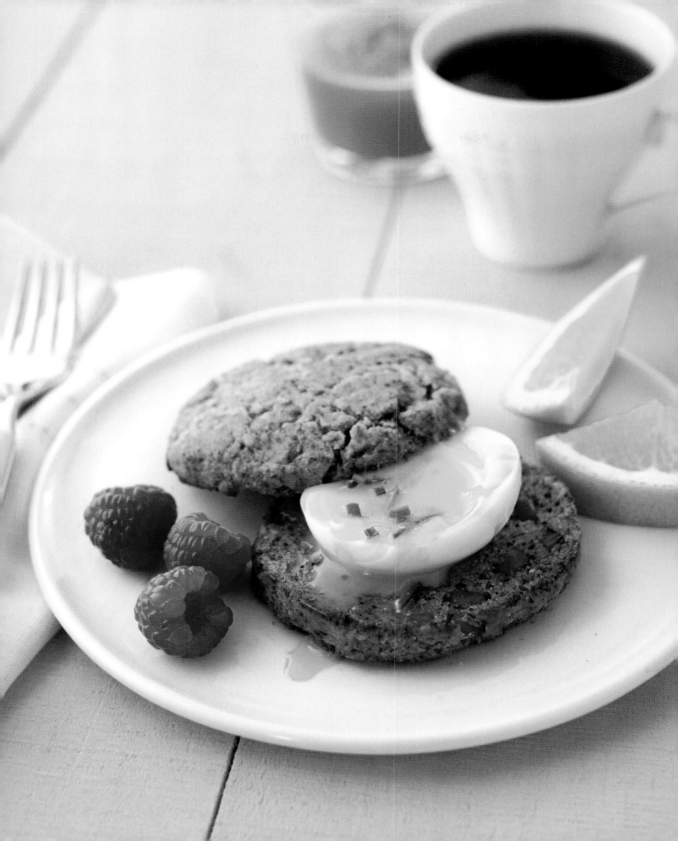

BELGIAN WAFFLES

HANDS-ON TIME: 25 MINUTES   TOTAL TIME: 25 MINUTES

PHASE 2

30 MINUTES OR LESS

The combination of buckwheat flour and teff flour produces a filling, fiber-rich, gluten-free waffle that's surprisingly light and fluffy. Top each waffle with ½ cup fresh berries or chopped fresh nectarines or peaches, or with ½ cup strawberry-apple purée (follow the instructions for the purée in Strawberry-Apple Breakfast Fool, page 34). If you don't have a Belgian waffle iron, use a regular waffle iron and follow the manufacturer's directions for how much batter to use.

1½ cups 100% buckwheat flour

¼ cup coconut flour

¼ cup teff flour

2 tablespoons monk fruit natural no-calorie sweetener (baking formula)

2 teaspoons gluten-free baking powder

½ teaspoon salt

2 cups fat-free milk

1 tablespoon fresh lemon juice

1 large egg yolk

1 tablespoon extra-virgin olive oil

2 teaspoons pure vanilla extract

3 large egg whites (don't use liquid egg whites here)

Olive oil cooking spray

In a medium bowl, whisk together the buckwheat flour, coconut flour, teff flour, monk fruit sweetener, baking powder, and salt.

In a separate medium bowl, whisk together the milk, lemon juice, egg yolk, oil, and vanilla. Mix the wet ingredients into the dry ingredients.

In another bowl, with an electric mixer at high speed, beat the egg whites until stiff peaks form. Gently fold the egg whites into the batter.

Preheat a Belgian waffle iron. Lightly spray the waffle iron with olive oil. Fill the waffle iron about two-thirds full with the batter and cook until golden brown (timing may vary with the waffle iron you are using). Repeat until all of the batter is used.

MAKES 6 WAFFLES (1 per serving) ▶ **Per waffle:** 217 calories, 5.5 g fat, 1.5 g saturated fat, 10 g protein, 33 g carbohydrate, 6.5 g fiber, 453 mg sodium

◀MAKE AHEAD▶ Make the entire batch of waffles and refrigerate for up to 1 week or freeze for up to 3 months. To freeze, arrange on a small nonstick baking sheet and freeze solid, then transfer to a freezer container. Reheat in a toaster oven to crisp up (from either refrigerated or frozen).

COCONUT-APPLE MUFFINS

HANDS-ON TIME: 10 MINUTES   TOTAL TIME: 35 MINUTES

For a healthy breakfast, enjoy the muffin with a scrambled egg and a glass of tomato juice. You can experiment with the spices here, adjusting the amounts to your own taste.

Olive oil cooking spray

1 cup sorghum flour

¼ cup coconut flour

¼ cup flaxseed meal

¼ cup monk fruit natural no-calorie sweetener (baking formula)

2 teaspoons gluten-free baking powder

1½ teaspoons ground cinnamon

¼ teaspoon ground ginger

¼ teaspoon grated nutmeg

¾ cup 1% milk

2 teaspoons extra-virgin olive oil

2 teaspoons pure vanilla extract

1½ cups grated carrots

½ cup grated green apple

½ cup grated red apple

½ cup unsweetened shredded coconut

3 large egg whites (don't use liquid egg whites here)

Preheat the oven to 350°F. Line a standard 12-cup muffin tin with paper liners and lightly spray with olive oil.

In a medium bowl, whisk together the sorghum flour, coconut flour, flaxseed meal, monk fruit sweetener, baking powder, cinnamon, ginger, and nutmeg.

In a bowl, with an electric mixer on low speed, beat together the milk, oil, and vanilla. With the mixer running, add the flour mixture in 3 additions, mixing well after each addition. By hand, gently mix in the carrots, apples, and coconut.

In a separate bowl, with an electric mixer at high speed, beat the egg whites until stiff peaks form. Gently fold the egg whites into the batter.

Spoon the batter evenly into the muffin cups. Bake until a toothpick inserted in the center of a muffin comes out clean, 24 to 28 minutes.

MAKES 12 MUFFINS (1 per serving) ▌ **Per muffin:** 120 calories, 5 g fat, 3 g saturated fat, 4 g protein, 16 g carbohydrate, 4 g fiber, 128 mg sodium

◀MAKE AHEAD▶ **You can make the muffins ahead and refrigerate for up to 1 week or freeze for up to 3 months. To freeze, arrange on a small baking sheet and freeze solid, then transfer to a freezer container. Thaw at room temperature and reheat, if desired.**

GINGERBREAD MUFFINS

HANDS-ON TIME: 10 MINUTES   TOTAL TIME: 35 MINUTES

PHASE
2

Buckwheat flour and sorghum flour are both exceptionally hearty flours, which makes them good companions to the dark and spicy flavors of ginger, cinnamon, and allspice. Enjoy one of these muffins as an accompaniment to scrambled eggs or egg whites, along with a slice of gluten-free Canadian bacon.

Olive oil cooking spray

¾ cup 100% buckwheat flour

¼ cup coconut flour

¼ cup sorghum flour

¼ cup flaxseed meal

2 teaspoons gluten-free baking powder

2 teaspoons ground cinnamon

2 teaspoons ground ginger

¼ teaspoon ground allspice

½ teaspoon salt

⅓ cup 1% milk

¼ cup unsweetened applesauce

3 tablespoons extra-virgin olive oil

1 large egg

¼ cup monk fruit natural no-calorie sweetener (baking formula)

2 tablespoons agave nectar

½ teaspoon pure vanilla extract

Preheat the oven to 400°F. Lightly spray a standard 12-cup muffin tin with olive oil.

In a medium bowl, whisk together the buckwheat flour, coconut flour, sorghum flour, flaxseed meal, baking powder, cinnamon, ginger, allspice, and salt.

In a large bowl, with an electric mixer at low speed, beat together the milk, applesauce, oil, egg, monk fruit sweetener, agave nectar, and vanilla. With the mixer running, gradually add the dry ingredients to the wet ingredients and beat until well combined.

Divide the batter evenly among the muffin cups. Bake until a toothpick inserted in the center of a muffin comes out clean, 19 to 22 minutes. Serve warm or at room temperature.

MAKES 12 MUFFINS (1 per serving) ❚ **Per muffin:** 110 calories, 5.5 g fat, 1 g saturated fat, 3 g protein, 14 g carbohydrate, 3 g fiber, 203 mg sodium

◀MAKE AHEAD▶ **You can assemble the dry ingredients ahead of time for convenience and refrigerate for up to 2 months. Or you can bake the whole batch and freeze the muffins for up to 3 months. To freeze, arrange on a small baking sheet and freeze solid, then transfer to a freezer container. Thaw at room temperature and reheat, if desired.**

PEANUT BUTTER–BANANA PANCAKES

HANDS-ON TIME: 25 MINUTES   TOTAL TIME: 25 MINUTES

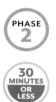

Peanut butter and banana are naturals together, and here they partner in pancakes that have good amounts of both protein and fiber. You can use either crunchy or smooth natural peanut butter—look for a brand with 1 gram of sugar or less per serving. Because the bananas are naturally sweet and moist, you won't need to add any sugar-free syrup or other topping.

1¾ cups 100% buckwheat flour

¼ cup coconut flour

2 teaspoons monk fruit natural no-calorie sweetener (baking formula)

1 teaspoon baking soda

½ teaspoon ground cinnamon

¼ teaspoon salt

2 cups plus 2 tablespoons fat-free milk

1 large egg

1 tablespoon all-natural peanut butter

1 tablespoon extra-virgin olive oil

1 teaspoon pure vanilla extract

Olive oil cooking spray

2 medium bananas, thinly sliced

In a large bowl, combine the buckwheat flour, coconut flour, monk fruit sweetener, baking soda, cinnamon, and salt. Mix thoroughly.

In a separate bowl, whisk together the milk, egg, peanut butter, oil, and vanilla. Add the wet ingredients to the dry and mix well with a whisk until a smooth batter forms.

Lightly spray a large nonstick skillet with olive oil and heat over medium heat.

For each pancake, pour ¼ cup batter into the skillet. Place 3 slices of banana on each pancake. Cook until small bubbles form near the middle of the pancake and it is golden brown on the underside (take a peek), 1 to 2 minutes. Flip and cook until golden brown on the other side, another 1 to 2 minutes. Repeat until no batter remains (it should yield 12 pancakes).

MAKES 12 PANCAKES (2 per serving) ▶ **Per serving:** 253 calories, 6.5 g fat, 2 g saturated fat, 10 g protein, 42 g carbohydrate, 6.5 g fiber, 369 mg sodium

◀MAKE AHEAD▶ The dry mixture will keep in the refrigerator for up to 2 months. Or cook up the whole batch of pancakes and freeze for up to 2 months. To freeze the pancakes, spread them out on a parchment-lined baking sheet and freeze solid, then transfer to a freezer container. Reheat a single portion (2 pancakes) from frozen in a microwave for 30 to 45 seconds. Or, if reheating the whole batch, preheat the oven to 375°F, spread the frozen pancakes on a baking sheet, cover with foil, and bake until heated through, 8 to 10 minutes.

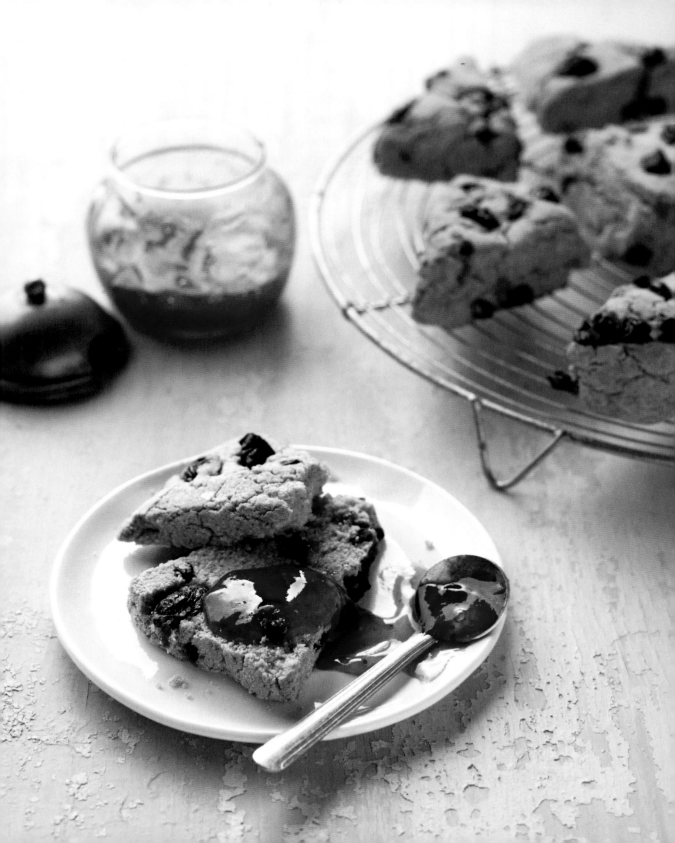

CINNAMON CHERRY SCONES

HANDS-ON TIME: 15 MINUTES   TOTAL TIME: 35 MINUTES

Look for dried Bing cherries, which are naturally sweet, and avoid dried tart cherries, which always have added sugar. Enjoy a scone with some sugar-free jam or a wedge of light spreadable cheese and a glass of fat-free or 1% milk for a healthy breakfast.

Olive oil cooking spray

1 cup gluten-free oat flour

½ cup almond flour

½ cup coconut flour

2 tablespoons monk fruit natural no-calorie sweetener (baking formula)

1 tablespoon gluten-free baking powder

1 teaspoon ground cinnamon

½ teaspoon salt

½ cup fat-free milk

1 large egg

1 teaspoon vanilla extract

1 teaspoon fresh lemon juice

½ cup chopped gluten-free all-natural, no-sugar-added dried cherries

Preheat the oven to 400°F. Line a baking sheet with foil (for easier cleanup) and lightly spray with olive oil.

In a large bowl, whisk together the oat flour, almond flour, coconut flour, monk fruit sweetener, baking powder, cinnamon, and salt.

In a separate bowl, whisk together the milk, egg, vanilla, and lemon juice. Stir the wet ingredients into the dry ingredients and mix until well combined. Fold in the dried cherries.

Divide the dough into 8 balls and place on the baking sheet. With moistened hands, flatten and shape the dough into 8 triangles, 1½ to 2 inches thick. Make sure the triangles are at least 2 inches apart.

Bake until lightly golden and a toothpick inserted in the center of a scone comes out clean, 15 to 20 minutes. Let cool on the pan.

MAKES 8 SCONES (1 per serving) ❭ **Per scone:** 164 calories, 6 g fat, 1.5 g saturated fat, 5 g protein, 22 g carbohydrate, 5 g fiber, 385 mg sodium

❬MAKE AHEAD❭ **The scones can be baked ahead and frozen for up to 3 months. To freeze, arrange on a small baking sheet and freeze solid, then transfer to a freezer container. Reheat in a microwave (30 to 45 seconds) or in a toaster oven (no need to thaw).**

AMARANTH, ALMOND, AND APRICOT BREAKFAST CEREAL

HANDS-ON TIME: 10 MINUTES   TOTAL TIME: 30 MINUTES

PHASE 2

30 MINUTES OR LESS

Toasting amaranth grains in a dry skillet before cooking brings out their nutty flavor. Agave nectar comes in both light (light in color, not calories) and dark, which has a more robust flavor. You can use whichever you have on hand.

1 cup amaranth

2 cups fat-free milk or unsweetened almond milk

2 tablespoons nonfat dry milk powder

½ teaspoon ground cinnamon

¼ teaspoon salt

4 teaspoons agave nectar

¼ cup sliced almonds

¼ cup gluten-free dried apricots, diced

In a medium saucepan, toast the amaranth over medium heat until lightly browned, about 3 minutes.

Meanwhile, in a small bowl, whisk together the milk, milk powder, cinnamon, and salt.

Add the milk mixture to the pan with the amaranth and bring to a simmer over medium heat. Cook, stirring occasionally, until the amaranth is tender but with a slight chew and the milk has been absorbed, about 15 minutes.

Spoon into 4 bowls (½ cup per serving). Drizzle each serving with 1 teaspoon agave nectar and top with the almonds and apricots.

MAKES 4 (½-cup) SERVINGS ▶ **Per serving:** 302 calories, 6.5 g fat, 1 g saturated fat, 13 g protein, 51 g carbohydrate, 4.5 g fiber, 212 mg sodium

OATMEAL BREAKFAST WEDGES

HANDS-ON TIME: 10 MINUTES   TOTAL TIME: 30 MINUTES

This may seem like a bread, but it's really just oatmeal in solid form. The sconelike wedges are sturdy and keep well, making them a perfect grab-and-go "cereal." Enjoy a wedge with ½ cup fat-free milk or top it with ¼ cup nonfat yogurt. To take the wedges in a different direction, make them with cashews and dried apricots or with almonds and unsweetened dried cherries instead of the pistachios and apples.

1½ cups gluten-free quick-cooking oats

½ cup finely chopped unsalted roasted pistachios (2 ounces)

¼ cup flaxseed meal

½ teaspoon baking soda

¼ teaspoon salt

2 pinches ground cinnamon

¼ cup finely chopped gluten-free dried apples

½ cup nonfat plain yogurt

2 tablespoons agave nectar

1 tablespoon extra-virgin olive oil

1 large egg

Preheat the oven to 350°F. Line a baking sheet with parchment paper. With a pencil, trace around a 9-inch round cake pan to make a circle on the parchment paper. Turn the paper over, but make sure you can still see the circle.

In a large bowl, stir together the oats, pistachios, flaxseed meal, baking soda, salt, and cinnamon until very well combined. Add the apples and use your fingers to pull the clumps of apple apart and evenly distribute them.

Make a well in the center of the oat mixture and add the yogurt, agave nectar, oil, and egg. Beat the wet ingredients together with a fork, then gradually stir in the oat mixture to form a wet dough.

Scrape the dough into the middle of the circle on the parchment paper and, with moistened hands, pat the dough into an even round the size of the circle. Bake until light golden but still nice and soft, 15 to 17 minutes.

Let cool on the pan for 2 minutes, then cut into 8 wedges. Transfer the wedges to a rack to cool slightly if serving warm, or cool completely if planning to eat later.

MAKES 8 WEDGES (1 per serving) ❯ **Per wedge:** 171 calories, 8 g fat, 1 g saturated fat, 6 g protein, 21 g carbohydrate, 3.5 g fiber, 174 mg sodium

❮MAKE AHEAD❯ You can make up the dry mixture and refrigerate for up to 2 months. Or bake the whole thing and freeze the wedges for up to 3 months. To freeze, spread the wedges out on a small baking sheet and freeze solid, then transfer to a freezer container. Reheat in the microwave to warm (30 to 45 seconds).

BANANA CREAM PIE BREAKFAST SHAKE

HANDS-ON TIME: 10 MINUTES   TOTAL TIME: 10 MINUTES

For this recipe use the sweetest, ripest banana you can find—it should be fully yellow with brown speckles on the skin. If you have bananas that are starting to brown before you get a chance to use them, pop them in the refrigerator, where they'll keep for several days without getting soft and overripe. The banana skins will turn completely black-brown, but the fruit inside will be fine. The addition of chia seeds boosts the fiber content of this shake.

1 very ripe small banana, cut into chunks

½ cup nonfat plain yogurt

2 tablespoons nonfat dry milk powder

2 teaspoons coconut flour

1 teaspoon chia seeds

1 teaspoon pure vanilla extract

¼ teaspoon ground nutmeg

5 ice cubes

In a blender, combine the banana, yogurt, milk powder, coconut flour, chia seeds, vanilla, nutmeg, and ice cubes. Blend until thick and smooth.

MAKES 1 SHAKE ❯ **Per shake:** 261 calories, 2.5 g fat, 1 g saturated fat, 11 g protein, 51 g carbohydrate, 6.5 g fiber, 131 mg sodium

BAKED BREAKFAST STACKS

HANDS-ON TIME: 10 MINUTES   TOTAL TIME: 30 MINUTES

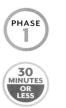

These stacks make a good carry-along breakfast or even lunch since they don't need to be refrigerated. Bake the egg, cheese, and bacon as directed. Cool to room temperature and wrap separately from the tomato and avocado. You can either stack and serve when ready or chop the tomato, toss it with the avocado along with 1 tablespoon of your favorite vinegar, and serve it as a salsa alongside the bacon/egg cup. With either approach, don't dice the avocado until ready to serve.

Olive oil cooking spray

4 slices (½ ounce each) gluten-free all-natural uncured Canadian bacon

4 large eggs

½ teaspoon coarse kosher salt

½ cup shredded reduced-fat Cheddar cheese (2 ounces)

1 large tomato, cut into 4 rounds

½ avocado, diced

Preheat the oven to 350°F. Spray four 6- to 10-ounce custard cups or ramekins with olive oil.

Place a slice of Canadian bacon in each cup or ramekin, pressing it down to line the cup. Crack the egg on top. Sprinkle with the salt and top evenly with the cheese.

Place the custard cups on a baking sheet and bake until the eggs are set, about 20 minutes.

Meanwhile, place a slice of tomato on each of 4 serving plates.

Run a knife around the edge of each custard cup or ramekin, lift the bacon and egg out, and place on top of a tomato slice. Top evenly with the avocado and serve hot.

MAKES 4 SERVINGS ❱ **Per serving:** 184 calories, 12 g fat, 4.5 g saturated fat, 13 g protein, 5 g carbohydrate, 1.5 g fiber, 550 mg sodium

STRAWBERRY-APPLE BREAKFAST FOOL

HANDS-ON TIME: 5 MINUTES   TOTAL TIME: 15 MINUTES PLUS COOLING TIME

We've given this popular British dessert a major health revamp. Instead of the traditional whipped cream and sugary fruit purée combination, we use high-protein Greek yogurt and a quick fiber-rich homemade applesauce blended with sweet strawberries. If using frozen strawberries, thaw them in a bowl so you don't lose any of the juices.

2 apples (your favorite variety), peeled and thinly sliced

10 strawberries (fresh or thawed frozen), thinly sliced; plus 4 small berries for garnish (optional)

2 tablespoons agave nectar

½ teaspoon pure vanilla extract

3 cups nonfat (0%) plain Greek yogurt

For the fruit purée: In a 1- or 2-quart microwave-safe bowl, combine the apples and 1 tablespoon water. Cover with a plate and microwave on high for 5 minutes. Add the strawberries, cover, and let stand for 5 minutes.

With an immersion blender (or in a standard blender), process the mixture to a purée (leave it a little chunky if you like). Let cool to room temperature.

Stir the agave nectar and vanilla into the yogurt. For each serving, spoon ¾ cup of the yogurt mixture into a small bowl or goblet, then swirl ½ cup of the strawberry-apple purée into the yogurt. Garnish with a small berry (if using).

MAKES 4 (1¼-cup) SERVINGS ❭ **Per serving:** 174 calories, 0 g fat, 0 g saturated fat, 16 g protein, 28 g carbohydrate, 2 g fiber, 64 mg sodium

❬**MAKE AHEAD**❭ **You can make the fruit purée up to 3 days ahead and refrigerate. Don't mix the yogurt and fruit until just before serving.**

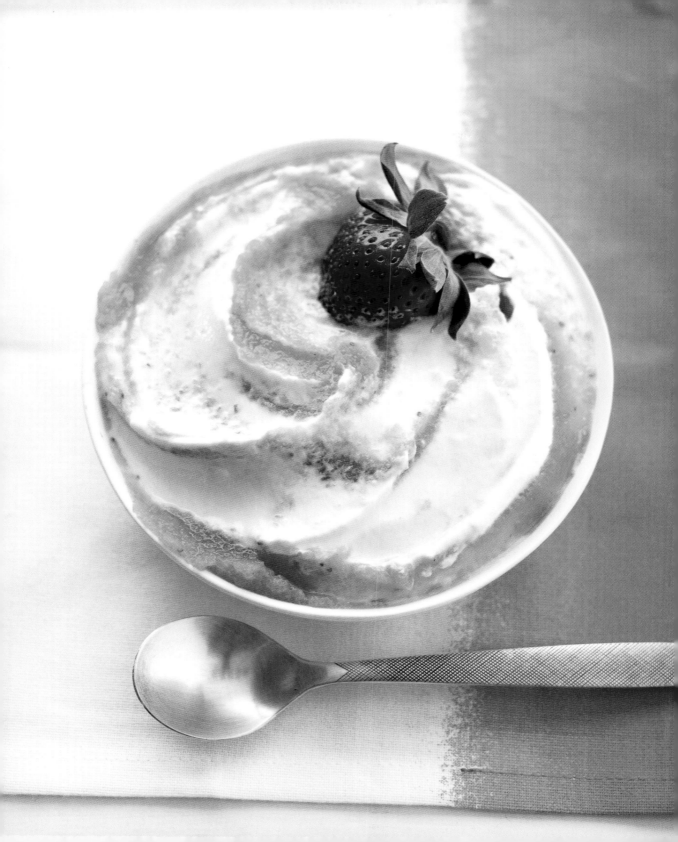

CREAMY 'N' CHEESY SCRAMBLED EGGS

HANDS-ON TIME: 10 MINUTES   TOTAL TIME: 10 MINUTES

Fat-free milk and light spreadable cheese make these eggs creamy. If you prefer your eggs a little drier, simply cook them longer. While we've used a light spreadable cheese with a hint of onion, you can change up the flavor with any of the other varieties available, such as chipotle or blue cheese.

4 large eggs	**1 tablespoon extra-virgin olive oil**
⅔ cup liquid egg whites	**1 wedge (¾ ounce) French onion–flavored light spreadable cheese, cut into small pieces**
¼ cup fat-free milk	
½ teaspoon salt	
¼ teaspoon freshly ground black pepper	

In a medium bowl, whisk together the whole eggs, egg whites, milk, salt, and pepper.

In a large nonstick skillet, heat the oil over medium-low heat. Pour the egg mixture into the skillet and scatter the cheese over the top. Cook, stirring constantly, until the eggs are just set and still creamy, about 2 minutes.

MAKES 4 (½-cup) SERVINGS ▶ **Per serving:** 133 calories, 8.5 g fat, 2.5 g saturated fat, 11 g protein, 2 g carbohydrate, 0 g fiber, 488 mg sodium

EGGS POACHED ON A BED
OF SAVORY VEGETABLES

HANDS-ON TIME: 15 MINUTES   TOTAL TIME: 25 MINUTES

Enjoy the poached egg and vegetables with an 8-ounce glass of fat-free or 1% milk to get an additional boost of filling protein and to work in some dairy for the day.

1 tablespoon plus 1 teaspoon extra-virgin olive oil

3 leeks, white and pale-green parts only, thinly sliced crosswise and well washed

2 packages (10 ounces each) cremini mushrooms, diced

½ teaspoon salt

¼ teaspoon red pepper flakes (optional)

3 tablespoons no-salt-added tomato paste

4 large eggs

Freshly ground black pepper

In a large nonstick skillet, heat the oil over medium-high heat. Add the leeks and cook, stirring, until softened, 3 to 5 minutes.

Add the mushrooms in a single layer and sprinkle with the salt and pepper flakes (if using). Cover and cook for 2 minutes without stirring. Stir the mushrooms into the leeks, cover, and cook until the mushrooms give up their liquid, about 2 minutes.

Meanwhile, in a small bowl, stir the tomato paste with 3 tablespoons water.

Stir the tomato paste mixture into the mushroom mixture and cook, uncovered, stirring occasionally, for 3 minutes to thicken the sauce and evaporate most of the mushroom liquid.

With a spoon, press 4 shallow wells into the mushroom mixture to hold the eggs. Crack an egg into each well. Reduce the heat to medium, cover the pan, and cook until the whites are set, 5 to 6 minutes (or a little longer if you want fully cooked yolks). Sprinkle some black pepper over the eggs.

MAKES 4 SERVINGS ❯ **Per serving:** 192 calories, 9.5 g fat, 2 g saturated fat, 11 g protein, 18 g carbohydrate, 2.5 g fiber, 391 mg sodium

◀**MAKE AHEAD**❯ The mushroom-leek mixture can be made 3 days ahead. For single breakfasts, simply divide it into equal portions and refrigerate. When ready to serve, gently reheat a portion of the vegetables in a small saucepan, adding a spoonful of water if necessary to loosen the mixture up. Bring it to a very gentle simmer, add an egg, cover, and cook as directed.

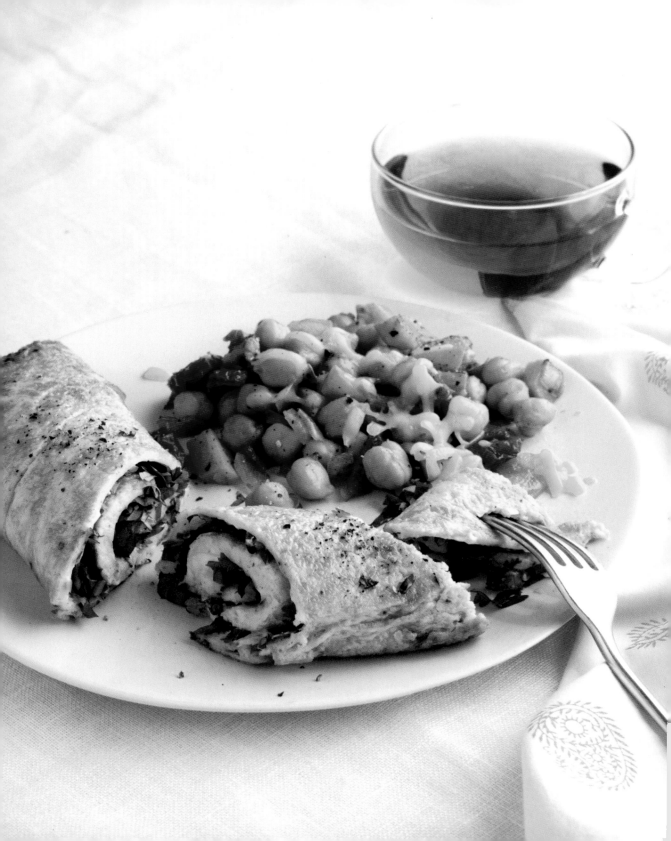

MEXICAN ROLLED OMELET

HANDS-ON TIME: 10 MINUTES   TOTAL TIME: 10 MINUTES

You can easily take this speedy single-serving omelet in different directions by changing up the type of spreadable cheese and the herbs and spices. If you're making omelets for multiple people, each person can have his or her own choice of seasonings. Having the cheese at room temperature makes it easier to spread on the hot omelet. Serve it with Chickpea Breakfast Hash (page 41).

1 large egg

2 large egg whites

1 tablespoon unsweetened almond milk, 1% dairy milk, or water

¼ teaspoon ground cumin

A large pinch dried oregano

A small pinch chipotle chile powder (optional)

Olive oil cooking spray

1 wedge (¾ ounce) chipotle-flavored light spreadable cheese, at room temperature

3 tablespoons chopped fresh cilantro, parsley, or scallion greens

In a small bowl, combine the whole egg, egg whites, milk, cumin, oregano, and chipotle powder (if using). Whisk well until just slightly frothy.

Spray a medium (10-inch) nonstick skillet with olive oil and heat over medium heat. Pour in the egg mixture and, as it cooks, pull it gently away from the sides of the pan to let the uncooked egg flow underneath. Cook until the eggs are mostly set, 1 to 2 minutes. Cover and cook until the top is set and the bottom is nicely browned, about 1 minute longer.

Loosen the edges and slide the omelet onto a plate. Spread the omelet with the cheese and sprinkle with the cilantro. Roll the omelet up and serve.

MAKES 1 OMELET ▌ **Per omelet:** 145 calories, 7 g fat, 2.5 g saturated fat, 16 g protein, 2 g carbohydrate, 0 g fiber, 453 mg sodium

GREEN EGGS AND HAM

HANDS-ON TIME: 15 MINUTES   TOTAL TIME: 15 MINUTES

PHASE
1

30
MINUTES
OR
LESS

If you're making breakfast just for yourself, simply divide the ingredients in half and use a medium skillet. Then enjoy half of the eggs immediately and refrigerate the other half for breakfast or lunch the next day. You can gently reheat the eggs or top them with a mixture of finely diced red bell peppers and celery and eat like a cold salad.

6 large eggs

⅔ cup liquid egg whites

¼ teaspoon salt

¼ teaspoon freshly ground black pepper

1 tablespoon plus 1 teaspoon extra-virgin olive oil

2 scallions, thinly sliced

2 ounces gluten-free all-natural uncured smoked ham, coarsely chopped

1 cup packed baby spinach, coarsely chopped (1 ounce)

½ cup chopped fresh parsley or cilantro

In a medium bowl, whisk together the whole eggs, egg whites, salt, and pepper.

In a large nonstick skillet, heat the oil over medium-high heat. Add the scallions and ham and cook for 1 minute to soften the scallions.

Add the egg mixture and sprinkle with the spinach and parsley. Let the eggs set around the edges, then begin pulling the cooked egg in from the edges with a silicone spatula to loosely scramble and incorporate the spinach and parsley. Cook to desired doneness of the eggs.

MAKES 4 SERVINGS ❙ **Per serving:** 187 calories, 12 g fat, 3 g saturated fat, 17 g protein, 3 g carbohydrate, 1 g fiber, 404 mg sodium

CHICKPEA BREAKFAST HASH

HANDS-ON TIME: 10 MINUTES   TOTAL TIME: 20 MINUTES

Shown pictured with Mexican Rolled Omelet on page 38.

PHASE 2

PHASE 1

SEE PHASE SWITCH

30 MINUTES OR LESS

Chickpeas replace the typical white potatoes in this healthy vegetarian hash, which can be enjoyed as a meal in itself or eaten as a side with eggs (in which case it will serve 6 people). The hash also makes delicious leftovers.

- 1 tablespoon plus 1 teaspoon extra-virgin olive oil
- 1 large sweet onion, diced
- ½ teaspoon ground cumin (optional)
- ¼ teaspoon salt
- ¼ teaspoon freshly ground black pepper
- 2 large carrots, cut into ½-inch cubes
- ⅓ cup chopped sun-dried tomatoes
- 1 can (15 ounces) gluten-free no-salt-added chickpeas, drained and rinsed
- ½ cup shredded reduced-fat sharp Cheddar cheese (2 ounces)

In a large nonstick skillet, heat the oil over medium-high heat. Add the onion, cumin (if using), salt, and pepper. Cook until the onion starts to soften, about 3 minutes.

Add the carrots, sun-dried tomatoes, and ½ cup water. Cover and cook until the carrots are crisp-tender, about 6 minutes.

Stir in the chickpeas and cook, uncovered and without stirring, until you hear the onions and carrots start to sizzle, about 5 minutes. Remove from the heat, sprinkle evenly with the cheese, and cover to let the residual heat melt the cheese.

MAKES 4 SERVINGS ▶ **Per serving:** 235 calories, 8.5 g fat, 2.5 g saturated fat, 11 g protein, 30 g carbohydrate, 6.5 g fiber, 321 mg sodium

◀PHASE SWITCH▶ **To make this a Phase 1 recipe, use 2 coarsely diced red bell peppers in place of the carrots and cook them only about 3 minutes.**

◀MAKE AHEAD▶ **This hash (without the cheese) keeps for up to 5 days in the refrigerator. Reheat the hash very gently in a nonstick skillet over medium-low heat (add a splash of water to the pan since the mixture may be a bit dry). When the hash is warmed through, top with the cheese and cover for a minute or so to melt.**

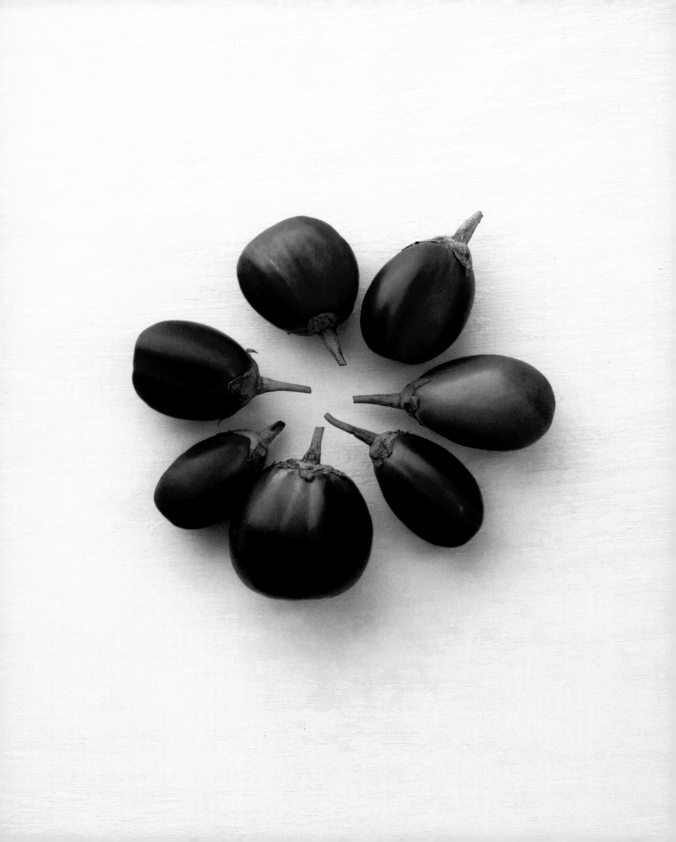

APPETIZERS AND SNACKS

Think appetizers and snacks and what comes to mind? Cheese and crackers, high-fat dips, pigs in white-bread blankets, pretzels, the vending machine. No wonder gluten overload is rampant. But you don't have to skip your midmorning or midafternoon snack or bypass the canapé tray just because you're avoiding gluten. Just nibble on our Mockamole, Coconut-Almond Chicken Strips, Spiced Peanut Wafers, or Spicy Chickpea "Nuts" or prepare one of the other taste-tempting recipes you'll find here.

LEMON ZUCCHINI BREAD

HANDS-ON TIME: 25 MINUTES
TOTAL TIME: 1 HOUR 35 MINUTES PLUS COOLING TIME

This is a great bread for an afternoon snack. Lightly toast a slice and spread it with a wedge of light spreadable cheese. Top the cheese with thinly sliced bell pepper for a little crunch. The egg whites in this recipe are beaten and folded into the batter to give the bread a lighter texture; don't substitute liquid egg whites, because they won't beat up as well.

Olive oil cooking spray

1 cup almond flour

½ cup coconut flour

2 tablespoons garbanzo bean flour

1 teaspoon gluten-free baking powder

½ teaspoon salt

¾ cup light sour cream

¼ cup fat-free milk

1 tablespoon fresh lemon juice

1 cup monk fruit natural no-calorie sweetener (baking formula)

2 tablespoons extra-virgin olive oil

¾ cup shredded zucchini

1½ tablespoons grated lemon zest

2 teaspoons poppy seeds

4 large egg whites (don't use liquid egg whites here)

Preheat the oven to 325°F. Spray a 9 × 5-inch loaf pan with olive oil.

In a medium bowl, sift together the almond flour, coconut flour, garbanzo flour, baking powder, and salt.

In a small bowl, whisk together the sour cream, milk, and lemon juice.

In a large bowl, with an electric mixer at medium speed, beat together the monk fruit sweetener and oil until crumbly, 2 to 3 minutes. With the mixer running, beat half the flour mixture into the oil mixture. Then beat in the sour cream mixture. Mix well. Add the remaining flour mixture and mix on low speed for 1 minute. Add the zucchini, lemon zest, and poppy seeds and gently mix on low speed just until evenly combined.

In a separate bowl, with the electric mixer at high speed, beat the egg whites until stiff peaks form. Gently fold the egg whites into the batter.

Pour the batter into the loaf pan and bake for 50 minutes. Cover the bread with foil and bake until a toothpick inserted in the center of the loaf comes out clean, about 20 minutes longer.

Cool in the pan on a rack for 20 minutes before turning out onto the rack to cool completely. The bread is best eaten the same day it is baked.

MAKES 16 SLICES (1 per serving) ▶ **Per slice:** 98 calories, 7 g fat, 2 g saturated fat, 4 g protein, 6 g carbohydrate, 2.5 g fiber, 142 mg sodium

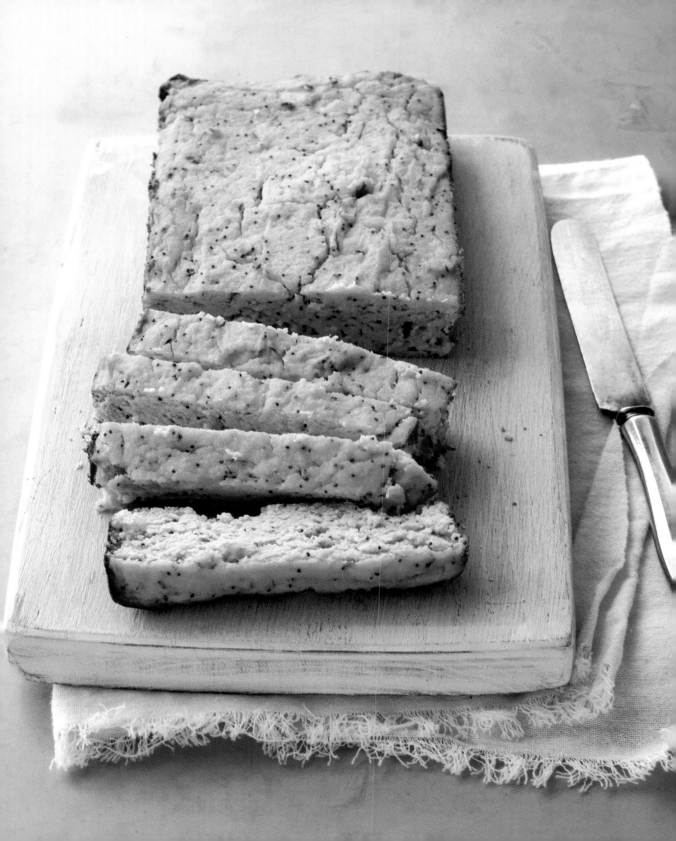

CHUNKY TOMATO AND
BLACK BEAN CHIPOTLE DIP

HANDS-ON TIME: 15 MINUTES   TOTAL TIME: 15 MINUTES

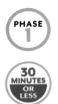

This spicy bean dip makes a delicious appetizer or satisfying midafternoon snack when served with veggie dippers or in endive leaves. It's also a fine topping for grilled steak or chicken breasts.

1 can (15 ounces) gluten-free no-salt-added black beans, drained and rinsed

2 teaspoons extra-virgin olive oil

1 teaspoon minced chipotle chile in adobo sauce

1 tablespoon fresh lime juice

1 teaspoon ground cumin

¾ teaspoon salt

½ teaspoon smoked paprika

1 cup diced fresh tomatoes

In a food processor, combine the beans, oil, chipotle, lime juice, cumin, salt, and paprika. Pulse to combine.

With the machine running, add water by the teaspoonful until the mixture is a smooth consistency. Add the tomatoes and pulse for 2 to 3 seconds, just to slightly break them up. Transfer to a bowl and serve at room temperature.

MAKES 6 (⅓-cup) SERVINGS ▶ **Per serving:** 81 calories, 1.5 g fat, 0 g saturated fat, 5 g protein, 12 g carbohydrate, 4 g fiber, 326 mg sodium

◀MAKE AHEAD▶ **You can refrigerate the dip for up to 3 days. Bring to room temperature before serving.**

ITALIAN WHITE BEAN AND ARTICHOKE DIP

HANDS-ON TIME: 15 MINUTES   TOTAL TIME: 15 MINUTES

PHASE
1

30
MINUTES
OR
LESS

This quick dip is a far healthier alternative to the typical artichoke dip, which is usually made with full-fat mayo and cheese. Serve it at your next party (or as a snack) with your choice of veggies (skip the carrots and gluten-free whole-grain crackers until Phase 2).

1 can (15 ounces) gluten-free no-salt-added cannellini beans, drained and rinsed

1 package (9 ounces) frozen artichoke hearts, thawed, quartered, and drained

½ cup fresh flat-leaf parsley leaves

2½ tablespoons fresh lemon juice

2 teaspoons extra-virgin olive oil

1½ teaspoons gluten-free Italian herb seasoning

1 teaspoon onion powder

¾ teaspoon garlic powder

¾ teaspoon salt

In a food processor, combine the beans, artichoke hearts, parsley, lemon juice, oil, Italian seasoning, onion powder, garlic powder, and salt. Pulse to combine.

With the machine running, add water by the teaspoonful until the mixture is a smooth consistency. Transfer to a bowl and serve at room temperature.

MAKES 6 (⅓-cup) SERVINGS ❱ **Per serving:** 97 calories, 2.5 g fat, 0 g saturated fat, 5 g protein, 15 g carbohydrate, 5.5 g fiber, 345 mg sodium

❮MAKE AHEAD❯ **You can refrigerate the dip for up to 3 days. Bring to room temperature before serving.**

CREAMY HOT BROCCOLI DIP

HANDS-ON TIME: 20 MINUTES   TOTAL TIME: 20 MINUTES

We've given this perennial party favorite a makeover by using broccoli (an antioxidant powerhouse) instead of the usual spinach and tweaking the other ingredients to cut the fat but still keep the dip tasting rich.

2 teaspoons extra-virgin olive oil

2 cloves garlic, minced

1 tablespoon garbanzo bean flour

½ cup fat-free milk

1 package (10 ounces) frozen chopped broccoli, thawed and squeezed dry

2 wedges (¾ ounce each) French onion–flavored light spreadable cheese, cut into small pieces

2 tablespoons mayonnaise (made with extra-virgin olive oil)

¼ cup grated Parmesan cheese

½ teaspoon hot sauce

¼ teaspoon salt

In a medium saucepan, heat the oil over low heat. Add the garlic and cook, stirring occasionally, until softened, about 2 minutes.

Whisk in the garbanzo flour. Gradually add the milk, stirring until smooth. Add the broccoli and cook, stirring occasionally, until tender, about 3 minutes.

Stir in the spreadable cheese, mayonnaise, Parmesan, hot sauce, and salt. Heat until the cheese has melted, about 3 minutes. Serve warm.

MAKES 4 (½-cup) SERVINGS ▶ **Per serving:** 116 calories, 7 g fat, 2 g saturated fat, 7 g protein, 7 g carbohydrate, 2.5 g fiber, 452 mg sodium

FAUX CAVIAR

HANDS-ON TIME: 15 MINUTES   TOTAL TIME: 15 MINUTES PLUS RESTING TIME

PHASE 1

Texas Caviar, Cowboy Caviar, and Poor Man's Caviar—these are just a few of the dips that are called caviar but don't have any actual fish eggs in them. Although the ingredients can vary, black beans are a must for these dishes because of their resemblance to black caviar. The crunch of pungent red onion and the fresh flavors of dill and lemon juice make this version particularly tasty.

1   **can (15 ounces) gluten-free no-salt-added black beans, drained and rinsed**

1   **can (15 ounces) gluten-free no-salt-added Great Northern or cannellini beans, drained and rinsed**

½   **cup finely diced red onion (1 small)**

¼   **cup minced fresh dill, plus small sprigs for garnish**

2   **tablespoons fresh lemon juice**

2   **tablespoons extra-virgin olive oil**

½   **teaspoon salt**

¼   **teaspoon freshly ground black pepper**

1   **English hothouse cucumber (at least 12 inches long), unpeeled, cut on an angle into about 32 (¼-inch-thick) slices**

½   **cup nonfat (0%) plain Greek yogurt**

Coarsely chop the beans by hand (not in a food processor, because you still want some texture).

In a medium bowl, combine the chopped beans, onion, dill, lemon juice, oil, salt, and pepper. If possible, let sit for at least 30 minutes to meld flavors.

Top each cucumber slice with a generous tablespoon of the bean mixture, a scant 1 teaspoon yogurt, and a teeny sprig of dill.

MAKES 32 PIECES (4 per serving) ❯ **Per serving:** 141 calories, 4 g fat, 0.5 g saturated fat, 7 g protein, 20 g carbohydrate, 7 g fiber, 178 mg sodium

◀MAKE AHEAD▶ **The "caviar" mixture can be made ahead and refrigerated for up to 2 days. Let return to room temperature for the best flavor, then slice the cucumber and assemble the canapés.**

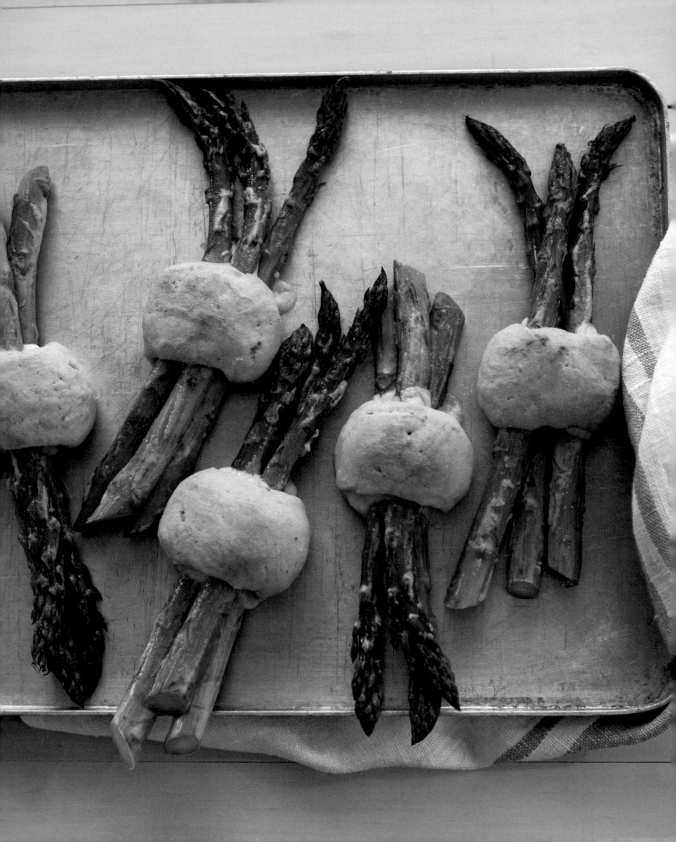

ASPARAGUS IN A BLANKET

HANDS-ON TIME: 10 MINUTES   TOTAL TIME: 30 MINUTES

Choose asparagus that are at least ½ inch across at the base. Really skinny (or really fat) asparagus won't work as well here. A typical pound of asparagus has 18 to 21 spears, and the ideal number of asparagus spears to wrap into a bundle is 3. So you may only get 6 bundles here instead of 7. If that's the case, divide the dough and cheese accordingly.

1 pound medium asparagus	3 tablespoons liquid egg whites
½ cup plus 2 tablespoons garbanzo bean flour	2 teaspoons extra-virgin olive oil
½ teaspoon gluten-free baking powder	2 slices (¾ ounce each) deli-sliced reduced-fat Swiss cheese, cut into a total of 7 thin strips
2 pinches salt	2 teaspoons Dijon mustard

In a steamer, cook the asparagus until still crisp but bright green in color, about 3 minutes. Remove from the steamer to a plate to cool.

Preheat the oven to 375°F. Line a small baking sheet or baking pan with parchment paper (or use a nonstick pan).

In a medium bowl, stir together the garbanzo flour, baking powder, and salt. Stir in the egg whites and 1 teaspoon of the oil. The dough should be like a slightly sticky pie dough.

Pinch off 1-inch balls of the dough and roll into logs about 3 inches long. Bundle 3 asparagus spears together, wrap a strip of cheese around the middle, and place the asparagus perpendicular to the log of dough. With moistened hands, wrap the dough around the cheese and form it into an even band, pressing it down to completely cover the cheese. Place the bundles on the baking sheet as you work.

In a small bowl, stir together the mustard and remaining 1 teaspoon oil. Brush the tops of the dough and the asparagus with the mustard mixture. Bake until the dough has puffed and browned, about 10 minutes. Serve warm or at room temperature.

MAKES 7 BUNDLES ▶ **Per bundle:** 81 calories, 3.5 g fat, 1 g saturated fat, 6 g protein, 8 g carbohydrate, 2 g fiber, 123 mg sodium

◀MAKE AHEAD▶ **You can steam the asparagus and assemble the bundles up to 4 hours ahead. Place on the baking sheet or in the baking pan, cover well, and refrigerate. Bring back to room temperature before baking.**

MOCKAMOLE

HANDS-ON TIME: 20 MINUTES   TOTAL TIME: 20 MINUTES

Serve on cucumber or jícama rounds on Phase 1 and with your own home-baked tortilla chips on Phase 2: Spray 100% corn tortillas lightly with olive oil and then add a squeeze of lime juice. Cut into wedges and bake in a 375°F oven until crisp, about 10 minutes.

1 cup frozen shelled edamame

½ cup fresh cilantro leaves and tender stems

1 medium fresh jalapeño, seeded and finely chopped (1 tablespoon)

1 tablespoon plus 1 teaspoon fresh lime juice

½ teaspoon salt

½ avocado, cut into large chunks

⅓ cup finely chopped onion

In a small pot of boiling water, cook the edamame until tender, about 4 minutes. Drain well and transfer to a food processor.

Add the cilantro, jalapeño, lime juice, salt, and 1 tablespoon water and pulse until the edamame and cilantro are coarsely ground. Add the avocado and onion and pulse until well combined.

MAKES 4 (6-tablespoon) SERVINGS ▶ **Per serving:** 86 calories, 4.5 g fat, 0.5 g saturated fat, 6 g protein, 7 g carbohydrate, 3.5 g fiber, 295 mg sodium

◀MAKE AHEAD▶ **You can make the mockamole a day ahead and refrigerate. Press a sheet of plastic wrap directly on the surface to keep it from turning dark. Serve chilled or at room temperature.**

CHEDDAR-ARUGULA PINWHEELS

HANDS-ON TIME: 15 MINUTES   TOTAL TIME: 25 MINUTES

Garbanzo–fava bean flour (a prepared mix of garbanzo and fava bean flours sometimes called Garfava flour) or white bean flour works just as well as fava bean or garbanzo bean flour in this recipe. To give the pinwheels a spicy kick, try shredded reduced-fat hot pepper cheese instead of the Cheddar.

Olive oil cooking spray

6 large eggs, separated, plus 2 large egg whites (don't use liquid egg whites here)

3 tablespoons fava bean flour or garbanzo bean flour

¼ teaspoon salt

¼ teaspoon freshly ground black pepper

¾ cup shredded reduced-fat Cheddar cheese (3 ounces)

2 cups torn arugula leaves

Preheat the oven to 350°F. Spray an 11 × 17-inch rimmed baking sheet with olive oil. Line the pan with parchment paper, leaving an overhang at both short ends, then spray the paper with olive oil. Set a clean large kitchen towel (at least 11 × 17 inches) out on a work surface.

In a large bowl, whisk together the 6 egg yolks, flour, salt, and pepper.

In a large bowl, with an electric mixer at high speed, beat the 8 egg whites until soft peaks form. Gently fold the egg whites into the yolk mixture.

Scrape the batter into the baking sheet and, with a spatula, spread to an even thickness. Bake until set and lightly browned, 9 to 10 minutes.

Immediately invert the egg cake onto the kitchen towel and scatter the cheese and arugula over it. Starting at one short end and using the towel to help, roll up the egg cake. To serve, cut crosswise into 12 pinwheels.

MAKES 12 PINWHEELS (2 per serving) ▌ **Per serving:** 145 calories, 8.5 g fat, 3.5 g saturated fat, 12 g protein, 4 g carbohydrate, 1 g fiber, 311 mg sodium

◀MAKE AHEAD▶ The pinwheels can be made up to 2 hours ahead and kept at room temperature. Leftovers can be refrigerated for up to 1 day and served either chilled or at room temperature.

BELGIAN ENDIVE WITH SCALLION-PEPPER CHEESE

HANDS-ON TIME: 20 MINUTES   TOTAL TIME: 20 MINUTES

PHASE 1

30 MINUTES OR LESS

The number of heads of Belgian endive you need will depend on their size. An average endive head will yield 10 to 12 largish spears; smaller endives may only have 8 "large" spears. You will have leftover endive—the small inner hearts. Cut them up and toss with a vinaigrette (about 1 teaspoon per cup of cut-up endive) and serve as a side salad with a main dish like Jerk Flank Steak (page 183). You can also use the scallion cheese as part of a snack roll-up (see Variation, below).

16 scallions; plus greens of 2 scallions for garnish (optional)

2 teaspoons extra-virgin olive oil

Coarse kosher salt

8 tablespoons (4 ounces) light cream cheese

¼ teaspoon freshly ground black pepper

24 large Belgian endive spears (2 or 3 endives)

Trim the scallions and cut off the tops where the pale green is turning dark green. Set the dark green tops aside. Thinly slice the scallion whites. Finely chop enough of the dark green tops to get 2 tablespoons.

In a medium nonstick skillet, heat the oil over medium heat. Add the scallion whites, sprinkle with a large pinch of salt, and cook, stirring, until the scallions are caramelized, 5 to 7 minutes. Scrape into a medium bowl and cool.

Add the cream cheese, pepper, and scallion greens to the caramelized scallions and beat together to combine. Refrigerate for up to 3 days if not using right away.

When ready to serve, spread 1 teaspoon of the scallion cheese into each endive spear. Garnish with thinly sliced scallion greens, if desired.

MAKES 6 (4-piece) SERVINGS ❯ **Per serving:** 71 calories, 4.5 g fat, 2 g saturated fat, 3 g protein, 6 g carbohydrate, 2.5 g fiber, 114 mg sodium

❮VARIATION❯ **TURKEY-SCALLION CHEESE SNACK (1 serving):** Halve a large stalk of celery crosswise. Spread each half with 2 teaspoons of the scallion-pepper cheese. Cut a slice of gluten-free lower-sodium deli turkey in half and wrap each celery stick with a piece of turkey.

PER (2-piece) SNACK: 102 calories, 4.5 g fat, 2 g saturated fat, 9 g protein, 6 g carbohydrate, 2 g fiber, 357 mg sodium

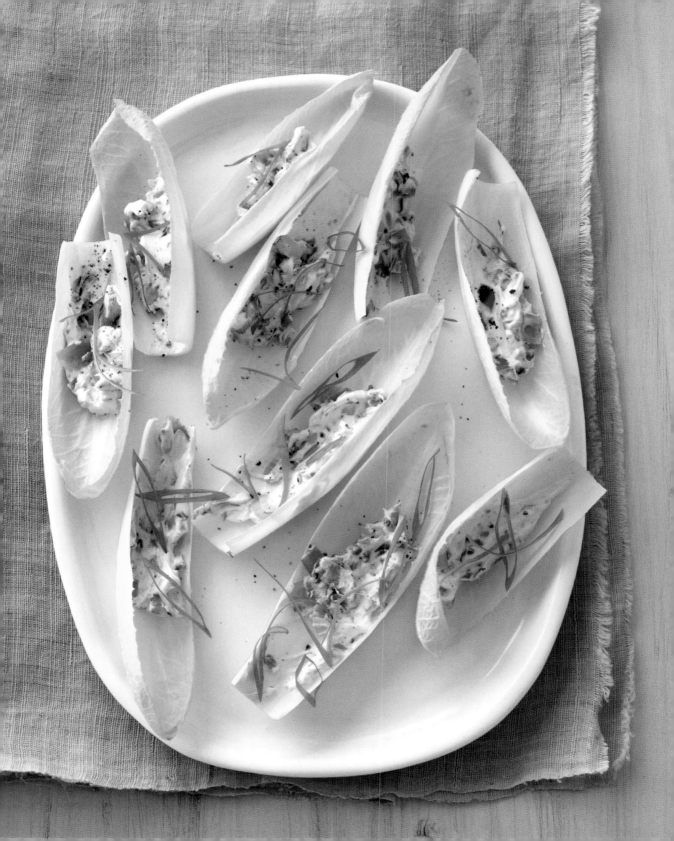

COCONUT-ALMOND CHICKEN STRIPS

HANDS-ON TIME: 15 MINUTES   TOTAL TIME: 20 MINUTES

You can make your own nut flour using whatever raw or dry-roasted nuts you favor, as long as they are unsalted. Just grind enough nuts in a mini food processor until powdery but not pasty to make ⅔ cup flour. For a snack, place a chicken strip on a butter lettuce leaf, squeeze a little lime juice over both, and roll up.

Olive oil cooking spray

½ pound thin-sliced chicken breast cutlets

⅔ cup almond flour

⅓ cup unsweetened shredded coconut

¼ teaspoon coarse kosher salt

1 large egg white

Hot sauce, for serving

Lime wedges, for serving

Preheat the broiler with the rack 6 inches from the heat. Line a baking sheet with foil (for easier cleanup) and lightly spray with olive oil.

With the flat side of a meat pounder or the bottom of a small heavy skillet, pound the chicken ⅛ inch thick. Cut lengthwise into strips 1½ to 2 inches wide.

In a bowl, whisk together the almond flour, coconut, and salt. Spread the mixture on a sheet of wax paper. In a shallow bowl or pie plate, beat the egg white with 1 teaspoon water. Dip the chicken in the egg white, then into the coconut mixture, turning to lightly coat both sides (it's not a solid or thick coating).

Place the strips on the baking sheet and broil for 3 minutes. Turn the chicken over and broil until the chicken is cooked through but still juicy, about 2 minutes.

Serve with hot sauce for sprinkling or dipping and lime wedges for squeezing.

MAKES 8 SERVINGS ❱ **Per serving:** 118 calories, 8 g fat, 2.5 g saturated fat, 9 g protein, 3 g carbohydrate, 1.5 g fiber, 104 mg sodium

◀MAKE AHEAD❱ **You can pound and slice the chicken and assemble the breading mixture up to 4 hours ahead. Refrigerate until ready to assemble and bake.**

SPANISH-SPICED TURKEY MEATBALLS

HANDS-ON TIME: 25 MINUTES   TOTAL TIME: 30 MINUTES

Ice cream scoops (also called dishers) come in a wide variety of sizes and are a great tool for shaping meatballs. Here you want a #30 ice cream scoop—which is about 2⅛ tablespoons, or the size a golf ball.

- 4 **100% corn tortillas (6-inch), torn into small pieces**
- 1¼ **pounds gluten-free ground turkey breast**
- 4 **tablespoons no-salt-added tomato paste**
- 1 **tablespoon mayonnaise (made with extra-virgin olive oil)**
- 2 **teaspoons smoked paprika**
- 1½ **teaspoons ground cumin**
- 1 **teaspoon ground coriander**
- ¾ **teaspoon dried oregano**
- ½ **teaspoon salt**
- 2 **large eggs**
- 2 **cups gluten-free low-sodium chicken broth**

In a food processor, coarsely grind the corn tortillas. Transfer the tortilla crumbs to a large bowl.

Add the turkey, 2 tablespoons of the tomato paste, the mayonnaise, paprika, cumin, coriander, oregano, and salt to the bowl. Add the eggs and gently mix to combine. Using a small ice cream scoop or your moistened hands, gently shape into 24 meatballs.

In a large skillet, combine the broth and remaining 2 tablespoons tomato paste. Bring to a simmer over medium heat. Add the meatballs and cook, turning the meatballs as they cook, until firm all over and just cooked through, 5 to 7 minutes.

With a slotted spoon, transfer the meatballs to a platter or serving bowl. Increase the heat under the broth to medium-high and cook until the broth has reduced by half, about 5 minutes. Pour over the meatballs and serve.

MAKES 8 (3-meatball) SERVINGS ❯ **Per serving:** 142 calories, 3 g fat, 0.5 g saturated fat, 21 g protein, 8 g carbohydrate, 1.5 g fiber, 239 mg sodium

❮MAKE AHEAD❯ **The shaped meatballs can be frozen for up to 3 months. To freeze, place the *uncooked* meatballs on a parchment-lined baking sheet and freeze solid; then transfer to a freezer container. Thaw in the refrigerator before using.**

SPICY CHICKPEA "NUTS"

HANDS-ON TIME: 5 MINUTES   TOTAL TIME: 45 MINUTES

PHASE 1

You can double this recipe to make more for a large group, but don't try to fit all the chickpeas on a single baking sheet or they'll be too crowded and steam instead of crisping. Instead, use two separate baking sheets (rotate the sheets from one rack to the other midway through the baking) or bake them in two batches.

1 tablespoon extra-virgin olive oil	2 pinches cayenne pepper
2 teaspoons grated lemon zest	1 can (15 ounces) gluten-free no-salt-added chickpeas, drained and rinsed
1½ teaspoons smoked paprika	
½ teaspoon coarse kosher salt	

Preheat the oven to 375°F. Line a rimmed baking sheet with parchment paper.

In a medium bowl, whisk together the oil, lemon zest, paprika, salt, and cayenne until well combined. Add the chickpeas and toss well to coat.

Transfer to the baking sheet and bake, shaking the pan once or twice, until dry and crunchy, about 40 minutes.

MAKES 6 (¼-cup) SERVINGS ▶ Per serving: 98 calories, 3 g fat, 0.5 g saturated fat, 4 g protein, 14 g carbohydrate, 3 g fiber, 178 mg sodium

◀MAKE AHEAD▶ Make the chickpea "nuts" ahead and store at room temperature for up to 2 days.

PEPPER TUNA ROLLS

HANDS-ON TIME: 25 MINUTES   TOTAL TIME: 25 MINUTES

PHASE
1

30
MINUTES
OR
LESS

If your pepper mill has a setting that lets you coarsely grind the pepper, use it here. Otherwise, you can either buy what's called "butcher's grind" pepper (in the spice aisle) or pour some peppercorns into a rimmed baking sheet and press on them with the flat side of a skillet or a meat mallet.

¼ cup nonfat (0%) plain Greek yogurt

1 tablespoon plus 1 teaspoon mayonnaise (made with extra-virgin olive oil)

1 tablespoon drained horseradish

2 teaspoons fresh lemon juice

½ teaspoon coarse kosher salt

½ teaspoon coarsely ground black pepper

1 tuna steak (8 ounces)

2 teaspoons extra-virgin olive oil

16 butter lettuce leaves

4 scallions, quartered lengthwise and cut crosswise into 1-inch lengths

1 small cucumber, halved lengthwise and thinly sliced crosswise

In a small bowl, whisk together the yogurt, mayonnaise, horseradish, lemon juice, and ¼ teaspoon of the salt.

Rub the remaining ¼ teaspoon salt and the pepper into both sides of the tuna. Rub the oil over both sides of the tuna.

Heat a grill pan over medium heat until hot but not smoking (a drop of water will sizzle in the pan). Place the tuna on the grill pan and cook about 2 minutes per side for medium-rare. Alternatively, place the tuna on a broiler pan set 4 inches from the heat and broil about 2 minutes per side for medium-rare. Transfer to a plate, cool to room temperature, then thinly slice.

Lay out the lettuce and divide the yogurt mixture among the leaves; spread to coat. Top evenly with sliced tuna, scallions, and cucumber and roll up.

MAKES 4 (4-roll) SERVINGS ❱ Per serving: 143 calories, 6.5 g fat, 1 g saturated fat, 16 g protein, 5 g carbohydrate, 1.5 g fiber, 329 mg sodium

❰MAKE AHEAD❱ The tuna can be cooked up to 1 day ahead and refrigerated. The horseradish cream can be made 1 or 2 days ahead and refrigerated.

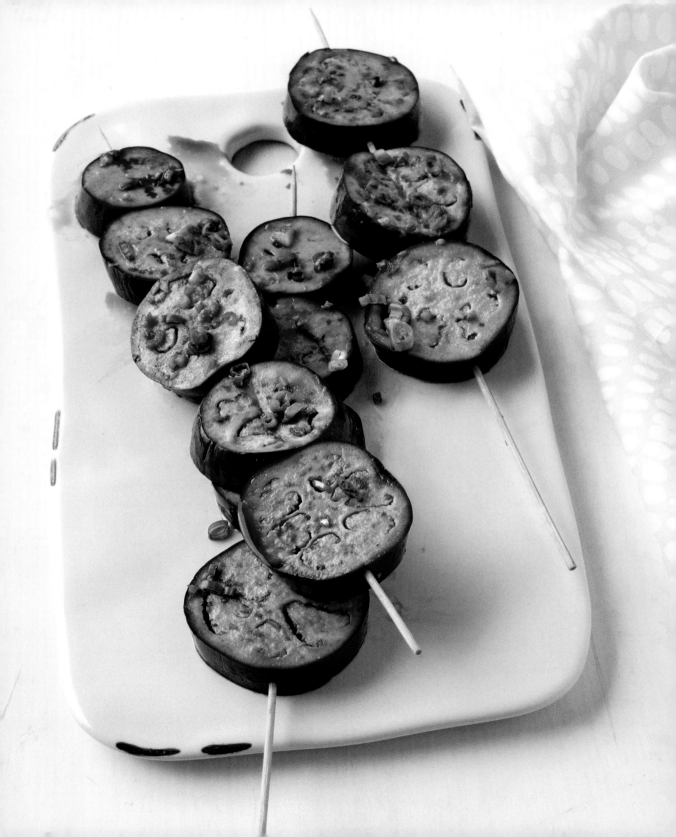

GINGER-GARLIC EGGPLANT SKEWERS

HANDS-ON TIME: 10 MINUTES
TOTAL TIME: 20 MINUTES PLUS MARINATING TIME

PHASE 1

If you're serving this as a party appetizer, you'll definitely want to make more than the 8 skewers, but this is an easy recipe to scale up. Double or triple the marinade accordingly, and make sure the container you use is big enough to let the eggplant rounds lie directly in the marinade.

- 8 baby Italian eggplants (5 inches long), 3 to 4 ounces each, unpeeled
- 1 tablespoon plus 1 teaspoon dark sesame oil
- 3 cloves garlic, minced
- 2 tablespoons minced fresh ginger
- 6 tablespoons gluten-free reduced-sodium tamari soy sauce
- 6 tablespoons apple cider vinegar
- Chopped scallions, for garnish (optional)

Cut the eggplants crosswise into ¾-inch-thick rounds. Thread the rounds onto eight 10- or 12-inch skewers (or 16 smaller skewers if your steamer won't accommodate the longer ones) with a skewer going through the skin on both sides of each round.

Working in batches if necessary, in a steamer, cook the eggplant skewers until tender, about 12 minutes.

Meanwhile, in a small saucepan, combine the sesame oil, garlic, and ginger and heat over medium heat for 1 to 2 minutes to flavor the oil and soften the garlic. Off the heat, stir in the tamari and vinegar and set aside.

Transfer the eggplant skewers to a baking pan or other shallow container that will hold the skewers snugly but in a single layer. Pour the ginger-garlic mixture over the skewers and turn to coat. Let marinate at room temperature for at least 30 minutes; the longer you can let them sit, the more flavor they will absorb. Turn the skewers every once in a while if you think of it. Serve 2 long skewers or 4 short skewers per person, at room temperature or chilled and garnished with the scallions (if using).

MAKES 4 SERVINGS ❱ Per serving: 82 calories, 2.5 g fat, 0.5 g saturated fat, 3 g protein, 13 g carbohydrate, 7 g fiber, 355 mg sodium

❰MAKE AHEAD❱ Preparing these up to a day ahead gives the flavors time to meld, so they taste even better. Serve chilled or at room temperatuve.

SPICED PEANUT WAFERS

HANDS-ON TIME: 15 MINUTES   TOTAL TIME: 25 MINUTES

PHASE
2

30
MINUTES
OR
LESS

For a party, serve these at room temperature with a little square of reduced-fat cheese (Cheddar would be great—just think of those peanut butter–cheese crackers we sometimes crave). Or serve them hot: Top each wafer with 1 tablespoon shredded reduced-fat Cheddar and bake in a 350°F oven until the cheese has melted. Look for sweet and spicy garam masala in the spice section of your supermarket or online (see page 295). It's typically a combo of cardamon, cloves, mace, cinnamon, cumin, fennel, black peppercorns, and fenugreek.

½ cup all-natural peanut butter

2 tablespoons coconut flour

2 large egg whites

1½ teaspoons monk fruit natural no-calorie sweetener (from packets)

½ teaspoon garam masala

½ teaspoon coarse kosher salt

¼ teaspoon cayenne pepper

Preheat the oven to 375°F. Line a large baking sheet with parchment paper.

In a large bowl, stir together the peanut butter, coconut flour, egg whites, monk fruit sweetener, garam masala, salt, and cayenne.

Shape the mixture into 18 walnut-size balls and drop onto the baking sheet, spacing them 1 inch apart. With the bottom of a glass, flatten each to a ¼-inch thickness. Bake until set, 10 to 12 minutes. Transfer to a rack to cool completely.

MAKES 18 WAFERS (2 per serving) ❱ **Per serving (without cheese):** 100 calories, 7 g fat, 1 g saturated fat, 4 g protein, 4 g carbohydrate, 1 g fiber, 122 mg sodium

SPINACH-STUFFED MUSHROOMS

HANDS-ON TIME: 15 MINUTES   TOTAL TIME: 50 MINUTES

For an elegant summer side dish, use the spinach stuffing to fill fresh tomatoes when they're in season. Cut a little off the tops of 6 medium or 4 large tomatoes, scoop out the centers, stuff, and bake as directed in the last step.

24 cremini mushrooms (about 20 ounces)

3 tablespoons fresh lemon juice

1 cup canned gluten-free no-salt-added cannellini beans or chickpeas, drained and rinsed

1 tablespoon extra-virgin olive oil

½ teaspoon dried oregano

¼ teaspoon freshly ground black pepper

1 package (10 ounces) frozen chopped spinach, thawed and squeezed dry

2 tablespoons almond flour

2 ounces reduced-fat Swiss cheese, coarsely chopped

Preheat the oven to 350°F.

Remove and discard the mushroom stems. In an ovenproof skillet or a pan large enough to hold the mushrooms in a single layer, stir together 1 tablespoon of the lemon juice and ⅓ cup water. Place the mushroom caps in the pan, stemmed side up. Place the pan in the oven and bake until the mushrooms are tender, about 20 minutes. Transfer the mushrooms to a plate but leave the oven on. Drain the liquid in the pan.

Meanwhile, in a medium bowl with a potato masher or a spoon, lightly mash the beans with the remaining 2 tablespoons lemon juice, the oil, oregano, and pepper. Add the spinach, almond flour, and cheese. Mix well to combine. Spoon a tablespoon of the bean mixture into each mushroom cap, mounding the filling.

Place the mushrooms on a baking sheet and bake until the filling is piping hot and the cheese has melted, about 15 minutes. Serve the mushrooms hot or at room temperature.

MAKES 6 (4-mushroom) SERVINGS ⏵ **Per serving:** 133 calories, 6 g fat, 1.5 g saturated fat, 9 g protein, 13 g carbohydrate, 4 g fiber, 93 mg sodium

◀MAKE AHEAD▶ **Precook the mushrooms and stuff them, then refrigerate for up to 24 hours before baking.**

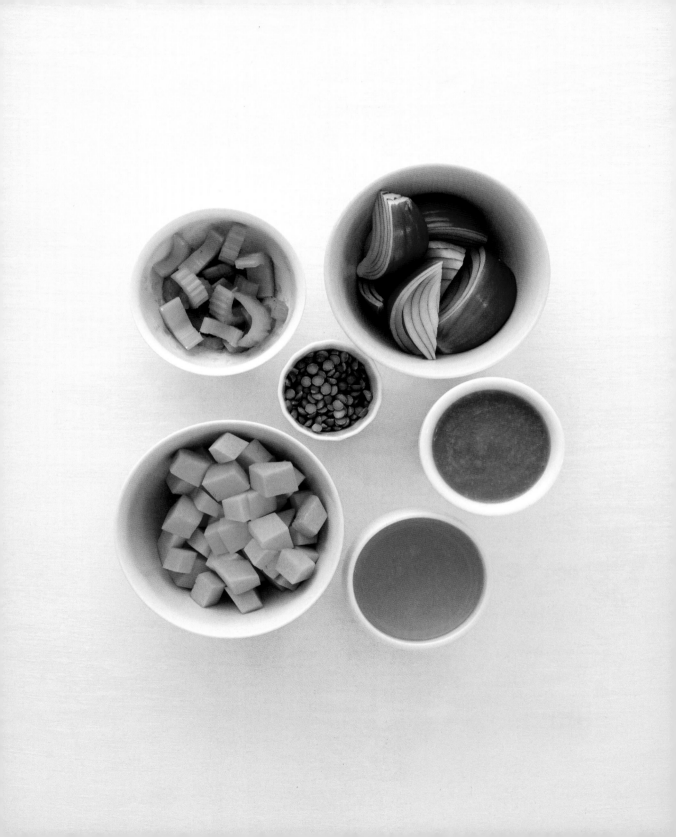

SOUPS AND SANDWICHES

Soups and sandwiches are some of the biggest offenders when you're trying to avoid gluten. Many canned soups contain wheat thickeners, and most breads are made with wheat or rye. Rather than take a chance, make your own gluten-free soups and breads. This chapter features satisfying main-dish soups, including Chicken Soup with Dumplings (made from almond and sorghum flour), as well as some innovative sandwiches featuring our own gluten-free breads or no bread at all (check out the Jícama Cheese Toasties, page 83).

CHICKEN, BUTTERNUT, AND QUINOA SOUP

HANDS-ON TIME: 15 MINUTES   TOTAL TIME: 40 MINUTES

Gluten-free, protein-rich, nutty-tasting quinoa subs for the usual wheat-based noodles in this hearty chicken soup. We like red quinoa, available at specialty markets, for the antioxidant-rich beta-carotene it provides, but you can use any type of quinoa here.

½ cup quinoa, preferably red

4 teaspoons extra-virgin olive oil

½ pound boneless, skinless chicken breasts, cut into ½-inch chunks

1 medium onion, chopped

3 cloves garlic, minced

2 cups gluten-free low-sodium chicken broth

1 cup carrot juice

2 teaspoons grated lemon zest

½ teaspoon salt

¼ teaspoon coarsely ground black pepper

1½ cups cubed (⅓-inch) butternut squash

Sliced scallion greens, for garnish

Lemon wedges, for serving

Soak the quinoa in a bowl of water to cover.

Meanwhile, in a large nonstick saucepan or Dutch oven, heat 2 teaspoons of the oil over medium-high heat. Add the chicken and cook until opaque all over (but still pink on the inside; it cooks more later), about 2 minutes. With a slotted spoon, transfer the chicken to a bowl.

Add the remaining 2 teaspoons oil, the onion, and garlic to the pan. Cook until the onion is softened and beginning to brown, 3 to 5 minutes.

Add the broth, carrot juice, lemon zest, salt, pepper, and 1 cup water. Bring to a simmer. Drain the quinoa, add to the soup, and bring to a boil. Reduce to a simmer, cover tightly, and cook for 5 minutes.

Add the butternut squash, re-cover, and simmer until the quinoa is tender, about 15 minutes. Stir in the chicken (and any juices) and cook for 2 minutes to finish cooking.

Divide the soup among 4 bowls, garnish with scallions, and serve with lemon wedges for squeezing.

MAKES 4 (1½-cup) SERVINGS ▌ **Per serving:** 265 calories, 7.5 g fat, 1 g saturated fat, 18 g protein, 33 g carbohydrate, 3.5 g fiber, 442 mg sodium

◀MAKE AHEAD▶ **The soup can be refrigerated for up to 2 days or frozen for up to 3 months. Bring back to room temperature before gently reheating.**

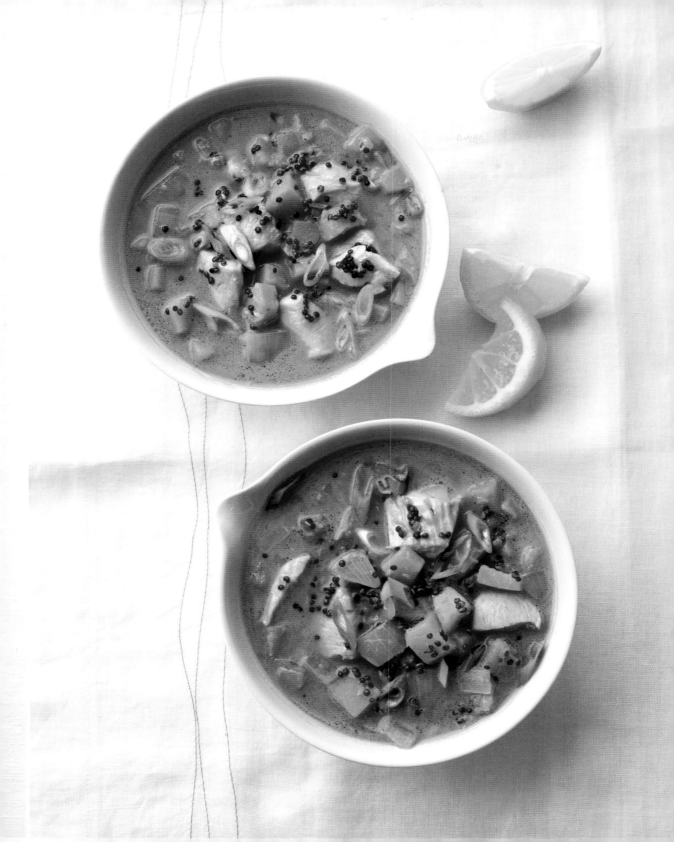

WEST AFRICAN–STYLE BEEF SOUP

HANDS-ON TIME: 35 MINUTES   TOTAL TIME: 35 MINUTES

PHASE
2

Peanut butter adds richness, protein, and healthy unsaturated fat to this soup. Though we tend to think of peanut butter and peanuts as distinctly American ingredients, the legume is actually West African in origin. When you're not in a rush, place the raw steak in the freezer for about 20 minutes to firm it up and make it easier to slice.

2 teaspoons extra-virgin olive oil

2 medium carrots, halved and thinly sliced

2 medium zucchini, halved and thinly sliced

3 cloves garlic, thinly sliced

3½ cups gluten-free low-sodium chicken broth

3 tablespoons creamy all-natural peanut butter

½ teaspoon salt

¼ teaspoon red pepper flakes

8 ounces flank steak, thinly sliced across the grain and then cut into bite-size pieces

In a large saucepan, heat the oil over medium-low heat. Add the carrots, zucchini, and garlic. Stir to coat. Add ¼ cup water and cook, stirring occasionally, until the vegetables are crisp-tender, about 5 minutes.

Add the broth, peanut butter, salt, and pepper flakes and bring to a boil. Reduce to a simmer, add the beef, and simmer until the meat is no longer pink and just cooked through, about 3 minutes. Serve hot.

MAKES 4 (1½-cup) SERVINGS ▶ **Per serving:** 219 calories, 12 g fat, 2.5 g saturated fat, 18 g protein, 10 g carbohydrate, 2.5 g fiber, 411 mg sodium

HEARTY TOMATO AND MEATBALL SOUP

HANDS-ON TIME: 30 MINUTES   TOTAL TIME: 45 MINUTES

Grated orange zest adds a little burst of sunshine to this cold-weather main-dish soup. Make sure the soup is simmering, not at a full boil, when you add the meatballs. This will ensure the meat will be tender, not tough.

1 tablespoon extra-virgin olive oil

1 medium onion, finely chopped

2 cloves garlic, thinly sliced

8 ounces extra-lean ground beef

⅓ cup grated Parmesan cheese

¼ cup chopped fresh flat-leaf parsley

3 tablespoons almond flour

½ teaspoon dried oregano

¼ teaspoon salt

2 tablespoons fat-free milk

1 large egg

3 cups gluten-free low-sodium beef broth

1 can (15 ounces) no-salt-added crushed tomatoes

2 teaspoons grated orange zest

In a large saucepan, heat the oil over medium heat. Add the onion, garlic, and ¼ cup water. Cook, stirring occasionally, until the onion is softened, about 7 minutes.

Meanwhile, in a medium bowl, combine the beef, Parmesan, parsley, almond flour, oregano, and salt. Add the milk and egg. Mix well. Shape into 12 walnut-size meatballs and transfer to a plate.

Add the broth, tomatoes, and orange zest to the pan and bring to a simmer. Add the meatballs, return to a simmer, cover, and cook until the meatballs are firm, about 12 minutes.

Divide the soup among 4 shallow bowls, serving each person 3 meatballs.

MAKES 4 SERVINGS ▶ Per serving: 249 calories, 12 g fat, 3.5 g saturated fat, 22 g protein, 12 g carbohydrate, 3 g fiber, 416 mg sodium

◀MAKE AHEAD▶ The soup and *uncooked* meatballs can be made ahead and refrigerated for 3 days or frozen for up to 3 months. Shape the meatballs, transfer them to a baking sheet, and freeze, then transfer to a freezer container. Freeze the soup base separately. When ready to serve, reheat the soup base to a simmer and add the meatballs (thawed in the refrigerator) and cook as directed.

NEW ENGLAND CHICKEN CHOWDER

HANDS-ON TIME: 25 MINUTES   TOTAL TIME: 35 MINUTES

PHASE 2

White bean flour helps give this soup its creamy base but has a mild enough flavor that the soup won't taste like a bean soup. Be sure to check the label on the Canadian bacon to make sure it's gluten free; some brands are not.

1 tablespoon plus 1 teaspoon extra-virgin olive oil	¾ pound boneless, skinless chicken breast, cut into ½-inch chunks
1 large onion, finely chopped	½ teaspoon salt
1½ ounces gluten-free all-natural uncured Canadian bacon, diced	¼ teaspoon freshly ground black pepper
¼ cup white bean flour	¼ teaspoon dried thyme
3 cups gluten-free low-sodium chicken broth	⅓ cup chopped fresh flat-leaf parsley

In a large saucepan, heat the oil over medium-low heat. Add the onion and Canadian bacon. Cook, stirring occasionally, until the onion is tender, about 7 minutes.

Stir in the bean flour and cook until the onion is well coated, about 1 minute. Gradually whisk in the broth until smooth. Bring to a boil, reduce to a simmer, and cook for 5 minutes to lightly thicken.

Add the chicken, salt, pepper, and thyme. Simmer until the chicken is cooked through but still juicy, about 5 minutes. Stir in the parsley and serve hot.

MAKES 4 (1¼-cup) SERVINGS ❱ **Per serving:** 210 calories, 7.5 g fat, 1.5 g saturated fat, 24 g protein, 10 g carbohydrate, 3 g fiber, 541 mg sodium

❰MAKE AHEAD❱ **The soup can be prepared through the second step and refrigerated for up to 2 days. Gently reheat and then start with the last step to complete.**

HOT AND SOUR CABBAGE SOUP WITH PORK

HANDS-ON TIME: 25 MINUTES   TOTAL TIME: 30 MINUTES

PHASE 1

30 MINUTES OR LESS

To cut the pork, thinly slice it crosswise (across the grain) and then cut each slice into thin strips. If you have the time, put the pork in the freezer for about 20 minutes to firm it up, which will make it easier to slice.

- 3 tablespoons apple cider vinegar
- 2 teaspoons gluten-free reduced-sodium tamari soy sauce
- 1 teaspoon dark sesame oil
- ½ teaspoon red pepper flakes
- ¾ pound pork tenderloin, cut into thin strips
- 1 tablespoon extra-virgin olive oil
- 1 medium green bell pepper, slivered

- 2 cloves garlic, grated on a rasp-style citrus zester
- 5 cups shredded red cabbage (about ½ small head)
- ½ teaspoon salt
- 4 cups gluten-free low-sodium chicken broth or vegetable broth

In a medium bowl, combine the vinegar, soy sauce, sesame oil, and pepper flakes. Add the pork and toss to coat. Let sit at room temperature while you prep the vegetables.

In a medium-large saucepan, heat the olive oil over medium-high heat. Add the bell pepper and garlic. Stir until the pepper is just beginning to soften, about 3 minutes.

Add the cabbage and salt and stir to coat. Stir in the pork (and its marinade). Add the chicken broth and bring to a simmer. Cook until the cabbage is tender, 3 to 5 minutes.

Taste and add more vinegar or pepper flakes, if desired. Divide among 4 bowls and serve hot.

MAKES 4 (2-cup) SERVINGS ▶ Per serving: 190 calories, 6.5 g fat, 1.5 g saturated fat, 22 g protein, 10 g carbohydrate, 2.5 g fiber, 548 mg sodium

◀**MAKE AHEAD▶ You can slice and marinate the pork ahead of time. It can sit at room temperature for 30 minutes, but if you're prepping well ahead, cover and refrigerate until about 30 minutes before you're ready to make the soup.**

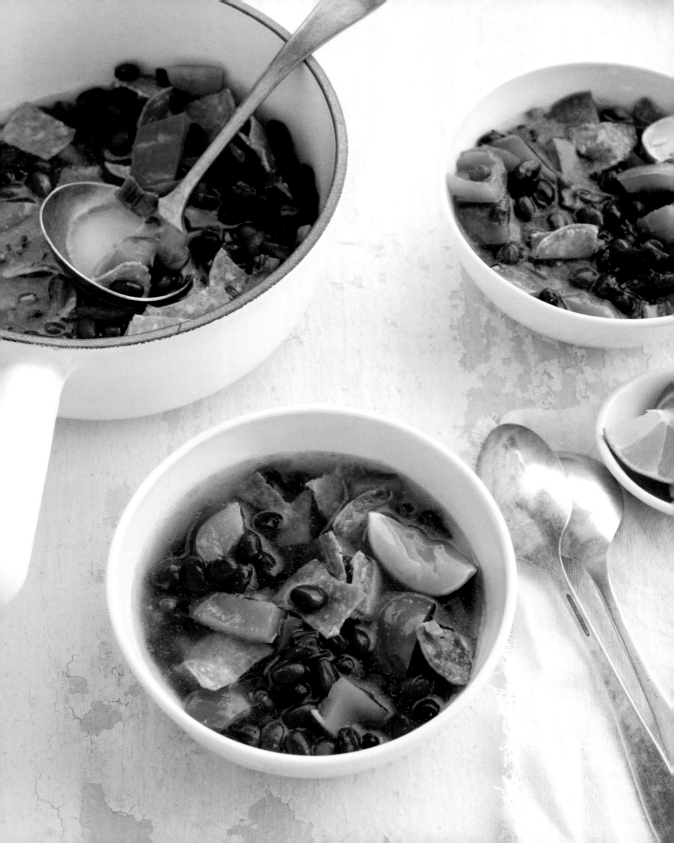

SPICY SAUSAGE, BLACK BEAN, AND PEPPER SOUP

HANDS-ON TIME: 20 MINUTES   TOTAL TIME: 30 MINUTES

Turn this hearty soup into a brown-bag lunch staple with this trick: Pack single portions of the soup into resealable freezer bags. Lay the bags on a baking sheet so that the soup freezes flat. Once frozen, you can stack the bags to save freezer space, and when you pop one in your lunch tote, it will thaw and be ready to reheat in the office microwave.

1 tablespoon extra-virgin olive oil

2 ounces gluten-free turkey pepperoni slices, quartered

6 scallions, thinly sliced

1 large green bell pepper, cut into ½-inch squares

1 teaspoon ground coriander

1 teaspoon ground cumin

¼ teaspoon salt

2 cans (15 ounces each) gluten-free no-salt-added black beans, drained and rinsed

3 cups gluten-free low-sodium chicken broth

Lime wedges, for serving

In a large saucepan, heat the oil over medium heat. Add the pepperoni, scallions, and bell pepper. Cook, stirring frequently, until the pepper is tender, about 7 minutes.

Stir in the coriander, cumin, and salt. Add the beans, broth, and 1 cup water and bring to a boil. Reduce to a simmer, cover, and cook for 10 minutes to develop the flavors.

Divide the soup among 4 serving bowls and serve hot with lime wedges for squeezing.

MAKES 4 (1¾-cup) SERVINGS ▌ **Per serving:** 270 calories, 5.5 g fat, 1 g saturated fat, 20 g protein, 37 g carbohydrate, 12 g fiber, 440 mg sodium

◀MAKE AHEAD▶ **The soup can be refrigerated for 3 days or frozen for 3 months. Let return to room temperature before gently reheating over medium-low heat.**

GREEK-STYLE TURKEY AND LENTIL SOUP

HANDS-ON TIME: 10 MINUTES   TOTAL TIME: 45 MINUTES

PHASE
1

The lentils may be tender somewhere around 40 minutes, but if you can spare the time, let them cook a little longer so that some of them break down and add body to the soup. And if you have access to fresh herbs, by all means use them here in place of the dried—1 tablespoon minced fresh mint and about 1½ teaspoons finely chopped fresh oregano.

5 cups gluten-free low-sodium chicken broth

¾ cup brown lentils

2 teaspoons grated lemon zest

1 teaspoon dried mint

¾ teaspoon dried oregano

½ teaspoon salt

4 teaspoons extra-virgin olive oil

1 large red bell pepper, diced

4 cloves garlic, minced

½ pound gluten-free ground turkey breast

2 tablespoons fresh lemon juice

¼ cup crumbled reduced-fat feta cheese (1 ounce)

In a medium saucepan, combine the broth, lentils, lemon zest, mint, oregano, and ¼ teaspoon of the salt. Bring to a boil, reduce to a simmer, cover, and cook until the lentils are tender, 40 to 45 minutes.

Meanwhile, in a large nonstick skillet, heat 2 teaspoons of the oil over medium-high heat. Add the bell pepper, garlic, and remaining ¼ teaspoon salt. Cook until the pepper is tender, about 3 minutes. Add the turkey and drizzle with the remaining 2 teaspoons oil. Cook, breaking the turkey up as it cooks, until mostly browned but still quite pink, about 1 minute. Set aside (in the skillet) until the lentils are done.

Once the lentils are tender, add the turkey mixture and cook to heat through. Stir in the lemon juice.

Divide the soup among 4 serving bowls, sprinkle each serving with 1 tablespoon of the feta, and serve hot.

MAKES 4 (1½-cup) SERVINGS ❯ **Per serving:** 278 calories, 6.5 g fat, 1.5 g saturated fat, 28 g protein, 27 g carbohydrate, 9.5 g fiber, 496 mg sodium

❮**MAKE AHEAD**❯ **The soup can be made 3 days ahead and refrigerated, or frozen for up to 3 months. Reheat gently over medium-low heat.**

KALE AND SMOKED TURKEY SOUP

HANDS-ON TIME: 30 MINUTES   TOTAL TIME: 45 MINUTES

PHASE
1

You can use another frozen green here, such as collards, but skip spinach, as this soup needs a sturdier green. The smoky flavor comes from both the paprika and the turkey, while the jalapeño gives a little heat. If you want a really spicy soup, choose a smoked paprika that's labeled *picante* (hot).

1 tablespoon plus 1 teaspoon extra-virgin olive oil

2 medium green bell peppers, cut into ½-inch squares

1 fresh jalapeño (seeded if desired for less heat), finely chopped

1½ teaspoons smoked paprika

5 cups gluten-free low-sodium chicken broth

1 can (15 ounces) gluten-free no-salt-added cannellini beans, drained and rinsed

1 package (10 ounces) frozen chopped kale, thawed and drained

4 ounces deli-sliced all-natural uncured mesquite-smoked turkey, cut into ½-inch-wide strips

2 plum tomatoes, diced

In a large saucepan, heat the oil over medium-low heat. Add the bell peppers and jalapeño. Cook, stirring occasionally, until the bell peppers are crisp-tender, about 7 minutes.

Stir in the smoked paprika. Add the broth, beans, kale, turkey, and tomatoes. Bring to a boil, then reduce to a simmer. Cover and cook until the kale is tender and the tomatoes have softened, about 15 minutes. Serve hot.

MAKES 4 (2-cup) SERVINGS ▶ **Per serving:** 222 calories, 6.5 g fat, 0.5 g saturated fat, 18 g protein, 25 g carbohydrate, 8 g fiber, 336 mg sodium

◀MAKE AHEAD▶ **This can be made ahead and refrigerated for up to 3 days or frozen for up to 3 months. Let return to room temperature before reheating gently over medium-low heat.**

CHICKPEA AND SWEET POTATO BISQUE

HANDS-ON TIME: 30 MINUTES
TOTAL TIME: 30 MINUTES PLUS COOLING AND CHILLING TIME

PHASE 2

This smooth, chilled soup makes a great summer lunch. Have it with Asparagus Salad with Feta and Roasted Nuts (page 111) and a slice of gluten-free multigrain toast. It also makes an elegant starter for a dinner party. Omit the walnuts and herb garnish and serve the soup in pretty teacups, so diners can sip it.

1 tablespoon extra-virgin olive oil

3 large or 2 small leeks, white and pale-green parts only, thinly sliced and well washed

1 can (15 ounces) gluten-free no-salt-added chickpeas, drained and rinsed

½ pound sweet potatoes, peeled and thinly sliced

¾ teaspoon salt

5 walnut halves

½ teaspoon crumbled dried tarragon

1 cup 1% or fat-free milk

1 cup fat-free evaporated milk, chilled

Chopped fresh flat-leaf parsley, cilantro, basil, or scallion greens, for garnish (optional)

In a medium saucepan, heat the oil over medium heat. Add the leeks and cook, stirring occasionally, until softened and beginning to brown, 5 to 7 minutes.

Add the chickpeas, sweet potatoes, salt, and 1½ cups water. Bring to a boil over high heat, then reduce to a simmer. Cover and cook until the sweet potatoes are very soft, about 15 minutes.

Meanwhile, in a toaster oven at 350°F or in a dry skillet over medium-low heat, cook the walnuts (stirring if in a skillet) until toasted and fragrant, 3 to 5 minutes. Immediately transfer to a cutting board to stop the cooking. When cool enough to handle, finely chop and set aside.

Transfer the sweet potato mixture to a food processor or blender. Purée until smooth. Add the tarragon and blend. With the machine running, gradually blend in the 1% milk. Transfer to a large bowl and let cool to room temperature. Cover and refrigerate until well chilled, at least 2 hours.

Stir in the evaporated milk and ladle into serving bowls. Top evenly with the toasted walnuts and chopped herbs (if using).

MAKES 4 (1⅓-cup) MAIN COURSE OR 8 (⅔-cup) STARTER SERVINGS ▶ Per main-course serving: 310 calories, 7 g fat, 1 g saturated fat, 15 g protein, 48 g carbohydrate, 7 g fiber, 588 mg sodium

Per starter serving (without walnuts): 147 calories, 2.5 g fat, 0.5 g saturated fat, 7 g protein, 24 g carbohydrate, 3.5 g fiber, 294 mg sodium

DOUBLE-MUSHROOM
CREAM OF MUSHROOM SOUP

HANDS-ON TIME: 15 MINUTES   TOTAL TIME: 25 MINUTES

After reconstituting dried mushrooms, you have to strain the soaking liquid because the mushrooms often have grit clinging to them. Any time you are soaking dried mushrooms, if you end up with more soaking liquid than you need for a recipe, freeze the extra after straining and use it in vegetarian dishes in place of a vegetable broth.

¼ ounce dried porcini mushrooms (¼ cup)

1 pound fresh white or cremini mushrooms

1 tablespoon plus 1 teaspoon extra-virgin olive oil

2 tablespoons black bean flour

2 cups fat-free milk

½ teaspoon dried rosemary

½ teaspoon salt

Freshly ground black pepper

2 wedges (¾ ounce each) light spreadable cheese, cut into small pieces

1 tablespoon fresh lemon juice

In a small bowl, combine the dried porcini and 1 cup hot water and let stand until softened, about 10 minutes. Using a slotted spoon, lift the mushrooms out of the soaking liquid. Reserve the liquid and coarsely chop the porcini. Line a fine-mesh strainer with dampened paper towels and strain the mushroom soaking liquid; reserve.

Thinly slice half the fresh mushrooms. In a food processor, pulse the remaining fresh mushrooms until very finely chopped.

In a large saucepan, heat the oil over medium heat. Add all of the fresh mushrooms and the porcini. Cook until the fresh mushrooms have softened, about 5 minutes.

Add the black bean flour and stir until the mushrooms are coated. Add the mushroom soaking liquid, milk, rosemary, salt, and a couple of pinches of pepper. Cook, stirring occasionally, until the soup is lightly thickened and the mushrooms are very soft, about 7 minutes.

Stir in the cheese and cook until melted, about 3 minutes. Stir in the lemon juice and serve hot.

MAKES 4 (1¼-cup) SERVINGS ▶ **Per serving:** 147 calories, 6 g fat, 1.5 g saturated fat, 11 g protein, 14 g carbohydrate, 2 g fiber, 479 mg sodium

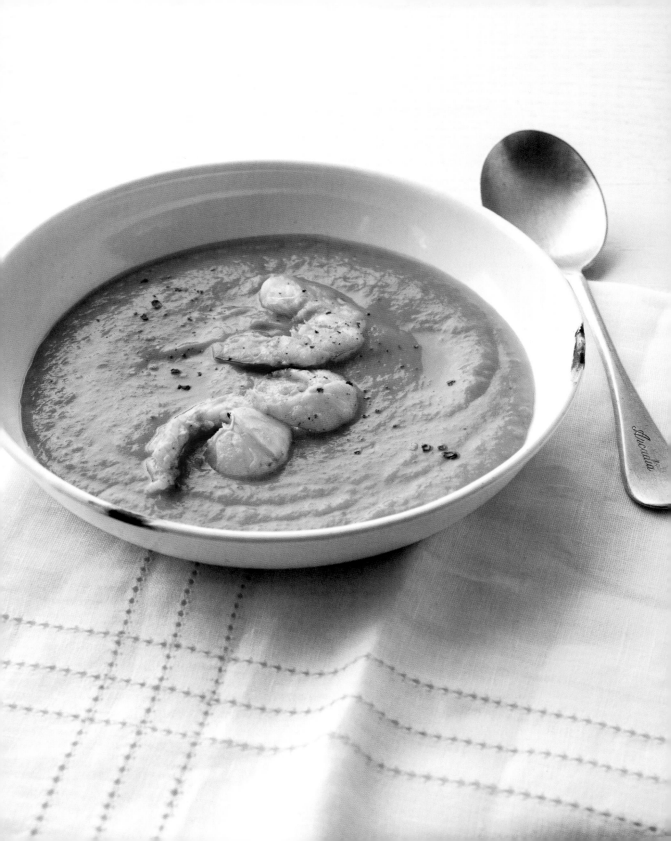

CREAMY ASPARAGUS-PEA SOUP WITH DEVILED SHRIMP

HANDS-ON TIME: 10 MINUTES   TOTAL TIME: 50 MINUTES

This pretty soup is filling enough to be served with just a side salad. One of our favorites is a tricolor mix of radicchio, arugula, and endive with a light vinaigrette of lemon juice and extra-virgin olive oil.

4 teaspoons extra-virgin olive oil

1 small red onion, coarsely chopped

1 pound asparagus, cut into 1-inch lengths

¾ cup green split peas

4 cups gluten-free low-sodium chicken broth

6 large shrimp (about ¼ pound), peeled, deveined, and halved horizontally

2 teaspoons Dijon mustard

1 teaspoon hot sauce

¼ cup grated Parmesan cheese

½ teaspoon salt

¼ cup finely chopped fresh flat-leaf parsley, for garnish (optional)

In a nonstick saucepan, heat 2 teaspoons of the oil over medium-high heat. Add the onion and cook until lightly browned, 3 to 5 minutes.

Add the asparagus, split peas, and broth. Bring to a boil, then reduce to a simmer. Cover and cook until the split peas are very tender and beginning to fall apart, 35 to 40 minutes.

Meanwhile, in a small bowl, toss the shrimp with 1 teaspoon of the mustard and the hot sauce. In a medium nonstick skillet, heat the remaining 2 teaspoons oil. Add the shrimp and toss until opaque throughout, 45 seconds to 1 minute. Transfer to a plate.

Carefully transfer the asparagus soup to a blender and purée (make sure you vent the top for steam). Add the Parmesan, salt, and remaining 1 teaspoon mustard. Purée again (the soup should still be hot enough to melt the cheese).

Divide the soup among 4 shallow bowls and top each serving with 3 shrimp halves and 1 tablespoon parsley (if using).

MAKES 4 (1½-cup) SERVINGS ▶ Per serving: 244 calories, 6.5 g fat, 1.5 g saturated fat, 17 g protein, 30 g carbohydrate, 12 g fiber, 586 mg sodium

◀MAKE AHEAD▶ **You can make the soup 2 days ahead and reheat, but the soup will thicken as it sits in the refrigerator, so loosen it up with a little chicken broth when you reheat. Don't cook the shrimp until just before serving.**

ITALIAN PUMPKIN SOUP

HANDS-ON TIME: 30 MINUTES   TOTAL TIME: 45 MINUTES

PHASE 2

When pumpkin isn't in season, substitute butternut squash, either fresh or frozen. You can find precut butternut squash in the produce department, often packaged in 1¼-pound bags or plastic containers.

1 tablespoon plus 1 teaspoon extra-virgin olive oil

3 cups chunks (1-inch) peeled fresh pumpkin

1 medium red bell pepper, cut into 1-inch squares

1 medium onion, finely chopped

3 cloves garlic, thinly sliced

4 cups gluten-free low-sodium chicken broth

2 cans (15 ounces each) gluten-free no-salt-added cannellini beans, drained and rinsed

½ teaspoon rubbed sage

½ teaspoon salt

⅓ cup grated Parmesan cheese

4 teaspoons hulled pumpkin seeds (pepitas)

In a large saucepan, heat the oil over medium heat. Add the pumpkin, bell pepper, onion, and garlic. Stir to coat. Add 1 cup water and cook, stirring occasionally, until the pumpkin is crisp-tender, about 10 minutes.

Add the broth, beans, sage, and salt and bring to a boil. Reduce to a simmer, cover, and cook, stirring once or twice, until the pumpkin is very soft, about 10 minutes.

Divide the soup among 4 bowls. Dividing evenly, sprinkle with the Parmesan and pumpkin seeds. Serve hot.

MAKES 4 (2-cup) SERVINGS ▶ **Per serving:** 345 calories, 9.5 g fat, 2 g saturated fat, 18 g protein, 49 g carbohydrate, 12 g fiber, 540 mg sodium

◀MAKE AHEAD▶ **The soup can be made ahead and either refrigerated for up to 2 days or frozen for up to 3 months. If you like, divide the soup into individual portions before freezing, then just reheat what you need.**

PASTA E FAGIOLI

PHASE 2

30 MINUTES OR LESS

A really easy way to get very finely "minced" garlic is to run it across a rasp-style citrus zester or the very fine holes of a box grater. The garlic will end up as more of a paste and will distribute easily through a soup.

1 tablespoon extra-virgin olive oil

4 cloves garlic, grated on a rasp-style citrus zester

¾ teaspoon dried oregano

¼ teaspoon freshly ground black pepper

4 cups gluten-free low-sodium chicken broth

½ teaspoon salt

4 ounces gluten-free quinoa elbow macaroni

1 can (15 ounces) gluten-free no-salt-added red kidney beans, drained and rinsed

1 can (14.5 ounces) no-salt-added diced tomatoes

1½ cups frozen small cauliflower florets, thawed

½ cup shredded fresh basil

⅓ cup grated Parmesan cheese

In a medium-large saucepan, heat the oil over medium heat. Add the garlic, oregano, and pepper. Cook until fragrant, about 30 seconds.

Add the broth and bring to a boil. Add the salt and macaroni and cook according to package directions until 2 minutes shy of done. Add the beans, diced tomatoes, and cauliflower. Return to a boil, then cook at a high simmer for 2 minutes to develop the flavors and heat through. Stir in the basil.

Divide the soup among 4 serving bowls. Dividing evenly, sprinkle with the Parmesan. Serve hot.

MAKES 4 (1¾-cup) SERVINGS ❯ **Per serving:** 305 calories, 6 g fat, 1.5 g saturated fat, 16 g protein, 48 g carbohydrate, 13 g fiber, 501 mg sodium

❮**MAKE AHEAD**❯ **You can make the soup 3 days ahead and refrigerate, but with these changes: Do not cook the pasta in the soup; instead when you reheat the made-ahead soup for serving, bring it to a simmer and then add the uncooked pasta and cook it. Do not add the fresh basil until just before serving.**

CHICKEN SOUP WITH DUMPLINGS

HANDS-ON TIME: 25 MINUTES   TOTAL TIME: 45 MINUTES PLUS CHILLING TIME

PHASE
2

These dumplings are made with a mix of almond and sorghum flour and get their fluffy texture from the addition of egg whites. Don't let dumpling-making intimidate you, it's easy!

1½ cups almond flour

1 cup sorghum flour

1 teaspoon garlic powder

1 teaspoon onion powder

1 teaspoon salt

2 large eggs

2 large egg whites

1 tablespoon extra-virgin olive oil

1 medium carrot, finely diced

1 small onion, finely diced

1 large stalk celery, finely diced

½ pound boneless, skinless chicken breasts, cut into 1-inch pieces

5 cups gluten-free low-sodium chicken broth

In a large bowl, combine the almond flour, sorghum flour, garlic powder, onion powder, and ½ teaspoon of the salt. Mix well.

In a bowl, with an electric mixer at medium speed, beat together the whole eggs and egg whites until the eggs are light and fluffy.

With the mixer at medium speed, gradually add the flour mixture to the egg mixture, mixing until well combined. Cover the bowl and refrigerate for 1 hour.

In a large nonstick saucepan, heat the oil over medium heat. Add the carrots, onion, and celery. Cook until the onions are translucent but not browned, 5 to 7 minutes.

Add the chicken and cook, stirring occasionally, until the chicken is lightly browned on all sides, about 5 minutes. Sprinkle with the remaining ½ teaspoon salt.

Add the broth and 5 cups water and bring to a simmer.

With moistened hands, shape the chilled batter into 12 balls. With a large spoon, gently lower the balls into the boiling soup, cover, reduce heat, and simmer until the dumplings firm up, about 20 minutes. If you like your dumplings very firm, do not cover the pot while cooking.

Divide the soup evenly among 6 bowls, serving each person 2 dumplings.

MAKES 6 SERVINGS ❱ **Per serving:** 369 calories, 20 g fat, 2 g saturated fat, 22 g protein, 29 g carbohydrate, 6.5 g fiber, 571 mg sodium

JÍCAMA CHEESE TOASTIES

HANDS-ON TIME: 15 MINUTES   TOTAL TIME: 35 MINUTES

PHASE 1

The skin of a jícama, a tuber with a sweet flavor and crunchy texture, is reminiscent of a potato. When searching for it in the market, chances are you'll find it near the potatoes. (But unlike the potato, the skin is not edible.) Here jícama serves as a sandwich "bread." If you've got any left over, dice and use it in a stir-fry, much like you would water chestnuts.

Olive oil cooking spray

1 medium-small jícama (at least 4 inches in diameter), peeled and cut into 8 thin rounds

4 teaspoons Dijon mustard

4 ounces deli-sliced reduced-fat provolone cheese

6 ounces deli-sliced gluten-free turkey breast

2 peperoncini (Italian pickled peppers), rinsed and sliced crosswise

Preheat the oven to 375°F. Spray a rimmed baking sheet with olive oil.

Place 4 jícama rounds on the baking sheet and brush with 2 teaspoons of the mustard. Top each with a slice of the provolone (trim to fit) and a slice of the turkey, then top evenly with the peperoncini. Brush one side of the remaining 4 slices of jícama with the remaining 2 teaspoons mustard and place them, mustard-side down, on top of the other rounds. Spray the tops with olive oil.

Bake for 10 minutes, then carefully turn the toasties over and bake until the tops are browned in spots and the sandwiches are piping hot, 5 to 7 minutes.

MAKES 4 SERVINGS ▶ Per serving: 169 calories, 6 g fat, 3.5 g saturated fat, 20 g protein, 7 g carbohydrate, 2.5 g fiber, 449 mg sodium

CAPRESE PANINI

HANDS-ON TIME: 15 MINUTES TOTAL TIME: 40 MINUTES

The flatbread, made with garbanzo flour and fresh basil, provides a nice amount of fiber per serving on its own: 7 grams. If you have a hinged electric grill or an electric sandwich press, you can use it here. When you don't want a whole sandwich, enjoy the bread as a snack: Toast a slice and then spread with 1 wedge light spreadable cheese or some all-natural peanut butter.

Olive oil cooking spray

1½ cups garbanzo bean flour

1 teaspoon gluten-free baking powder

⅓ cup minced fresh basil plus 12 large basil leaves

¼ teaspoon plus a pinch of salt

¼ teaspoon freshly ground black pepper

1 large egg white beaten with 2 tablespoons water

2 teaspoons extra-virgin olive oil

3 vine-ripened or 4 plum tomatoes, cut into ⅓-inch-thick slices

4 ounces thinly sliced part-skim mozzarella

Preheat the oven to 425°F. Line a 10 × 15-inch rimmed baking sheet with parchment paper to come up on the long sides. Spray the short sides of the pan with a little olive oil, then lightly spray the parchment paper.

In a medium bowl, whisk together the garbanzo flour, baking powder, minced basil, salt, and pepper. Add the beaten egg white, olive oil, and ¾ cup plus 3 tablespoons water. Stir to blend. The batter will be as thin as pancake batter.

Pour the batter into the center of the pan, spreading it evenly over the pan. Bake until the top of the bread is firm, about 15 minutes. Let cool for 5 minutes in the pan, then halve lengthwise and cut each half crosswise into quarters (8 pieces total).

Transfer the pieces to a work surface. (Note: The bread should not look "bready." It is on the moist side.) Spray the tops of the bread lightly with olive oil. Flip the pieces over so the oiled sides are down. Layer the tomato, mozzarella, and whole basil leaves on 4 of the slices and top with the remaining 4 slices, oiled side up.

Preheat a ridged grill pan or cast-iron skillet over medium-high heat. Add the sandwiches and top with another skillet to weight them down. Cook until the tomatoes are hot and the cheese starts to melt, flipping them once, 3 to 5 minutes total. Cut in half on the diagonal to serve.

MAKES 4 SERVINGS ❯ **Per serving:** 283 calories, 10.5 g fat, 3.5 g saturated fat, 18 g protein, 31 g carbohydrate, 8.5 g fiber, 518 mg sodium

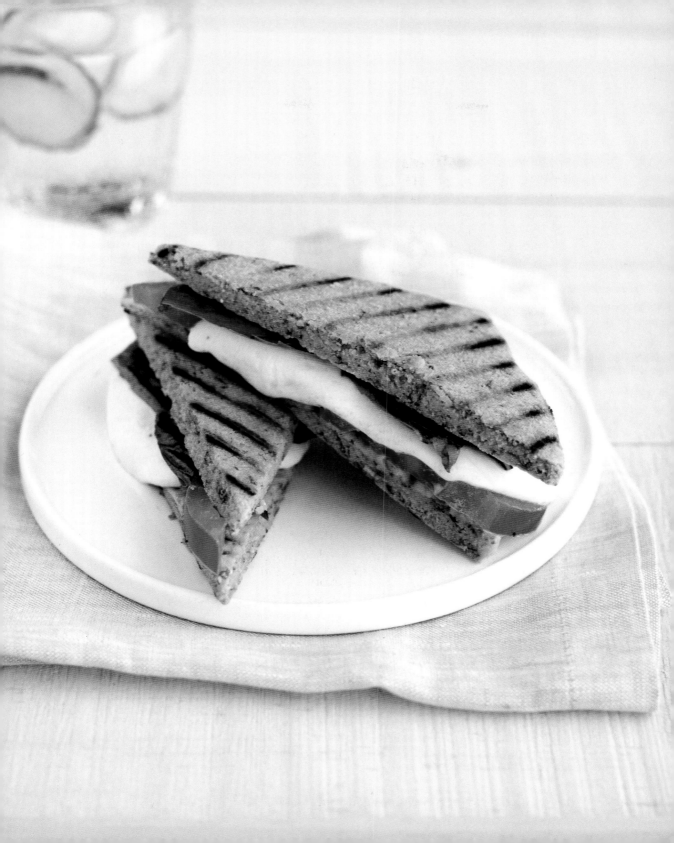

"EVERYTHING" OAT BREAD

HANDS-ON TIME: 15 MINUTES
TOTAL TIME: 1 HOUR 10 MINUTES PLUS COOLING TIME

Like the popular "everything" bagels so many New Yorkers enjoy, which have a mixture of nuts, seeds, and spices (and maybe some onion and garlic added, too), this bread features a wide array of ingredients, including a flavorful poppy seed and sesame seed topping. It makes delicious sandwiches or an accompaniment to your favorite soup.

⅔ cup gluten-free oat flour

½ cup almond flour

⅓ cup flaxseed meal

¼ cup coconut flour

1½ teaspoons gluten-free baking powder

½ teaspoon table salt

4 large eggs, separated, at room temperature

2 tablespoons agave nectar

2½ teaspoons apple cider vinegar

1 cup fat-free milk

1 teaspoon poppy seeds

1 teaspoon sesame seeds

¼ teaspoon coarse kosher salt

Preheat the oven to 300°F. Line a 9 × 5-inch loaf pan with parchment paper, leaving a bit of an overhang on the sides.

In a large bowl, combine the oat flour, almond flour, flaxseed meal, coconut flour, baking powder, and table salt. Whisk well.

In a medium bowl, beat together the egg yolks, agave nectar, and vinegar. Beat in the milk.

In a bowl, with an electric mixer at high speed, beat the egg whites until stiff peaks form.

Add the milk mixture to the flour mixture and beat to combine. Gently fold in the egg whites until fully combined.

Pour the batter into the pan and sprinkle the poppy seeds, sesame seeds, and coarse salt on top. Bake until the bread springs back when touched and a toothpick inserted in the center comes out clean, 50 to 55 minutes.

Let cool in the pan on a rack for 10 minutes, then turn out onto the rack to cool.

MAKES 12 SLICES (1 per serving) ❭ **Per slice:** 112 calories, 6 g fat, 1 g saturated fat, 5 g protein, 10 g carbohydrate, 3 g fiber, 245 mg sodium

❰MAKE AHEAD❱ **This bread will keep well in the freezer for up to 1 month. Cut the loaf into 12 slices, arrange them on a parchment-lined baking sheet, and freeze solid. Wrap each slice in plastic wrap and transfer to a freezer container. Thaw at room temperature.**

JOHNNYCAKE CHICKEN SANDWICHES

HANDS-ON TIME: 30 MINUTES   TOTAL TIME: 30 MINUTES

PHASE 2

30 MINUTES OR LESS

A johnnycake, a traditional New England "bread," is really just cornbread cooked pancake style. Johnnycakes are sturdy without being tough, making them a perfect substitute for sliced bread in a sandwich.

½ teaspoon crumbled dried rosemary

¼ teaspoon freshly ground black pepper

¾ pound boneless, skinless chicken breasts

5 teaspoons extra-virgin olive oil

¾ cup plus 2 tablespoons yellow cornmeal

½ teaspoon coarse kosher salt

1 cup fat-free milk

1 teaspoon agave nectar

2 teaspoons mayonnaise (made with extra-virgin olive oil)

4 lettuce leaves

1 vine-ripened tomato, cut into 4 slices

Preheat the broiler with the rack 4 inches from the heat. Sprinkle the rosemary and pepper over the chicken and rub it in. Rub 1 teaspoon of the oil over the chicken. Broil, turning the chicken over midway, until just cooked through but still juicy, about 10 minutes. Transfer to a cutting board to cool. When cool enough to handle, thinly slice the chicken across the grain.

Meanwhile, in a medium bowl, combine the cornmeal and salt. In a small saucepan, bring the milk to a simmer over medium-low heat. Stir the milk into the cornmeal, stirring until evenly moistened. Stir in the agave nectar.

In a large nonstick or cast-iron skillet, heat 2 teaspoons of the oil over medium heat. Using a scant ¼ cup batter for each, spoon 4 johnnycakes into the pan. Cook until bubbles appear on the surface, about 2 minutes. Turn the cakes over and cook until the undersides are golden brown, about 1 minute longer. Transfer to a rack to cool. Repeat with the remaining 2 teaspoons oil and remaining batter to make 8 johnnycakes.

Let the johnnycakes cool to room temperature. Spread the mayonnaise on one side of each of the johnnycakes. Top the mayo on 4 of the johnnycakes with a lettuce leaf and a slice of tomato. Top evenly with the chicken and then place the remaining 4 johnnycakes, mayo-side down, on tops to make sandwiches.

MAKES 4 SERVINGS ❱ **Per serving:** 315 calories, 9 g fat, 1.5 g saturated fat, 24 g protein, 33 g carbohydrate, 2 g fiber, 333 mg sodium

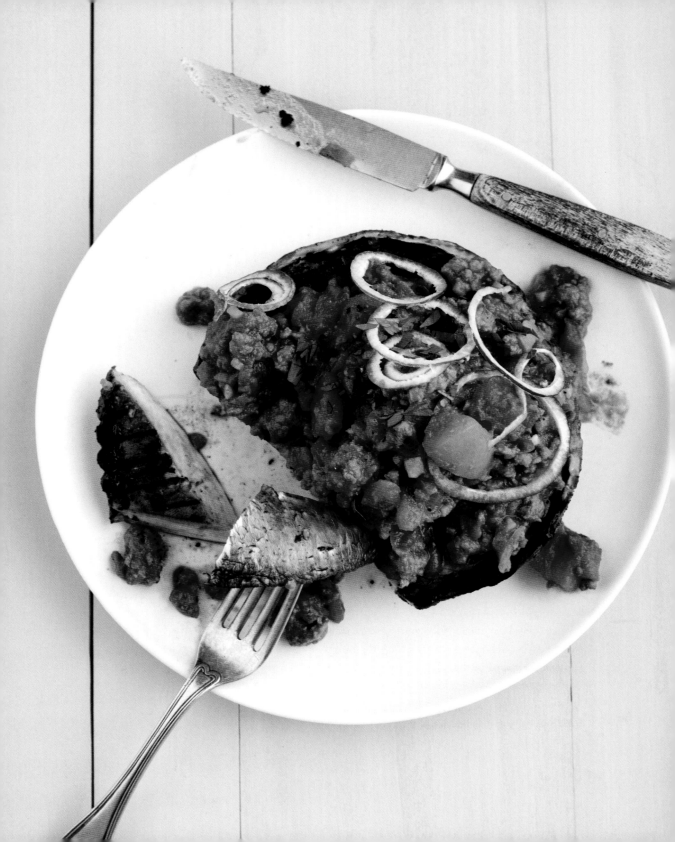

SMOKED PORTOBELLO SLOPPY JOES

HANDS-ON TIME: 20 MINUTES   TOTAL TIME: 30 MINUTES

Portobello mushrooms make great gluten-free "buns" for this popular sandwich filling. The portobello gills do not contribute any flavor and release a slightly gritty black liquid if cooked, so it's usually better to scrape them out (simply use a teaspoon for scraping).

1 tablespoon plus 1 teaspoon extra-virgin olive oil

1 large red onion, finely chopped; plus ½ small red onion, sliced, for garnish (optional)

3 cloves garlic, minced

1 teaspoon gluten-free chili powder

¼ teaspoon salt

1 pound lean ground sirloin

1 can (14.5 ounces) no-salt-added diced tomatoes

3 tablespoons no-salt-added tomato paste

1 tablespoon gluten-free Worcestershire sauce

4 smoked or regular portobello mushroom caps (4 inches across)

Olive oil cooking spray

In a large nonstick skillet, heat the oil over medium heat. Add the onion, garlic, chili powder, and salt. Cook, stirring occasionally, until the onion is softened, about 5 minutes.

Add the beef to the skillet and cook, breaking it up with a spoon, until almost all browned but still a little pink, about 3 minutes.

Stir in the diced tomatoes, tomato paste, and Worcestershire sauce. Simmer until the sauce is thickened and flavorful, 15 to 20 minutes. It should be wet but not soupy.

Meanwhile, scrape the black gills out of the mushroom caps and cut the stems flush with the mushrooms. Spray the mushrooms inside and out lightly with olive oil. Cook the mushrooms in a sandwich press, hinged electric grill, or on a preheated stovetop grill pan until tender (but not shriveled), 6 to 8 minutes, depending on the thickness of the mushrooms.

To serve, place a portobello cap gilled-side up on a plate and top with a generous ¾ cup of the sloppy Joe mixture. Garnish with onion slices, if desired.

MAKES 4 SERVINGS ▸ Per serving: 278 calories, 10 g fat, 3 g saturated fat, 28 g protein, 22 g carbohydrate, 5 g fiber, 301 mg sodium

◀MAKE AHEAD▶ **The sloppy Joe mixture can be cooked 3 days ahead and refrigerated. Reheat gently over medium-low heat, adding a splash of water to loosen the mixture if it's too thick.**

OAT CAKE QUESADILLAS

HANDS-ON TIME: 25 MINUTES   TOTAL TIME: 30 MINUTES

PHASE 2

30 MINUTES OR LESS

These are delicious as a light lunch, perhaps with a fresh tomato salsa, but they can also serve as the starting point for a more substantial meal: Layer in sliced cooked beef or poultry, chopped tomato, scallion greens, and some cooked kale—all would marry well with the cheese.

1¼ cups nonfat plain yogurt

1 large egg

1 large egg white

¼ cup chopped fresh dill or parsley; plus dill sprigs for garnish (optional)

2 cloves garlic, minced

1 teaspoon grated lemon zest

¼ teaspoon salt

1 cup gluten-free rolled oats

3 tablespoons gluten-free oat bran

3 teaspoons extra-virgin olive oil

¾ cup shredded reduced-fat Mexican blend cheese (3 ounces)

Preheat the oven to 350°F.

In a large bowl, whisk together the yogurt, whole egg, egg white, dill, garlic, lemon zest, and salt. Stir in the oats, oat bran, and 3 tablespoons water until well combined.

In a medium nonstick skillet, heat 1½ teaspoons of the oil over medium heat. Drop a generous ⅓ cup of the batter for each of 2 oat cakes into the pan and cook until bubbles appear on the surface and the undersides are golden brown, about 1 minute. Carefully turn the oat cakes over and cook until the undersides are golden brown, about 30 seconds. Repeat with the remaining 1½ teaspoons oil and batter to make 2 more oat cakes.

Place 2 oat cakes on a baking sheet and divide the cheese between them. Top with the remaining 2 oat cakes and bake until the cheese has melted, about 5 minutes. Cut each into 4 wedges. Serve each person 2 wedges and garnish with a dill sprig, if desired.

MAKES 4 (2-wedge) SERVINGS ❱ **Per serving:** 236 calories, 11 g fat, 3.5 g saturated fat, 15 g protein, 23 g carbohydrate, 3 g fiber, 380 mg sodium

❰MAKE AHEAD❱ The oat cakes can be refrigerated for up to a day or frozen for up to 3 months. If freezing, arrange on a small baking sheet and freeze solid, then transfer to a freezer container. To reheat, place the oat cakes on a baking sheet and cover with foil. Reheat in a 350°F oven for about 10 minutes.

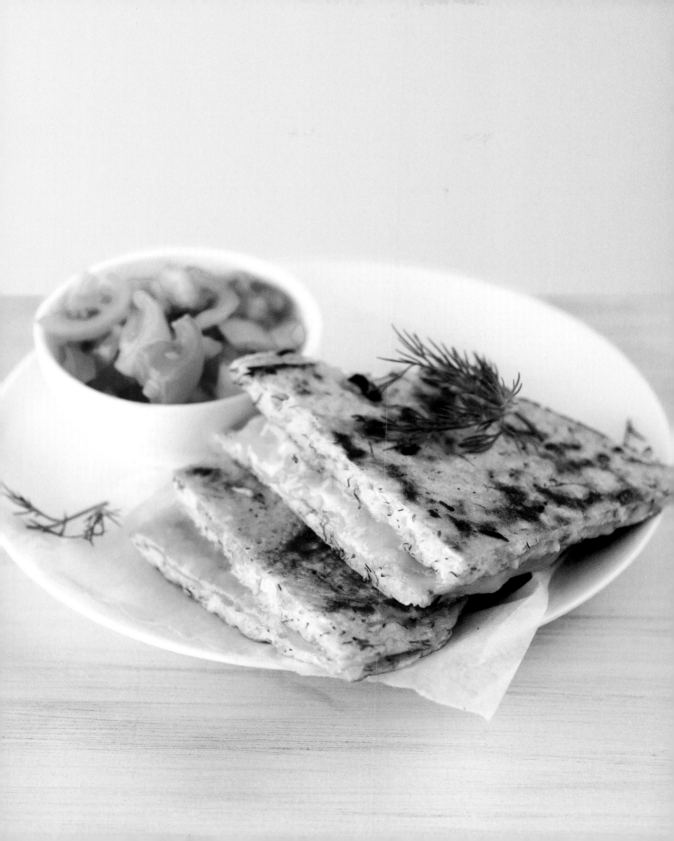

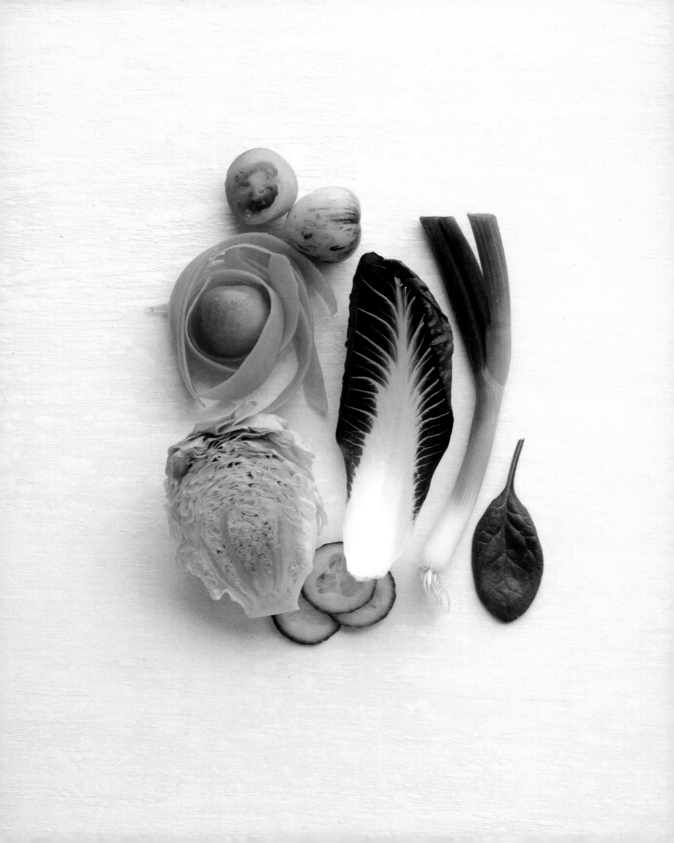

SALADS

Nutrient-rich salads are a South Beach Diet staple. But watch out for those commercial salad dressings. Many contain gluten and sugar, so it's best to make your own, as we do with each of the salads featured here. You'll find main-dish poultry, beef, and pork salads; seafood, pasta, and bean salads; and side salads, too. One of our favorites: the Gluten Solution SuperSalad, which has 20 grams of filling protein and 8 grams of fiber!

LATIN AMERICAN CHICKEN AND CABBAGE SALAD

HANDS-ON TIME: 35 MINUTES   TOTAL TIME: 40 MINUTES

PHASE
1

Cilantro and chili powder give gusto to this refreshing salad. Here the crunchy slawlike salad is served topped with thinly sliced chicken, but you could also dice the chicken and toss it into the salad. And for more variations, try this same idea with roasted pork tenderloin or grilled shrimp in place of the chicken.

2½ teaspoons gluten-free chili powder

½ teaspoon coarse kosher salt

1¼ pounds boneless, skinless chicken breasts

1 tablespoon plus 2 teaspoons extra-virgin olive oil

1 tablespoon apple cider vinegar

¾ pound cabbage, cut into ½-inch-wide strips about 2 inches long

½ cup cilantro leaves

4 radishes, halved and thinly sliced

1 stalk celery, thinly sliced

In a small bowl, stir together 1½ teaspoons of the chili powder and the salt. Rub the mixture into both sides of the chicken. Brush the chicken with 1 teaspoon of the oil.

Heat a grill pan over medium heat and cook the chicken, turning it over as it gets grill marks, until the chicken is cooked through but still juicy, 10 to 12 minutes. Alternatively, preheat the broiler with the rack 4 inches from the heat and broil the chicken until just cooked through but still juicy, about 10 minutes, turning it over midway. Transfer to a cutting board to cool. When cool enough to handle, thinly slice crosswise.

In a large bowl, whisk together the remaining 1 tablespoon plus 1 teaspoon oil, the remaining 1 teaspoon chili powder, and the vinegar. Add the cabbage, cilantro, radishes, and celery. Toss to combine.

Spoon the cabbage salad onto 4 plates. Dividing evenly, top with the chicken.

MAKES 4 SERVINGS ❯ **Per serving:** 245 calories, 10 g fat, 1.5 g saturated fat, 31 g protein, 6 g carbohydrate, 3 g fiber, 462 mg sodium

❮**MAKE AHEAD**❯ **When served freshly made, the cabbage salad is crisp, but you can make it up to a day ahead and refrigerate it, which changes the texture slightly (and pleasantly) as the cabbage softens up a bit. Cook the chicken shortly before you're ready to serve.**

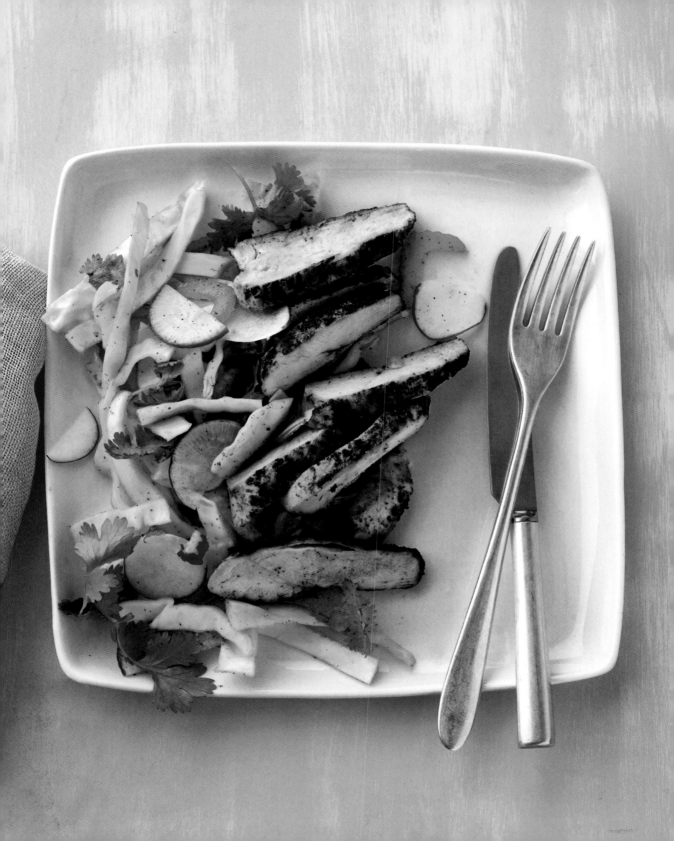

CHICKEN AND SWEET POTATO SALAD WITH SPICY PEANUT DRESSING

HANDS-ON TIME: 15 MINUTES   TOTAL TIME: 25 MINUTES

This Thai-inspired salad can turn Mexican just by switching out the basil and mint for cilantro. And as long as you're headed in that direction, add a minced pickled jalapeño, too.

1 pound sweet potatoes, peeled and cut into ½-inch cubes

3 cloves garlic, peeled and halved

1¼ pounds boneless, skinless chicken breasts

3 tablespoons creamy all-natural peanut butter

2 tablespoons fresh lime juice

1 teaspoon hot sauce

½ teaspoon salt

¼ cup chopped fresh basil

¼ cup chopped fresh mint

1 pound plum tomatoes, cut into bite-size chunks

In a steamer, cook the sweet potatoes until firm-tender, about 10 minutes. Let cool, then transfer to a large salad bowl.

Meanwhile, in a large skillet, combine the garlic and 3 cups of water and bring to a boil. Add the chicken and reduce to a simmer. Cover and cook until the chicken is just cooked through but still juicy, turning over once midway, about 10 minutes.

Reserving the cooking liquid, remove the garlic and set aside. Transfer the chicken to a cutting board. When cool enough to handle, cut the chicken across the grain into bite-size pieces. Add to the sweet potatoes.

Place the garlic in a small bowl. Whisk in ¼ cup of the reserved cooking liquid, the peanut butter, lime juice, hot sauce, and salt. Stir in the basil and mint.

Add the peanut dressing and tomatoes to the salad bowl. Toss to combine. Serve at room temperature.

MAKES 4 (2-cup) SERVINGS ❯ **Per serving:** 333 calories, 10 g fat, 1.5 g saturated fat, 35 g protein, 25 g carbohydrate, 5 g fiber, 494 mg sodium

❮MAKE AHEAD❯ You can prepare some of the ingredients a day ahead (cook the sweet potatoes and chicken, cut up the tomatoes) and refrigerate. Or you can assemble the entire salad ahead and refrigerate; bring back to room temperature before serving.

ROSEMARY CHICKEN SALAD
WITH GOAT CHEESE

HANDS-ON TIME: 10 MINUTES TOTAL   TIME: 20 MINUTES PLUS COOLING TIME

PHASE
1

30
MINUTES
OR
LESS

Instead of using reduced-fat goat cheese in this recipe, try reduced-fat feta. You can buy it precrumbled in most supermarkets. You can also use a mix of halved red and yellow grape tomatoes instead of cherry tomatoes.

1¼ pounds boneless, skinless chicken breasts

½ teaspoon crumbled dried rosemary

½ teaspoon coarse kosher salt

¼ teaspoon freshly ground black pepper

   Olive oil cooking spray

2 tablespoons balsamic vinegar

1 tablespoon extra-virgin olive oil

3 cups arugula

3 cups packed baby spinach (about 3 ounces)

2 cups cherry tomatoes, halved

3 ounces reduced-fat goat cheese, crumbled

Preheat the broiler with the rack 4 inches from the heat. Rub the chicken all over with the rosemary, ¼ teaspoon of the salt, and the pepper. Lightly spray both sides with olive oil.

Broil the chicken until cooked through but still a little pink, 3 to 4 minutes per side (depending on the thickness of the chicken breasts). Transfer to a cutting board and when cool enough to handle, cut the chicken into bite-size pieces.

In a large bowl, whisk together the vinegar, oil, and remaining ¼ teaspoon salt. Add the chicken, arugula, spinach, and tomatoes to the dressing. Toss well to coat.

Divide the chicken mixture among 4 plates. Dividing evenly, sprinkle the goat cheese over the salads.

MAKES 4 (2-cup) SERVINGS ❱ **Per serving:** 267 calories, 10 g fat, 2.5 g saturated fat, 35 g protein, 8 g carbohydrate, 2 g fiber, 521 mg sodium

❰MAKE AHEAD❱ **You can make the vinaigrette and broil the chicken several hours ahead and let sit, covered, at room temperature.**

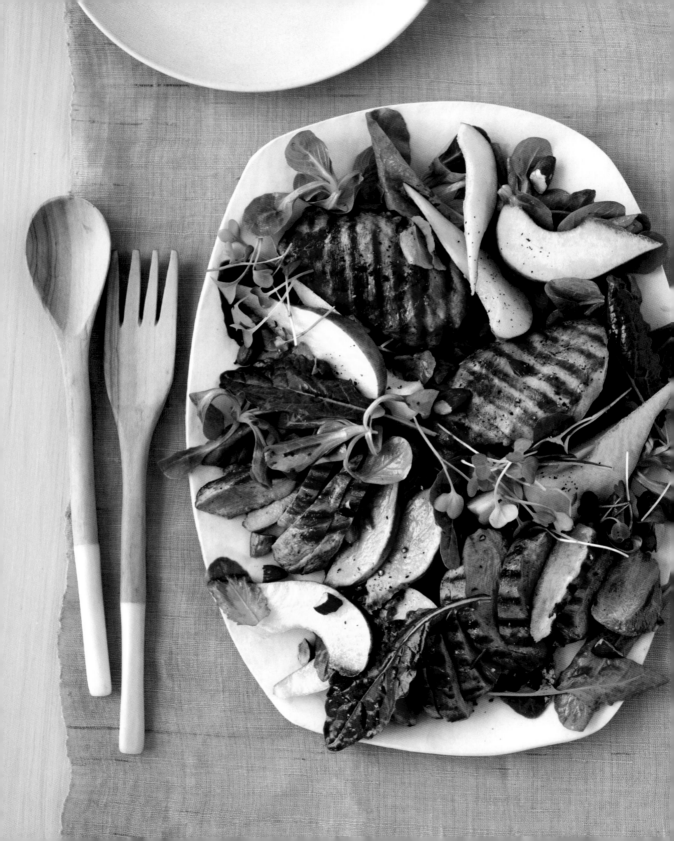

GRILLED DUCK AND PEAR SALAD
WITH ALMONDS

HANDS-ON TIME: 20 MINUTES   TOTAL TIME: 25 MINUTES

PHASE 2

PHASE 1

SEE PHASE SWITCH

30 MINUTES OR LESS

Duck breasts rarely come skinless, and a substantial amount of the weight is actually in the fat and skin. So be sure that you buy breast halves that weigh about 8 ounces. Once you discard the skin and the thick layer of fat underneath, you'll have about 4 ounces of lean duck. If you'd like, you can cook the breasts on an outdoor grill. The timing should be the same, but check after 2 minutes per side in case your grill runs hot.

1½ tablespoons gluten-free reduced-sodium tamari soy sauce

1½ tablespoons sherry vinegar or white wine vinegar

1 tablespoon plus 2 teaspoons extra-virgin olive oil

4 boneless Long Island (Pekin) duck breast halves (8 ounces each), skinned

Freshly ground black pepper

8 cups field greens

2 pears, such as Bosc, halved lengthwise, cored, and thinly sliced lengthwise

4 tablespoons coarsely chopped unsalted roasted almonds

In a small bowl, whisk together the soy sauce, vinegar, and 1 tablespoon of the oil. Set the dressing aside.

Heat a grill pan or cast-iron skillet over medium-high heat. Rub both sides of each duck breast with the remaining 2 teaspoons oil and sprinkle both sides with pepper. Cook, turning once, for 2 to 3 minutes per side for rare or 1 minute longer per side for medium-rare. (Unlike other poultry, duck breast can be cooked to rare or medium-rare, just like beef.) Transfer to a cutting board and let rest for 5 minutes before thinly slicing across the grain.

In a large bowl, toss the field greens with all but about 2 tablespoons of the dressing.

Divide the greens among 4 plates. Dividing evenly, top with the duck and pears, then drizzle each serving with any juices from the cutting board and the reserved dressing. Sprinkle each serving with 1 tablespoon almonds.

MAKES 4 SERVINGS ❱ **Per serving:** 318 calories, 15 g fat, 2.5 g saturated fat, 27 g protein, 21 g carbohydrate, 6.5 g fiber, 368 mg sodium

❰PHASE SWITCH❱ **To have this on Phase 1, leave out the pears and serve with 1 large slivered yellow bell pepper instead.**

WARM BEEF AND BROCCOLI ROMESCO SALAD

HANDS-ON TIME: 20 MINUTES   TOTAL TIME: 30 MINUTES

PHASE 1

30 MINUTES OR LESS

The Spanish-style dressing for this salad is a variation on traditional Romesco sauce and would work equally well as a topping for chicken, fish, or even gluten-free pasta. Look for roasted red peppers jarred or from a salad bar.

1½ cups roasted red peppers

¼ cup raw (skin-on) almonds

1½ tablespoons no-salt-added tomato paste

1½ tablespoons red wine vinegar

1½ teaspoons paprika

1 tablespoon plus 1 teaspoon extra-virgin olive oil

½ teaspoon coarse kosher salt

1 head broccoli (about 1 pound)

1 pound sirloin steak

In a food processor, purée the roasted peppers, almonds, tomato paste, vinegar, paprika, 1 tablespoon of the oil, ¼ teaspoon of the salt, and 2 tablespoons water. Transfer the dressing to a bowl and set aside.

Separate the broccoli florets from the stalks. Trim off the very bottoms of the stalks. Peel the stalks and cut crosswise into ½-inch-thick slices. Cut the broccoli into smaller florets.

In a large skillet, bring 3 inches of water to a boil. Add the broccoli florets and the stalks. Cook, uncovered, until crisp-tender, about 5 minutes. Drain and run under cold water to stop the cooking. Drain again.

Preheat the broiler with the rack 4 inches from the heat.

Sprinkle the steak with the remaining ¼ teaspoon salt and brush with the remaining 1 teaspoon oil. Broil until cooked to the desired degree of doneness, about 3 minutes per side for medium-rare. Transfer to a cutting board and when cool enough to handle, thinly slice.

Divide the beef among 4 plates and top with the broccoli. Dividing evenly, spoon the dressing on top. Serve warm or at room temperature.

MAKES 4 SERVINGS ▌ Per serving: 293 calories, 14 g fat, 2.5 g saturated fat, 30 g protein, 12 g carbohydrate, 4 g fiber, 436 mg sodium

◀**MAKE AHEAD**▶ **The Romesco dressing will keep in the refrigerator for up to 3 days. Let the dressing return to room temperature before spooning it over the beef and broccoli.**

MUSTARD-ROASTED PORK
AND APPLE SALAD

HANDS-ON TIME: 20 MINUTES   TOTAL TIME: 50 MINUTES

PHASE
2

PHASE
1

SEE PHASE
SWITCH

We've used sweet apples, but a tarter apple such as Granny Smith would work equally as well here, too.

3 tablespoons Dijon mustard

4 tablespoons apple cider vinegar

2½ teaspoons agave nectar

½ teaspoon coarse kosher salt

1¼ pounds cabbage, cut into large chunks

1 tablespoon plus 2 teaspoons extra-virgin olive oil

¼ teaspoon freshly ground black pepper

1 pound pork tenderloin

2 apples (such as Fuji, Braeburn, or Pink Lady), thinly sliced

Preheat the oven to 400°F.

In a large bowl, whisk together the mustard, 3 tablespoons of the vinegar, the agave nectar, and ¼ teaspoon of the salt. Measure out ¼ cup of the dressing to use for the pork and set the large bowl aside.

Place the cabbage in a roasting pan. Drizzle with the 1 tablespoon oil and sprinkle with the pepper and remaining ¼ teaspoon salt. Toss to coat.

Place the pork on top of the cabbage mixture and spoon the ¼ cup of the dressing over the top of the pork. Roast until the pork is just cooked through and an instant-read thermometer inserted in the center registers 145°F, about 30 minutes. Transfer the pork to a cutting board and when cool enough to handle, thinly slice crosswise.

Add the remaining 1 tablespoon vinegar, remaining 2 teaspoons oil, the sliced pork, roasted cabbage, and apples to the large bowl with the dressing. Toss to combine.

Divide the salad among 4 plates and serve at room temperature or chilled (see Make Ahead, below).

MAKES 4 (2-cup) SERVINGS ▮ **Per serving:** 278 calories, 9 g fat, 2 g saturated fat, 23 g protein, 25 g carbohydrate, 4.5 g fiber, 591 mg sodium

◀PHASE SWITCH▶ **To make this a Phase 1 dish, use 2 sliced bell peppers (1 red, 1 yellow) in place of the apples.**

◀MAKE AHEAD▶ **The salad can be made several hours ahead of time, tossed together, and chilled until ready to serve.**

GARLICKY ROAST PORK
AND TOMATO SALAD

HANDS-ON TIME: 20 MINUTES   TOTAL TIME: 45 MINUTES

If you're a fan of pungent greens, make this with half romaine and half arugula and/or watercress. At the height of summer, use the ripest tomatoes you can find. Heirloom tomatoes such as Black Krim, Green Zebra, Brandywine, or Big Pink would make a colorful and flavorful addition.

6 plum tomatoes (about 1½ pounds)

2 small cloves garlic

4 teaspoons plus 1 tablespoon extra-virgin olive oil

½ teaspoon coarse kosher salt

   Freshly ground black pepper

¼ teaspoon paprika (optional)

1 pound pork tenderloin

1 small red onion, finely minced

1 teaspoon grated lemon zest

1 tablespoon fresh lemon juice

8 cups chopped romaine lettuce (about 1 large head)

Preheat the oven to 400°F. Line a rimmed baking sheet with foil (for easier cleanup).

Quarter the tomatoes lengthwise and scrape the seeds and center core into a strainer set over a small bowl. Press the flesh and seeds to get the juice out and set aside to drain. Place the tomato quarters in a medium bowl.

Grate the garlic (on a rasp-style citrus zester or the finest holes of a box grater) into a small bowl. Add 4 teaspoons of the oil, ¼ teaspoon of the salt, ¼ teaspoon pepper, and the paprika (if using). Stir to combine.

Rub half of the garlic mixture over the pork tenderloin and place the pork on one side of the baking sheet. Add the remaining garlic mixture to the quartered tomatoes and toss well. Arrange the tomatoes next to the pork.

Roast until the pork is cooked through but still juicy and an instant-read thermometer inserted in the center registers 145°F, 20 to 25 minutes (the tomatoes will also be done by that time). Transfer the pork to a cutting board and let rest for 10 minutes before thinly slicing crosswise at a steep angle (to get long oval slices).

While the pork is cooking, make the vinaigrette: Measure out 3 tablespoons of the strained tomato juice and place in a screw-top jar (discard any remaining juice or save it for a soup broth). Add the onion, lemon zest, lemon juice, the remaining 1 tablespoon oil and ¼ teaspoon salt, and a pinch of pepper. Shake well.

Just before serving, in a large bowl, toss the romaine with the dressing.

Divide the romaine among 4 plates. Dividing evenly, top the romaine with the sliced pork and roasted tomatoes. Drizzle any juices from the cutting board over the meat and tomatoes. Serve warm or at room temperature (see Make Ahead, below).

MAKES 4 SERVINGS ❱ **Per serving:** 251 calories, 12 g fat, 2.5 g saturated fat, 24 g protein, 13 g carbohydrate, 4.5 g fiber, 424 mg sodium

❰MAKE AHEAD❱ **The pork and tomatoes can be roasted several hours ahead. The dressing can also be made ahead. Keep everything at room temperature and don't chop or dress the greens until ready to serve.**

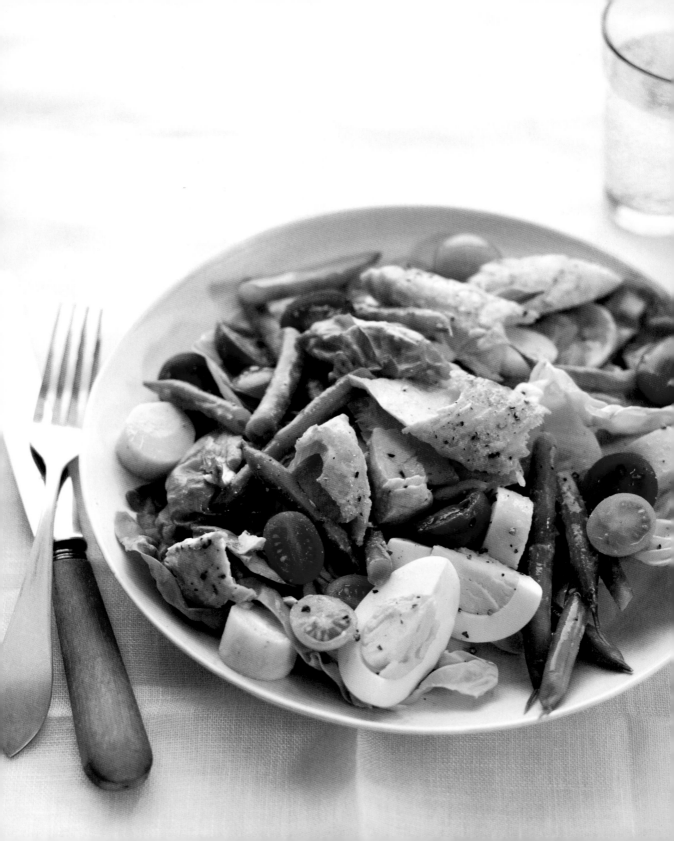

SALMON SALADE NIÇOISE

HANDS-ON TIME: 25 MINUTES   TOTAL TIME: 25 MINUTES

PHASE 1

30 MINUTES OR LESS

Hearts of palm stand in for the traditional potatoes in this classic dish, making it a perfect entrée for Phase 1 dieters. While the method for cooking the hard-boiled eggs may seem unusual, it makes for tender whites and creamy yolks. Your best bet when making hard-boiled eggs is to start with eggs that aren't past their sell-by date, but aren't superfresh either; this makes peeling them easier.

- 2 large eggs
- ¾ pound skin-on salmon fillet
- ½ pound green beans, halved crosswise
- 2 tablespoons fresh lemon juice
- 1 tablespoon plus 1 teaspoon extra-virgin olive oil
- 1 tablespoon Dijon mustard
- ½ teaspoon coarse kosher salt
- 1½ cups grape tomatoes, halved
- 1 cup canned hearts of palm (from a 14.5-ounce can), rinsed and cut crosswise into ½-inch slices
- 1 head Boston lettuce, torn into bite-size pieces

Preheat the oven to 400°F.

In a small saucepan, combine the eggs and cold water to cover. Bring to a boil over high heat. Remove from the heat, cover, and let stand for 12 minutes, then run under cold water. Peel and cut each egg into quarters.

Meanwhile, place the salmon, skin-side down, on a rimmed baking sheet. Bake until opaque throughout but still moist, about 10 minutes. With a thin-bladed metal spatula, lift the salmon off the baking sheet, leaving the skin behind. Break the salmon into large chunks.

While the eggs and salmon cook, fill a large skillet with about 2 inches of water. Add the beans and bring to a boil. Cover and cook until the beans are crisp-tender, about 3 minutes (timing will vary depending on size and age of the beans). Transfer to a colander and run under cold water to stop the cooking.

In a large bowl, whisk together the lemon juice, oil, mustard, and salt. Add the green beans, tomatoes, hearts of palm, and lettuce. Toss to combine.

Divide the lettuce mixture among 4 plates. Dividing evenly, top each with the quartered eggs and chunks of salmon.

MAKES 4 SERVINGS ❯ **Per serving:** 306 calories, 19 g fat, 4 g saturated fat, 23 g protein, 11 g carbohydrate, 3.5 g fiber, 576 mg sodium

❮MAKE AHEAD❯ **The green beans can be cooked, rinsed under cold water, dried, and refrigerated in a paper towel–lined container up to a day ahead. The eggs can be cooked several days ahead and refrigerated unpeeled.**

ARTICHOKE, EDAMAME, AND WALNUT SALAD

HANDS-ON TIME: 10 MINUTES   TOTAL TIME: 15 MINUTES

Edamame, buttermilk, walnuts, and reduced-fat Gouda cheese all bring protein to this meatless main-dish salad. Buttermilk is a great low-fat ingredient, but often after using some in a recipe, you'll find yourself with lots left over. The good news is that buttermilk freezes well, so pour leftovers into 1-cup portions and freeze until needed. Thaw in the refrigerator or on the kitchen counter.

2 tablespoons fresh lemon juice

1 tablespoon extra-virgin olive oil

½ teaspoon salt

1 package (12 ounces) frozen shelled edamame, thawed (about 2½ cups)

1 package (9 ounces) frozen artichoke hearts, thawed

⅓ cup walnuts, coarsely chopped

½ cup light (1.5%) buttermilk

½ cup shredded reduced-fat Gouda cheese (2 ounces)

In a large saucepan, bring ½ cup water, the lemon juice, oil, and salt to a boil over high heat. Add the edamame and artichoke hearts, cover, and cook until the artichokes are tender, 5 to 6 minutes.

Meanwhile, in a mini food processor, pulse the walnuts until finely ground. Transfer to a large bowl and whisk in the buttermilk.

Add the edamame mixture (along with any cooking liquid) to the bowl and toss to combine.

Divide the salad among 4 plates and sprinkle each with 2 tablespoons of cheese. Serve the salad warm, at room temperature, or lightly chilled (no longer than 1 hour in the refrigerator).

MAKES 4 (1¼-cup) SERVINGS ▶ **Per serving:** 276 calories, 17 g fat, 3 g saturated fat, 18 g protein, 16 g carbohydrate, 8.5 g fiber, 566 mg sodium

MEXICAN BEAN AND CHEESE SALAD

HANDS-ON TIME: 20 MINUTES   TOTAL TIME: 20 MINUTES

It may come as a surprise that both the leaves and the stems of cilantro are edible, which makes for little waste. (Even the roots of the cilantro plant are edible; if you're lucky enough to find them, save them for flavoring stocks and soups.) The creamy avocado dressing is a natural on this salad, but can made on its own for other uses: Swap it in for mayo in your favorite tuna salad, serve it as a dip for crudités, or drizzle some over sliced summer tomatoes.

1½ cups light (1.5%) buttermilk

½ avocado, cut into chunks

¼ cup cilantro leaves and tender stems

1 tablespoon plus 1 teaspoon fresh lime juice

¼ teaspoon salt

2 cans (15 ounces each) gluten-free no-salt-added pinto beans, drained and rinsed

6 radishes, thinly sliced

4 cups shredded romaine lettuce

1 cup shredded reduced-fat Mexican blend cheese (4 ounces)

2 tablespoons hulled pumpkin seeds (pepitas)

In a food processor, purée the buttermilk, avocado, cilantro, lime juice, and salt.

Transfer the avocado dressing to a large bowl and add the beans, radishes, and lettuce. Toss to combine.

Divide the salad among 4 plates and top each serving with ¼ cup cheese and 1½ teaspoons pumpkin seeds.

MAKES 4 (1½-cup) SERVINGS ▶ **Per serving:** 362 calories, 12 g fat, 4.5 g saturated fat, 24 g protein, 41 g carbohydrate, 13 g fiber, 429 mg sodium

◀MAKE AHEAD▶ **The dressing can be made a day ahead and refrigerated. Serve chilled or at room temperature.**

GLUTEN SOLUTION SUPERSALAD

HANDS-ON TIME: 10 MINUTES   TOTAL TIME: 35 MINUTES

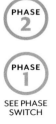

PHASE 2

PHASE 1

SEE PHASE
SWITCH

The fun (and high-protein) part of this pasta, black bean, and vegetable salad is the baked egg cubes. Here we season them with a little tomato paste and smoked paprika, but you can take them in all sorts of flavor directions: Give them a Mexican flair with cumin, oregano, and a tablespoon of minced pickled jalapeños. Or give them a French twist with a little dried tarragon and a couple of teaspoons of chopped capers.

3 large eggs

1 cup liquid egg whites

2 tablespoons no-salt-added tomato paste

1 tablespoon plus 3 teaspoons extra-virgin olive oil

½ teaspoon smoked paprika

½ teaspoon salt

2 tablespoons red wine vinegar

1 tablespoon Dijon mustard

¼ teaspoon freshly ground black pepper

1 can (15 ounces) gluten-free no-salt-added black beans, drained and rinsed

1 medium zucchini, cut into ½-inch chunks

4 ounces gluten-free multigrain penne pasta

4 cups baby arugula or baby spinach (about 4 ounces)

Preheat the oven to 375°F. Line a 9 × 5-inch loaf pan with parchment paper that comes at least 3 inches up the sides of the pan.

In a bowl, with a whisk or an electric mixer at medium speed, beat together the whole eggs, egg whites, tomato paste, 1 teaspoon of the oil, the smoked paprika, and ¼ teaspoon of the salt until the tomato paste is very evenly combined (no streaks of egg white). Pour the mixture into the loaf pan and bake until the eggs are puffed and set, 20 to 25 minutes. Using the parchment paper, pull the egg cake out of the pan to cool slightly (the egg cake will collapse as it cools), then cut into ¾-inch cubes.

Meanwhile, in a screw-top jar, combine the vinegar, mustard, pepper, the remaining 1 tablespoon plus 2 teaspoons oil, and the remaining ¼ teaspoon salt. Shake the dressing well.

In a medium bowl, toss the beans and zucchini with 3 tablespoons of the dressing. Let sit while you cook the pasta.

In a saucepan of boiling water, cook the penne according to package directions. Drain and rinse under cool water. Add to the beans and zucchini and toss to coat.

Toss the arugula with the remaining dressing and make a bed of the greens on 4 plates. Dividing evenly, top with the bean and pasta mixture and then the egg cubes.

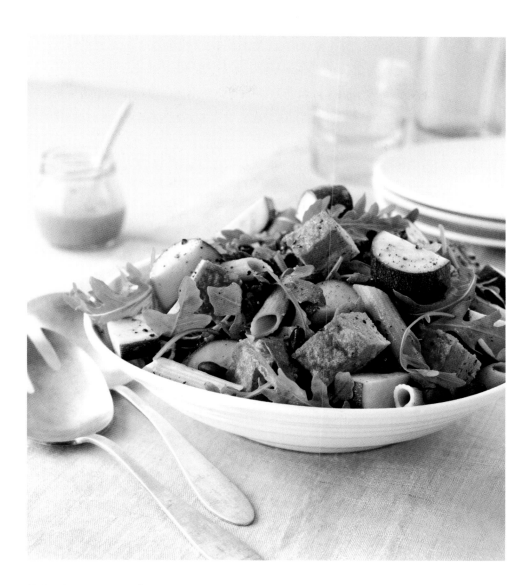

MAKES 4 SERVINGS ❱ **Per serving:** 355 calories, 12 g fat, 2 g saturated fat, 20 g protein, 45 g carbohydrate, 8 g fiber, 546 mg sodium

❰PHASE SWITCH❱ **To make this a Phase 1 recipe, use 1 can (15 ounces) no-salt-added chickpeas in place of the penne.**

❰MAKE AHEAD❱ **You can make the egg cubes ahead of time and refrigerate for up to 2 days. They may release moisture as they sit in the fridge, so blot them dry and let them return to room temperature before adding to the salad.**

SALSA GRILLED TURKEY AND MACARONI SALAD

HANDS-ON TIME: 10 MINUTES   TOTAL TIME: 25 MINUTES

PHASE
2

30
MINUTES
OR
LESS

When you choose a jarred salsa for this salad, look for a gluten-free brand that also contains no added sugar.

2 **medium bell peppers (1 red, 1 green)**

4 **ounces gluten-free quinoa elbow macaroni**

1 **teaspoon ground coriander**

1 **teaspoon ground cumin**

¼ **teaspoon salt**

1 **pound turkey breast cutlets or steaks, about ½ inch thick**

Olive oil cooking spray

1 **cup mild or medium-hot gluten-free salsa (from a jar)**

1 **avocado, diced**

⅓ **cup chopped fresh cilantro**

Preheat the broiler with the rack 4 inches from the heat.

Stand the peppers stem up and slice them vertically into 4 (or 5, depending on the shape of the pepper) flat panels. Place the pepper pieces skin-side up on a broiler pan and broil until the skin is charred all over, about 12 minutes. Remove from the broiler and turn the pepper pieces skin-side down on the broiler pan to cool. When cool enough to handle, pull off the skins and cut the peppers into 1-inch squares.

Meanwhile, in a medium pot of boiling water, cook the macaroni according to package directions. Drain and rinse under cool water.

In a small bowl, combine the coriander, cumin, and salt. Rub the spice mixture into both sides of the turkey.

Spray a grill pan or cast-iron pan lightly with olive oil and heat over medium-high heat. Place the turkey in the pan and cook, flipping once, until cooked through but still juicy, about 3 minutes per side. Transfer to a cutting board and let sit for at least 5 minutes before cutting into cubes.

In a large serving bowl, toss together the turkey, macaroni, peppers, salsa, avocado, and cilantro.

Divide the salad among 4 plates and serve at room temperature.

MAKES 4 (1½-cup) SERVINGS ❭ **Per serving:** 343 calories, 7 g fat, 1 g saturated fat, 31 g protein, 33 g carbohydrate, 5.5 g fiber, 574 mg sodium

❬MAKE AHEAD❭ **You can roast the peppers ahead and refrigerate for up to 2 days.**

ASPARAGUS SALAD WITH FETA AND TOASTED NUTS

HANDS-ON TIME: 20 MINUTES   TOTAL TIME: 20 MINUTES

When toasting nuts, watch carefully, because they can go from toasted to burned in a flash.

¼ cup walnuts or pecans

4 teaspoons extra-virgin olive oil

1 large red bell pepper, cut into 2-inch-long slivers

2 cloves garlic, minced

1 tablespoon plus 1 teaspoon balsamic vinegar

1 pound asparagus, cut on an angle into 2-inch pieces

4 cups field greens

Pinch of coarse kosher salt

¼ cup crumbled reduced-fat feta cheese (1 ounce)

In a toaster oven at 350°F or in a small dry skillet over medium-low heat, cook the walnuts (stirring if in a skillet) until toasted and fragrant, 3 to 5 minutes. Immediately transfer to a cutting board to stop the cooking. When cool enough to handle, coarsely chop.

In a large nonstick skillet, heat 2 teaspoons of the oil over medium-high heat. Add the bell pepper, garlic, and 1 tablespoon of the vinegar. Cook until the pepper is crisp-tender, about 4 minutes. Remove from the heat.

Meanwhile, in a steamer, cook the asparagus until crisp-tender, 3 to 5 minutes. Transfer to the skillet and toss to combine.

In a medium bowl, toss the greens with the remaining 2 teaspoons oil, remaining 1 teaspoon vinegar, and the salt.

Divide the greens among 4 salad plates. Dividing evenly, top the greens with the asparagus-pepper mixture, then sprinkle each with 1 tablespoon each of the feta and nuts.

MAKES 4 SERVINGS ❱ **Per serving:** 141 calories, 10 g fat, 1.5 g saturated fat, 5 g protein, 9 g carbohydrate, 3.5 g fiber, 167 mg sodium

❰MAKE AHEAD❱ **You can make the asparagus-pepper combo a couple of hours ahead of time and serve at room temperature, if you like.**

CELERY AND CELERY LEAF SALAD

HANDS-ON TIME: 10 MINUTES   TOTAL TIME: 10 MINUTES

PHASE
1

30
MINUTES
OR
LESS

When buying celery look for stalks with leaves attached. The leaves have a mild celery flavor and a delicate texture. No leaves, no worries; the salad is still tasty without them.

2 teaspoons Dijon mustard

2 tablespoons fresh lemon juice

1 tablespoon extra-virgin olive oil

¼ cup grated Parmesan cheese

¼ teaspoon salt

8 stalks celery with leaves, stalks cut crosswise into ½-inch slices, leaves left whole

2 tablespoons sliced almonds

In a large bowl, whisk together the mustard, lemon juice, and oil. Whisk in the Parmesan and salt until well combined. Add the celery and leaves and toss well.

Divide the salad among 4 salad plates. Sprinkle each with ½ tablespoon (1½ teaspoons) almonds.

MAKES 4 (1-cup) SERVINGS ❱ **Per serving:** 85 calories, 6.5 g fat, 1.5 g saturated fat, 3 g protein, 4 g carbohydrate, 1.5 g fiber, 346 mg sodium

FRESH CUCUMBER-DILL SALAD

HANDS-ON TIME: 10 MINUTES   TOTAL TIME: 10 MINUTES PLUS CHILLING TIME

PHASE 1

Serve this tangy and slightly sweet cucumber salad (it tastes a little like bread-and-butter pickles) as a side dish, or tuck the cucumbers into a sandwich.

- 1 pound kirby cucumbers
- ⅓ cup apple cider vinegar
- 1 tablespoon agave nectar
- ½ teaspoon salt
- ¼ teaspoon freshly ground black pepper
- ⅓ cup chopped fresh dill

With a vegetable peeler, peel the cucumbers in lengthwise stripes, leaving some of the skin on. Halve lengthwise, remove the seeds with a small spoon, and thinly slice crosswise.

In a medium bowl, whisk together the vinegar, agave nectar, salt, and pepper. Add the cucumbers and dill. Toss to combine. Refrigerate for at least 1 hour before serving to let the flavors meld (see Make Ahead, below).

MAKES 4 (¾-cup) SERVINGS ▶ **Per serving:** 36 calories, 0 g fat, 0 g saturated fat, 1 g protein, 8 g carbohydrate, 0.5 g fiber, 294 mg sodium

◀MAKE AHEAD▶ **The cucumbers can be refrigerated for up to 3 days.**

GREEN LENTIL SALAD

HANDS-ON TIME: 10 MINUTES   TOTAL TIME: 50 MINUTES

French green lentils (sometimes sold as petite or Puy lentils) hold their shape much better than other lentils and do well in salads such as this.

¾ cup small French green lentils (Puy)

2 cloves garlic, minced

2 teaspoons grated lemon zest

¼ teaspoon salt

¼ teaspoon freshly ground black pepper

¾ cup chopped fresh flat-leaf parsley

⅓ cup finely diced red onion

1 tablespoon plus 1 teaspoon fresh lemon juice

1 tablespoon extra-virgin olive oil

In a medium saucepan, combine the lentils, garlic, lemon zest, salt, pepper, and 2 cups water. Bring to a boil over high heat, then reduce to a simmer. Cover and cook until the lentils are just tender, 35 to 40 minutes.

Drain any excess liquid and transfer the lentils to a large bowl. Add the parsley, onion, lemon juice, and oil. Toss well.

Divide the salad among 4 salad plates and serve warm or at room temperature.

MAKES 4 (½-cup) SERVINGS ❭ **Per serving:** 156 calories, 4 g fat, 0.5 g saturated fat, 8 g protein, 23 g carbohydrate, 6 g fiber, 156 mg sodium

❰VARIATION❱ **GREEN LENTIL AND PORK SALAD (4 servings): For a main dish, add ½ pound cooked pork loin or tenderloin cut into cubes along with 1 cup finely chopped fresh fennel to the lentil salad. Season with a little hot sauce, if desired.**

Per serving: 284 calories, 10 g fat, 2.5 g saturated fat, 25 g protein, 25 g carbohydrate, 7 g fiber, 196 mg sodium

RAINBOW CHARD SALAD
WITH SESAME-CARROT DRESSING

HANDS-ON TIME: 10 MINUTES   TOTAL TIME: 30 MINUTES

So-called rainbow chard isn't a variety unto itself, but rather three different types of chard sold together: regular Swiss chard (with white stalks), red chard, and golden chard. Each color brings its own flavor quality to the table: Swiss chard has a slightly tannic, mineral flavor; red is slightly sweet; and golden is sweeter than the red. If you can't find rainbow chard, use regular Swiss chard.

1¼ cups thinly sliced carrots

2 cloves garlic, thinly sliced

1 tablespoon dark sesame oil

2 teaspoons red wine vinegar

¼ teaspoon salt

2 bunches rainbow Swiss chard (about 1 pound), stems and leaves cut crosswise into ½-inch pieces

1 teaspoon sesame seeds

In a small saucepan, bring the carrots, garlic, and 1 cup water to a boil over high heat. Reduce to a simmer, cover, and cook until the carrots are very soft, about 20 minutes. Transfer the carrots, garlic, and any liquid remaining in the pan to a food processor. Add the sesame oil, vinegar, and salt. Purée until smooth.

While the carrots are cooking, in a large skillet, bring ½ cup water to a boil over high heat. Add the chard and reduce the heat to medium. Cover and cook until the chard is tender, about 5 minutes. Rinse under cold water, drain well, and pat dry.

Transfer the Swiss chard to a large salad bowl, spoon the puréed carrot mixture over it, and toss to coat. Sprinkle evenly with the sesame seeds.

MAKES 4 (1-cup) SERVINGS ▶ **Per serving:** 75 calories, 4.5 g fat, 0.5 g saturated fat, 3 g protein, 9 g carbohydrate, 3 g fiber, 414 mg sodium

◀ MAKE AHEAD ▶ **The carrot dressing can be made up to 3 days ahead and refrigerated.**

CHOPPED SALAD WITH BAKED TOFU AND TOMATOES

HANDS-ON TIME: 15 MINUTES   TOTAL TIME: 35 MINUTES

PHASE 1

Store-bought baked tofu is usually not gluten-free and is often swimming in a high-sugar marinade. The solution is to make your own home-baked tofu cubes, as we do here, marinating the tofu in some vegetable juice blend before baking.

¾ cup or 1 can (5.5 ounces) low-sodium vegetable juice blend

1 tablespoon fresh lemon juice

1 teaspoon hot sauce (optional)

1 tablespoon plus 1 teaspoon extra-virgin olive oil

1 container (14 ounces) extra-firm tofu, drained

Olive oil cooking spray

½ teaspoon coarse kosher salt

20 walnut halves (a generous ⅓ cup)

5 cups coarsely chopped romaine lettuce

1 bunch watercress (about 6 ounces), tough stems trimmed, coarsely chopped

1 cup grape tomatoes, finely chopped

2 ounces reduced-fat feta cheese, crumbled

In a small bowl, whisk together the vegetable juice blend, lemon juice, hot sauce (if using), and 1 teaspoon of the oil.

Halve the block of tofu horizontally, then cut each slab into 20 cubes (for a total of 40). Transfer the cubes to a container big enough to hold them snugly in a single layer and pour ½ cup of the vegetable juice mixture over them. Let the tofu stand while you preheat the oven.

Whisk the remaining 1 tablespoon oil into the remaining vegetable juice mixture and set the dressing aside.

Preheat the oven to 400°F. Line a baking sheet with foil (for easier cleanup). Lightly spray the foil with olive oil.

Spread the tofu cubes on the baking sheet. Drizzle each cube with a little of the marinade left in the container. Roast until firm and beginning to brown at the edges, about 30 minutes. Transfer to a medium bowl and sprinkle with the salt. Toss well and let cool slightly.

Meanwhile, in a toaster oven at 350°F or in a small dry skillet over medium-low heat, cook the walnuts (stirring if in a skillet) until toasted and fragrant, 3 to 5 minutes. Immediately transfer to a cutting board to stop the cooking. When cool enough to handle, coarsely chop.

In a salad bowl, toss together the walnuts, lettuce, watercress, tomatoes, feta, and all but 2 tablespoons of the reserved dressing.

Divide the lettuce mixture among 4 plates. Top each serving with 10 tofu cubes. Drizzle the tofu with the reserved dressing (about 1½ teaspoons per serving).

MAKES 4 SERVINGS ❱ **Per serving:** 265 calories, 18 g fat, 3 g saturated fat, 17 g protein, 11 g carbohydrate, 4.5 g fiber, 487 mg sodium

❰MAKE AHEAD❱ **The tofu can be baked several hours ahead of time. In fact its flavor improves if it gets a chance to sit for awhile at room temperature.**

SOUTHWESTERN CAESAR SALAD

The quality of a Caesar salad can live and die on the freshness of the Parmesan cheese used. Ideally you should grate the cheese yourself, from a block of Parmesan. Next-best choice is to buy a tub of refrigerated grated Parmesan. But it would really be best to avoid the cans of shelf-stable grated Parmesan for this salad. As veteran South Beach dieters know, we've never been big on croutons, as they're usually made from white bread, but these cornmeal croutons have way more nutrients and fiber and are a healthy option for the gluten sensitive.

CROUTONS

- 6 tablespoons yellow cornmeal
- ¼ teaspoon gluten-free baking powder
- ¼ teaspoon chipotle chile powder
- ¼ teaspoon garlic powder
- ¼ teaspoon salt
- 3 tablespoons liquid egg whites
- Olive oil cooking spray

DRESSING AND SALAD

- 2 tablespoons mayonnaise (made with extra-virgin olive oil)
- 1 tablespoon fresh lemon juice
- 1 to 2 teaspoons chopped pickled jalapeño (to taste)
- ¼ teaspoon ground cumin
- 1 head romaine lettuce, cut crosswise into strips (8 cups)
- ¼ cup freshly grated Parmesan cheese

For the croutons: Preheat the oven to 350°F. Line a rimmed baking sheet with parchment paper.

In a small bowl, stir together the cornmeal, baking powder, chipotle powder, garlic powder, and salt. Whisk in the egg whites and 2 tablespoons water.

Place the dough on the baking sheet and pat to a 5-inch square (about ¼ inch thick). Bake until set, about 10 minutes. Remove from the oven (but leave the oven on). Spray the top of the cornbread lightly with olive oil, then flip over and lightly spray the bottom. Cut the squares into ½- to ¾-inch cubes and separate so air can circulate round them. Return to the oven and bake until crisp and dry, 8 to 10 minutes longer. Let cool slightly on the pan.

Meanwhile, for the dressing: In a small bowl, whisk together the mayonnaise, lemon juice, jalapeño, cumin, and 1 tablespoon water.

In a large bowl, toss the romaine with the dressing.

Divide the romaine among 4 salad plates. Dividing evenly, top with the croutons and sprinkle with the Parmesan.

MAKES 4 SERVINGS ❯ **Per serving:** 129 calories, 5 g fat, 1 g saturated fat, 5 g protein, 17 g carbohydrate, 2.5 g fiber, 339 mg sodium

◀MAKE AHEAD▶ You can make the croutons ahead and store them at room tempera-ture in an airtight container for up to a week. Just before assembling the salad, re-crisp the croutons in a toaster oven or regular oven at 325°F (3 to 5 minutes in the toaster oven; 5 to 7 minutes in the regular oven).

WINTER SQUASH SALAD

HANDS-ON TIME: 15 MINUTES   TOTAL TIME: 25 MINUTES

PHASE 2

30 MINUTES OR LESS

This is like a potato salad . . . but without the potatoes. If you can find kuri squash (often sold in farmers' markets in the fall and early winter), definitely give it a try. It has an almost nutty flavor; in fact the French call this squash *potimarron*, which loosely translated means chestnut squash.

4 cups peeled and cubed (¾-inch) winter squash (kuri, kabocha, acorn, or butternut)

¼ cup finely diced red onion

2 teaspoons apple cider vinegar

½ teaspoon coarse kosher salt

¼ teaspoon freshly ground black pepper

1 large stalk celery, finely diced

½ cup chopped fresh flat-leaf parsley, cilantro, or a combo

3 tablespoons mayonnaise (made with olive oil)

In a steamer, cook the squash until firm-tender, about 15 minutes.

Meanwhile, in a large bowl, combine the onion, vinegar, salt, and pepper.

Transfer the hot squash to the bowl with the onion and toss to coat. Stir in the celery, parsley, and mayonnaise. Toss to coat.

Serve warm, at room temperature, or chilled (see Make Ahead, below).

MAKES 4 (1-cup) SERVINGS ▶ **Per serving:** 107 calories, 3 g fat, 0 g saturated fat, 2 g protein, 20 g carbohydrate, 3.5 g fiber, 334 mg sodium

◀MAKE AHEAD▶ **You can make the salad several hours ahead and keep at room temperature or make it up to 3 days ahead and refrigerate. As the salad sits, the dressing will be absorbed into the sweet potatoes, so add a little 1% milk to the salad and toss together before serving to loosen it up a little.**

ZUCCHINI CEVICHE

PHASE 1

30 MINUTES OR LESS

For a colorful variation, use a combo of zucchini and yellow squash. This salad can also be dolled up with some roasted red bell pepper.

- 2 tablespoons plus 2 teaspoons fresh lime juice
- 1 tablespoon plus 1 teaspoon extra-virgin olive oil
- ¼ teaspoon salt

- 1 pound zucchini, thinly sliced
- ¼ cup finely chopped red onion
- 2 large green olives, pitted and chopped

In a large shallow bowl, whisk together the lime juice, oil, and salt. Add the zucchini and toss to coat.

Using a slotted spoon, remove the zucchini from the lime mixture and arrange on 4 salad plates. Dividing evenly, scatter the onion and olives on top. Drizzle any lime mixture remaining in the bowl over each.

MAKES 4 (¾-cup) SERVINGS ▶ **Per serving:** 68 calories, 5 g fat, 1 g saturated fat, 2 g protein, 5 g carbohydrate, 1.5 g fiber, 176 mg sodium

◀**MAKE AHEAD**▶ **The zucchini can be dressed up to a day ahead and refrigerated, but don't add the onion and olives any sooner than 2 hours before serving. Serve chilled or at room temperature.**

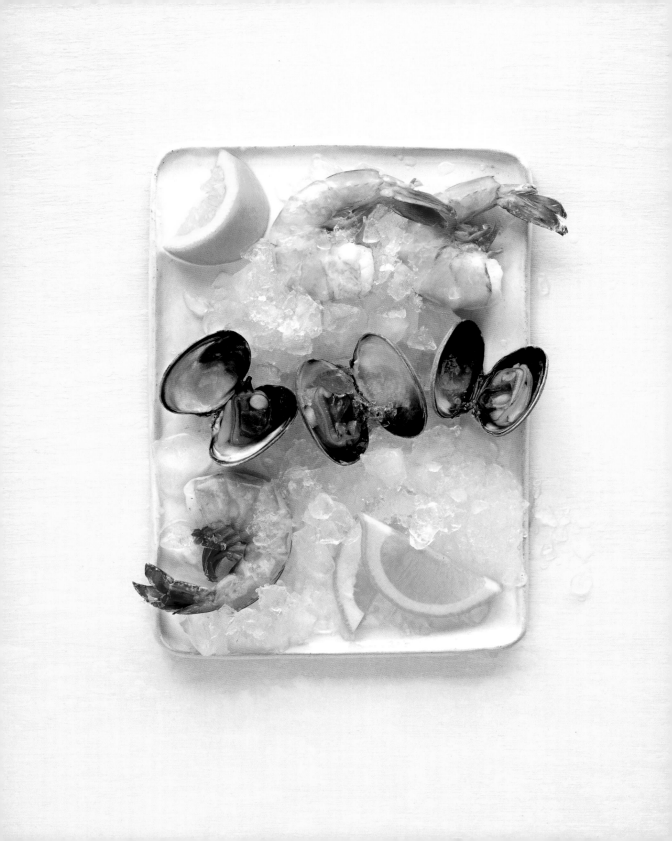

FISH AND SHELLFISH

Batter-Baked Cod with Mango Chutney. California Fish Tacos. Fish Cakes with Pepper Salsa. Baked Salmon with Spinach and Couscous. Who would believe these taste-tempting recipes could be gluten free? Just page through this chapter and you'll see how. Whether you're a fan of tuna, salmon, cod, clams, shrimp, or all of them, you won't go wrong with seafood, an important source of lean protein, B vitamins, potassium, iron, and omega-3 fatty acids. Choose the freshest fish available and substitute in a recipe, when necessary.

"SPAGHETTI" WITH RED CLAM SAUCE

HANDS-ON TIME: 30 MINUTES   TOTAL TIME: 30 MINUTES

Mild-tasting spaghetti squash picks up the flavor of the sauce it's tossed with. Be sure to buy a ripe one; look for a squash with a bright or golden yellow skin—not a greenish hue. You can keep the squash in a cool, dry spot for a couple of months. Manila clams are small, sweet (as in not too briny) clams that may be found wild, but in general are sustainably farmed and available at most good fish markets.

1 **spaghetti squash (about 3 pounds)**

1 **tablespoon extra-virgin olive oil**

3 **shallots, minced**

2 **cloves garlic, minced**

2 **tablespoons fresh lemon juice**

4 **dozen Manila clams, in the shell**

1 **can (15 ounces) no-salt-added crushed tomatoes**

½ **teaspoon coarse kosher salt**

Pinch red pepper flakes

¼ **cup chopped fresh flat-leaf parsley**

With a paring knife, pierce the spaghetti squash in several places. Microwave on high until the squash is tender but not collapsed, 10 to 12 minutes. Let cool several minutes, then halve the squash lengthwise. Holding a squash half with an oven mitt, scrape out the seeds. Then use a fork and scrape lengthwise to pull out the strands of squash into a bowl. Repeat with the other half.

While the squash is cooking, in a large skillet, heat the oil over medium heat. Add the shallots and garlic. Cook, stirring frequently, until softened, about 5 minutes. Add ½ cup water and the lemon juice. Bring to a boil. Add the clams, cover, and cook until the clams pop open, about 3 minutes (some will open before others; remove them as they do, and transfer to a large bowl).

Add the spaghetti squash, tomatoes, salt, and pepper flakes to the pan. Cook until the squash is piping hot, about 5 minutes. Return the clams (either in or out of the shell) to the pan and toss to combine and reheat briefly. Divide the "spaghetti" and clams among 4 bowls and sprinkle with the parsley.

MAKES 4 SERVINGS ❱ **Per serving:** 283 calories, 6.5 g fat, 1 g saturated fat, 22 g protein, 36 g carbohydrate, 5.5 g fiber, 379 mg sodium

❰MAKE AHEAD❱ The squash can be cooked and the strands scraped out a day or two ahead. Refrigerate the squash and bring back to room temperature before heating in the sauce in the last step.

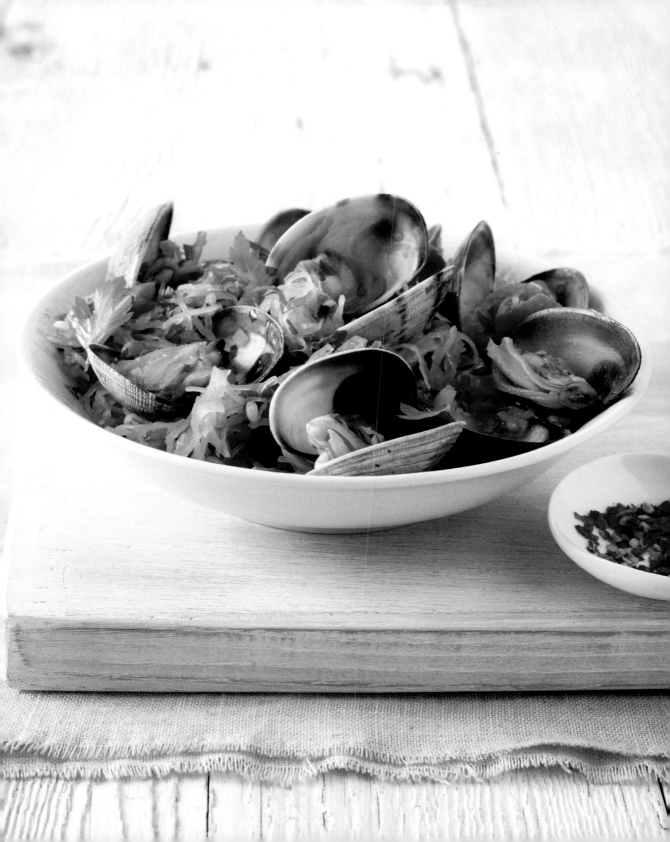

BATTER-BAKED COD WITH HOMEMADE MANGO CHUTNEY

HANDS-ON TIME: 20 MINUTES   TOTAL TIME: 30 MINUTES

To peel and chunk any type of mango, cut off both "cheeks," getting as close to the pit as possible. With a paring knife, make several parallel cuts (about ½ inch apart) into the fruit side of the "cheeks," stopping short of the skin. Then make another set of parallel cuts perpendicular to the first set. Press on the skin to invert it and then use the knife to cut underneath the fruit and pop out the chunks. Serve this dish with Celery and Celery Leaf Salad (page 112), if you like.

2 large egg whites

4 skinless cod fillets (6 ounces each)

3 tablespoons coconut flour

Olive oil cooking spray

½ teaspoon coarse kosher salt

1 mango (about 12 ounces), cut into ½-inch chunks

1 tablespoon no-salt-added tomato paste

1 tablespoon apple cider vinegar

2 teaspoons agave nectar

1 scallion, thinly sliced

Preheat the oven to 375°F.

In a wide shallow bowl, whisk together the egg whites and 2 teaspoons water (skip the water if you're using liquid egg whites). Dip the fish in the egg whites, shaking off the excess, then sprinkle the tops of the fish with the coconut flour, patting to adhere. Place the fish on a baking sheet, lightly spray the fish with olive oil, and sprinkle the salt evenly over the top of the fillets. Bake for 10 minutes, then turn the oven to broil and cook until lightly golden, about 2 minutes.

Meanwhile, in a medium bowl, combine the mango, tomato paste, vinegar, agave nectar, and scallion.

Place the fish on 4 plates and top each serving with ½ cup of the mango chutney.

MAKES 4 SERVINGS ❭ **Per serving:** 213 calories, 3 g fat, 1 g saturated fat, 30 g protein, 16 g carbohydrate, 3 g fiber, 374 mg sodium

❬MAKE AHEAD❭ **The mango chutney can be made up to 3 days ahead and refrigerated. Bring it to room temperature before serving.**

BROILED MAHI MAHI WITH
SIZZLING SCALLION OIL

HANDS-ON TIME: 10 MINUTES TOTAL TIME: 20 MINUTES

Also sold as dolphin fish or dorado, mahi mahi is a mild-tasting, meaty fish that's the perfect complement to Asian-inspired scallion oil. Serve the fish with Roasted Baby Bok Choy and Peppers (page 231) to keep the Asian theme going.

4 skinless Atlantic mahi mahi fillets (6 ounces each)

5 teaspoons gluten-free reduced-sodium tamari soy sauce

1 tablespoon extra-virgin olive oil

1 teaspoon dark sesame oil

4 scallions, thinly sliced

Line a baking sheet with foil (for easier cleanup). Place the fish, skinned-side down, on the baking sheet and brush the tops with 4 teaspoons of the tamari. Let sit while you preheat the broiler.

Preheat the broiler with the rack 4 inches from the heat.

Broil the fish until it pulls apart in flakes, but still looks moist, about 10 minutes.

Meanwhile, in a small saucepan, combine the olive oil, sesame oil, remaining 1 teaspoon tamari, and the scallions. Cook over medium heat until the scallions are at a high sizzle, about 1 minute.

Place the fish on 4 plates and drizzle each serving evenly with the scallion oil.

MAKES 4 SERVINGS ▶ **Per serving:** 190 calories, 5.5 g fat, 1 g saturated fat, 31 g protein, 2 g carbohydrate, 0.5 g fiber, 438 mg sodium

CALIFORNIA FISH TACOS

HANDS-ON TIME: 30 MINUTES   TOTAL TIME: 30 MINUTES PLUS CHILLING TIME

While many chili powders are a blend of chiles and other spices, ancho chile powder is made from only one chile—dried poblano peppers—without any other seasonings. The flavor is both smoky and hot, yet not overpowering. Pure chile powders are gluten free; blends may not be, so check labels carefully.

4 cups shredded cabbage (about ¾ pound)

1 small red onion, halved and thinly sliced

2 tablespoons fresh lime juice

6 teaspoons extra-virgin olive oil

1 pound skinless grouper fillets, cut into 1-inch pieces

1 teaspoon ancho chile powder

¾ teaspoon coarse kosher salt

3 tablespoons sorghum flour

8 100% corn tortillas (6-inch)

½ cup nonfat (0%) plain Greek yogurt

½ avocado, cut into ½-inch chunks

In a medium bowl, combine the cabbage, onion, lime juice, and 2 teaspoons of the oil. Refrigerate the cabbage slaw for at least 1 hour.

Sprinkle the fish with the chile powder and salt to evenly coat, then sprinkle evenly with the flour, patting to adhere.

In a large nonstick skillet, heat 2 teaspoons of the oil over medium heat. Add half the fish and cook, turning once, until golden brown and opaque throughout but still moist, about 2 minutes per side (timing will vary depending on the thickness of the fish). Transfer to a plate. Repeat with the remaining 2 teaspoons oil and remaining fish.

In a large dry skillet, heat the tortillas over medium heat until soft and pliable, about 10 seconds each. (Alternatively, wrap the tortillas in microwave-safe paper towels and microwave until hot, about 15 seconds, or wrap them in foil and bake in a 400°F oven for 10 minutes.)

Dividing evenly, spread the yogurt over all the tortillas, leaving a 1-inch border all around. Place 2 tortillas on each of 4 plates. Divide half the cabbage slaw among the tortillas. Dividing evenly, top with the fish, the remaining cabbage slaw, and the avocado. Roll up.

MAKES 4 (2-taco) SERVINGS ❱ Per serving: 377 calories, 12 g fat, 2 g saturated fat, 30 g protein, 39 g carbohydrate, 7 g fiber, 463 mg sodium

❰MAKE AHEAD❱ **The cabbage slaw can be made up to a day ahead and refrigerated. Serve chilled or at room temperature.**

LEMON-BAKED TROUT WITH GREEN GODDESS SAUCE

HANDS-ON TIME: 15 MINUTES   TOTAL TIME: 25 MINUTES

This recipe borrows some of the flavors (but way less fat) from the traditional Green Goddess salad dressing to make a creamy sauce for rich-tasting brook trout. With its tangy, herbal taste, our Green Goddess would also work well as a dip for vegetables or as a salad dressing.

⅔ cup nonfat (0%) plain Greek yogurt

1 tablespoon mayonnaise (made with extra-virgin olive oil)

2 tablespoons fresh lemon juice

¼ cup chopped fresh flat-leaf parsley

1 scallion, thinly sliced

1 teaspoon dried tarragon

2 whole boned brook trout (about 14 ounces each), heads and tails removed

2 teaspoons extra-virgin olive oil

½ teaspoon coarse kosher salt

Preheat the oven to 400°F. Line a rimmed baking sheet with foil (for easier cleanup).

In a small bowl, stir together the yogurt, mayonnaise, 1 tablespoon of the lemon juice, the parsley, scallion, and tarragon. Refrigerate until ready to use (see Make Ahead, below).

Open the trout so they lie flat and place on the baking sheet, skin-side down. Drizzle evenly with the oil and remaining 1 tablespoon lemon juice. Sprinkle evenly with the salt. Bake until the fish can be easily pierced with a fork, about 10 minutes.

To serve, halve each fish lengthwise, then run a knife under the flesh of the fish to separate it from the skin. Carefully lift the fish onto 4 serving plates. Serve each with 3 tablespoons of the sauce on the side.

MAKES 4 SERVINGS ▶ **Per serving:** 284 calories, 12 g fat, 3 g saturated fat, 39 g protein, 3 g carbohydrate, 0.5 g fiber, 375 mg sodium

◀MAKE AHEAD▶ The sauce will keep in the refrigerator for up to 3 days. If storing for longer than a day, omit the scallion and add it up to 4 hours before serving.

MANHATTAN FISH STEW

HANDS-ON TIME: 35 MINUTES   TOTAL TIME: 35 MINUTES

Fennel is also known as anise because of its mild licorice-like taste. If the fennel bulb you buy still has its green, leafy fronds, save them to garnish the stew—they too have a mild licorice flavor. When striped bass isn't available, use another white, firm-fleshed fish such as grouper. Or swap in cod; its texture will be somewhat softer than the striped bass or grouper, but its flavor will still be delicious.

1 small fennel bulb, thinly sliced

2 medium bell peppers (1 green, 1 red), cut into ½-inch squares

1 small onion, halved and thinly sliced

3 cloves garlic, thinly sliced

1 tablespoon plus 1 teaspoon extra-virgin olive oil

1 cup chopped fresh tomatoes or canned no-salt-added diced tomatoes

¾ teaspoon salt

4 striped bass fillets (6 ounces each)

1½ tablespoons almond flour

In a large nonstick saucepan, over medium heat, combine the fennel, bell peppers, onion, garlic, and oil. Cook, stirring frequently, until the onion is softened, about 10 minutes.

Add the tomatoes, salt, and ¾ cup water. Bring to a boil. Top with the fish, reduce to a simmer, cover, and cook until the fish pulls apart in flakes but is still moist, about 5 minutes.

With a slotted spoon or spider, lift out the fish and vegetables, dividing among 4 shallow bowls.

Stir the almond flour into the liquid remaining in the pan until well combined. Spoon about ½ cup of the thickened broth over each serving of the fish and vegetables.

MAKES 4 (1½-cup) SERVINGS ▶ **Per serving:** 272 calories, 10 g fat, 1.5 g saturated fat, 33 g protein, 12 g carbohydrate, 4 g fiber, 590 mg sodium

◀MAKE AHEAD▶ The vegetables in the first step can be cooked up to a day ahead and refrigerated before adding the tomatoes and proceeding with the recipe.

FISH CAKES WITH PEPPER SALSA

HANDS-ON TIME: 35 MINUTES   TOTAL TIME: 35 MINUTES

PHASE 1

To make the garlic that goes into the fish cakes less sharp than raw garlic (but still garlicky) the cloves are cooked for 2 minutes in boiling water. A salsa of crunchy cucumbers and red bell pepper along with olive oil, lemon juice, and Old Bay is a nice foil for the tender cakes.

3 cloves garlic, peeled

¾ pound skinless cod, striped bass, grouper, or tilefish fillets, cut into large chunks

½ pound peeled and deveined shrimp, cut into large pieces

½ cup fresh flat-leaf parsley leaves

2 shallots, thickly sliced

5 tablespoons fresh lemon juice

1 large egg

1 teaspoon 30% less sodium Old Bay seasoning

2 kirby cucumbers or 1 regular cucumber, peeled, quartered lengthwise, and thinly sliced

1 medium red bell pepper, cut into ¼-inch dice

6 teaspoons extra-virgin olive oil

In a small saucepan of boiling water, cook the garlic 2 minutes to blanch. Drain and transfer the garlic to a food processor.

Add the cod, shrimp, parsley, shallots, 3 tablespoons of the lemon juice, the egg, and ¾ teaspoon of the Old Bay to the food processor. Pulse until the fish is finely chopped.

Using a ⅓-cup measure, scoop out 8 portions of fish, place on a baking sheet, and flatten to a 1-inch thickness.

For the salsa: In a small bowl, combine the cucumbers, bell pepper, 2 teaspoons of the oil, the remaining 2 tablespoons lemon juice, and the remaining ¼ teaspoon Old Bay.

In a large nonstick or cast-iron skillet, heat 2 teaspoons of the oil over medium heat. Add 4 fish cakes and cook until lightly browned on one side, about 2 minutes. Turn the fish cakes over and cook until just firm to the touch and cooked through, about 1 minute longer. Repeat with the remaining 2 teaspoons oil and remaining 4 fish cakes.

Place 2 fish cakes on each of 4 plates and top each serving with ½ cup salsa.

MAKES 4 SERVINGS ❱ **Per serving:** 249 calories, 11 g fat, 2 g saturated fat, 26 g protein, 12 g carbohydrate, 2 g fiber, 503 mg sodium

❰MAKE AHEAD❱ **The fish cakes can be formed and refrigerated for up to 8 hours or frozen for up to 3 months. If freezing, wrap individually in wax paper and then foil. Thaw in the refrigerator before cooking.**

SESAME SALMON FINGERS WITH LEMON-DILL CREAM

HANDS-ON TIME: 10 MINUTES   TOTAL TIME: 20 MINUTES

If your market has a fish counter, ask for a single piece of center-cut salmon so that the fish is 1 to 1½ inches thick (and have it skinned if it isn't already). If precut salmon with the skin on is your only choice, buy a little more than a pound (again, making sure you're getting thickish pieces) and then slice the fish off the skin with a sharp flexible knife. Save any leftover cooked fish and lemon-dill cream to turn into a lunch salad (see Variation).

¾ cup nonfat (0%) plain Greek yogurt

3 tablespoons chopped fresh dill

2 teaspoons grated lemon zest

Salt

Freshly ground black pepper

1 large egg white

2 teaspoons fresh lemon juice

1 pound skinless center-cut salmon fillet, cut into ¾ × 2-inch strips

6 tablespoons sesame seeds

In a small bowl, stir together the yogurt, dill, lemon zest, and a generous pinch each of salt and pepper.

Preheat the oven to 375°F. Line a baking sheet with parchment paper or use a non-stick baking sheet.

In a medium bowl, beat together the egg white, lemon juice, and a generous pinch of pepper. Add the fish and toss to coat.

Spread the sesame seeds on a plate or in a shallow bowl. One at a time, lift a fish finger out of the egg white and let the excess drip off. Lightly coat 2 sides of each fish finger (not all 4 sides) in the sesame seeds and place on the baking sheet with one of the sesame sides down. (Discard any unused sesame seeds.)

Bake until the fish is opaque throughout but still moist, about 10 minutes.

Divide the fish among 4 plates and serve with the lemon-dill cream on the side (about 3 tablespoons per serving).

MAKES 4 SERVINGS ❱ **Per serving:** 271 calories, 14 g fat, 2 g saturated fat, 32 g protein, 3 g carbohydrate, 1 g fiber, 137 mg sodium

◀**VARIATION**❱ **Salmon-Cucumber Salad (to serve 1): Cut 3 cooked fish fingers into coarse chunks and toss with 2 mini (or Persian) cucumbers (sliced) and 2 tablespoons of the lemon-dill cream thinned with a little lemon juice to the consistency of salad dressing. Add some more fresh dill if you have any left over.**

Per serving: 204 calories, 9 g fat, 1.5 g saturated fat, 24 g protein, 6 g carbohydrate, 2 g fiber, 110 mg sodium

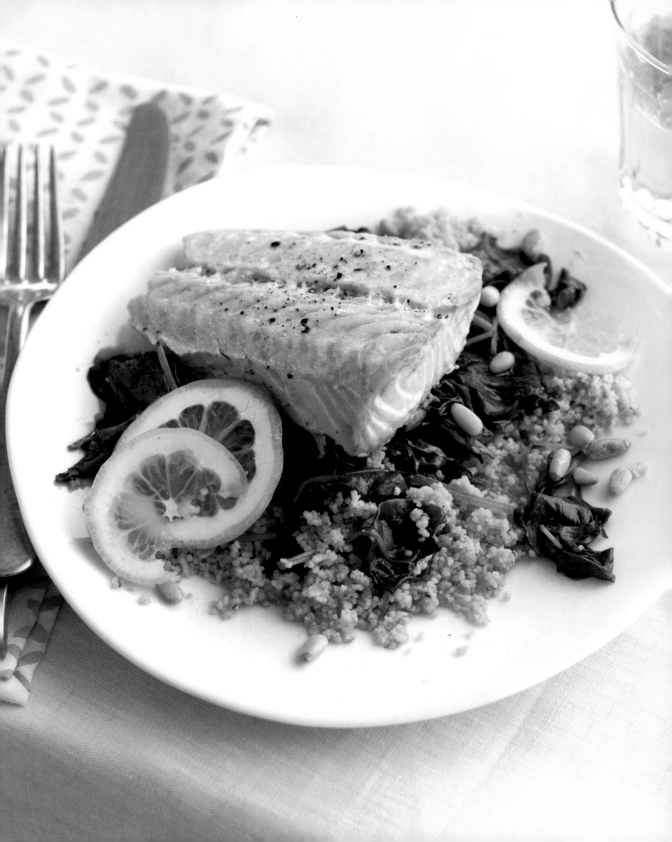

BAKED SALMON WITH SPINACH AND COUSCOUS

HANDS-ON TIME: 10 MINUTES   TOTAL TIME: 25 MINUTES

PHASE 2

PHASE 1

SEE PHASE SWITCH

30 MINUTES OR LESS

Couscous is usually relegated to side dish status, but here it's used as a bed for baking spinach and salmon for a nice one-dish meal. Unlike wheat-based couscous, which is prepared by soaking in boiling water for just 5 minutes off the heat, gluten-free brown rice couscous takes longer to get tender, making it the perfect candidate for some time in the oven. Any leftovers make a delicious cold lunch.

½ cup brown rice couscous

1⅓ cups boiling water

2 tablespoons fresh lemon juice

1 teaspoon dried tarragon or oregano, crumbled

½ teaspoon salt

2 packages (5 ounces each) fresh baby spinach

1 skinless salmon fillet (1 pound)

2 teaspoons extra-virgin olive oil

1 tablespoon toasted pine nuts

Lemon slices for garnish (optional)

Preheat the oven to 400°F.

In a 9 × 13-inch baking dish, stir together the couscous, boiling water, 1 tablespoon of the lemon juice, the tarragon, and salt. Top with the spinach and the salmon.

Cover with foil and bake until the salmon pulls apart in flakes but is still moist and the couscous is tender, about 12 minutes.

Lift the salmon out of the pan and place on a cutting board. Add the remaining 1 tablespoon lemon juice, the oil, and pine nuts to the couscous-spinach mixture and fluff with a fork.

Divide the couscous-spinach mixture among 4 plates. Cut the salmon into 4 pieces and place on top. Garnish with lemon slices, if desired.

MAKES 4 SERVINGS ❭ Per serving: 376 calories, 20 g fat, 4 g saturated fat, 27 g protein, 26 g carbohydrate, 5 g fiber, 470 mg sodium

◀PHASE SWITCH▶ To make this Phase 1, omit the couscous and boiling water. In a 9 × 13-inch baking dish, toss the spinach with the lemon juice, tarragon, and salt. Top with the salmon and cook, uncovered, until the salmon is still moist and just cooked through, about 10 minutes.

MINI SALMON LOAVES

HANDS-ON TIME: 10 MINUTES   TOTAL TIME: 40 MINUTES

PHASE
1

Drain the salmon, but don't discard any little pieces of bone; they're edible (they get softened during processing) and they add calcium to the dish. Pink salmon is the most readily available and the least expensive of the canned salmons. If you don't have jumbo muffin tins, you can make these loaves in standard muffin tins—you'll get about 6.

Olive oil cooking spray

1 can (14.75 ounces) pink or sockeye salmon, drained

2 tablespoons mayonnaise (made with extra-virgin olive oil)

1 large egg

½ cup chopped fresh cilantro

3 scallions, thinly sliced

2 teaspoons grated fresh ginger

2 teaspoons Dijon mustard

¼ teaspoon salt

Lemon wedges, for serving

Preheat the oven to 350°F. Spray 4 cups of a jumbo muffin tin with olive oil.

In a medium bowl, combine the salmon, mayonnaise, egg, cilantro, scallions, ginger, mustard, and salt. Stir until well combined. Divide the mixture among the muffin cups and bake until set and lightly browned around the edges, about 30 minutes.

Run a knife around the edge of each cup and invert the loaves onto 4 plates. Serve with lemon wedges for squeezing.

MAKES 4 MINI LOAVES ▶ **Per mini loaf:** 190 calories, 7.5 g fat, 1 g saturated fat, 28 g protein, 3 g carbohydrate, 0.5 g fiber, 523 mg sodium

◀MAKE AHEAD▶ The mini loaves can be shaped, baked, and then frozen for up to 3 months. Wrap them individually in foil before freezing. Thaw in the fridge before reheating in a 350°F oven for about 20 minutes.

MISO-GLAZED TILAPIA

HANDS-ON TIME: 5 MINUTES   TOTAL TIME: 10 MINUTES

Miso is a fermented soybean paste generally sold in resealable packages or plastic or glass containers in Japanese groceries as well as in most health food stores and many larger supermarkets. In general, the lighter in color the miso, the less salty it is. "White" miso is actually golden yellow in color and has a sweet flavor. Read the label carefully, though, because some misos can contain barley or wheat, and thus gluten. Unopened miso will keep indefinitely at room temperature; once opened, tightly close and refrigerate (it should be good for at least a year).

1 tablespoon plus 1 teaspoon white miso paste

1 tablespoon agave nectar

1½ teaspoons dark sesame oil

4 skinless tilapia fillets (6 ounces each)

1 scallion, thinly sliced

Preheat the broiler with the rack 4 inches from the heat.

In a small bowl, whisk together the miso, agave nectar, sesame oil, and 1 tablespoon water. Place the tilapia fillets on a broiler pan and brush the miso mixture evenly over the tops. Broil until the miso glaze has browned in spots and the tilapia is easily pierced with a fork and still moist, about 5 minutes.

Place the fish on 4 plates and scatter the sliced scallion evenly over each.

MAKES 4 SERVINGS ❯ **Per serving:** 205 calories, 4.5 g fat, 1 g saturated fat, 35 g protein, 6 g carbohydrate, 1 g fiber, 269 mg sodium

GREEN CURRY WITH SCALLOPS AND PEPPERS

HANDS-ON TIME: 15 MINUTES   TOTAL TIME: 25 MINUTES

The flavor in Thai-style curries comes from a savory herb/spice paste that infuses the oil used to sauté the other ingredients. In this green curry, the paste is made with scallions, cilantro, garlic, ginger, and lime juice. A Thai curry paste is a useful thing to keep in the fridge (it will last at least a week in an airtight container): Put a little bit in a skillet before making scrambled eggs, or add it when you're stir-frying vegetables for a side dish.

8 scallions, thickly sliced (including some of the dark green)

½ cup firmly packed fresh cilantro sprigs

¼ cup fresh lime juice (2 or 3 limes)

4 cloves garlic, peeled

2 tablespoons coarsely chopped fresh ginger

1 tablespoon plus 1 teaspoon extra-virgin olive oil

2 large green bell peppers, cut into small squares

Coarse kosher salt

1 can (15 ounces) gluten-free no-salt-added cannellini beans, drained and rinsed

¾ cup lite coconut milk

¾ pound bay scallops (leave whole), or sea scallops, quartered

In a food processor, combine the scallions, cilantro, lime juice, garlic, and ginger. Process to a smooth paste.

In a large nonstick saucepan or Dutch oven, heat the oil over medium heat. Add the bell peppers and sprinkle with a generous pinch of salt. Cook, stirring frequently, until beginning to soften, about 3 minutes. Add the scallion paste and cook until fragrant, about 3 minutes.

Stir in the beans, coconut milk, ¼ teaspoon salt, and 2 cups water. Mash some of the beans against the side of the pot to thicken the stew slightly. Bring to a boil and stir in the scallops. Cover, reduce to a simmer, and cook until the scallops are opaque throughout, 5 to 7 minutes. Divide among 4 shallow bowls and serve hot.

MAKES 4 (1⅔-cup) SERVINGS ▶ **Per serving:** 248 calories, 9 g fat, 3.5 g saturated fat, 17 g protein, 26 g carbohydrate, 6.5 g fiber, 561 mg sodium

◀ MAKE AHEAD ▶ **You can make the scallion paste in the first step and cut up the bell peppers several hours ahead and refrigerate.**

SHRIMP AND CHICKEN PAD THAI

HANDS-ON TIME: 40 MINUTES   TOTAL TIME: 40 MINUTES

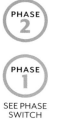

PHASE 2

PHASE 1

SEE PHASE SWITCH

You can buy shrimp already peeled and deveined in the freezer section of the supermarket. Once you've opened the bag, return what you haven't used to the freezer. Halving the shrimp horizontally makes it seem like you have double the amount of shrimp, and cutting the chicken into small bites means they'll both cook in the same amount of time. While pad Thai is usually served hot, you can refrigerate any leftovers and enjoy them for lunch the next day, either chilled or at room temperature.

4 ounces gluten-free brown rice linguine or spaghetti

2 tablespoons fresh lime juice

1 tablespoon gluten-free reduced-sodium tamari soy sauce

2 teaspoons agave nectar

1 tablespoon plus 1 teaspoon extra-virgin olive oil

½ pound large peeled and deveined shrimp, halved horizontally

¼ pound boneless, skinless chicken breast, cut into ½-inch dice

2 cloves garlic, thinly sliced

8 ounces cremini or white mushrooms, thinly sliced

1 large egg, lightly beaten

3 scallions, thinly sliced

2 tablespoons unsalted dry-roasted peanuts, coarsely chopped

In a large pot of boiling water, cook the pasta according to package directions.

Meanwhile, in a medium bowl, stir together the lime juice, tamari, and agave nectar.

Drain the pasta and add to the lime juice mixture, tossing well to coat.

In a large nonstick skillet, heat 1 tablespoon of the oil over medium heat. Add the shrimp, chicken, and garlic. Cook, stirring frequently, until both the chicken and shrimp are opaque throughout, about 3 minutes. Transfer to a medium bowl.

Add the remaining 1 teaspoon oil to the skillet along with the mushrooms and cook, stirring occasionally, until tender, about 4 minutes.

Add the pasta to the pan and cook until heated through, about 1 minute. Return the shrimp and chicken to the pan, add the egg, and toss to coat (and cook the egg).

Transfer the mixture to a platter and scatter the scallions and peanuts over the top.

MAKES 4 (1¼-cup) SERVINGS ▶ Per serving: 297 calories, 11 g fat, 2 g saturated fat, 21 g protein, 31 g carbohydrate, 2 g fiber, 560 mg sodium

◀PHASE SWITCH▶ To make this a Phase 1 dish, omit the pasta and just serve as a shrimp and chicken stir-fry.

QUINOA PASTA SALAD WITH SHRIMP

HANDS-ON TIME: 30 MINUTES   TOTAL TIME: 30 MINUTES

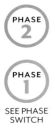

PHASE 2

PHASE 1

SEE PHASE SWITCH

30 MINUTES OR LESS

Although you can find bell peppers and yellow squash in the supermarket year-round, this colorful salad is at its best in summer, when these vegetables are at their peak. In season, look for deep, golden yellow squash—they tend to be sweeter than their paler cousins.

4 ounces gluten-free quinoa pasta, such as shells, rotelle, or garden pagodas (radiatore), or elbow macaroni

1 tablespoon plus 2 teaspoons extra-virgin olive oil

1 medium red bell pepper, cut into ½-inch squares

1 yellow squash, quartered lengthwise and thinly sliced crosswise

¾ pound peeled and deveined shrimp

3 cloves garlic, thinly sliced

¼ cup fresh lemon juice

¼ teaspoon coarse kosher salt

1 can (15 ounces) gluten-free no-salt-added chickpeas, drained and rinsed

In a medium pot of boiling water, cook the penne according to package directions. Drain and rinse under cold water.

Meanwhile, in a large nonstick skillet, heat 1 tablespoon of the oil over medium-high heat. Add the bell pepper and squash. Cook, stirring frequently, until the squash is almost tender, about 3 minutes.

Add the shrimp and garlic to the pan. Cook, tossing frequently, until the shrimp are opaque throughout and just cooked through, 3 to 4 minutes.

In a large bowl, whisk together the remaining 2 teaspoons oil, the lemon juice, and salt. Add the vegetable-shrimp mixture, the pasta, and chickpeas. Toss to combine.

Divide the salad among 4 plates and serve warm or at room temperature.

MAKES 4 (2-cup) SERVINGS ❱ **Per serving:** 379 calories, 7.5 g fat, 0.5 g saturated fat, 30 g protein, 48 g carbohydrate, 7.5 g fiber, 394 mg sodium

❰PHASE SWITCH❱ **For Phase 1, omit the pasta and increase the yellow squash to about 10 ounces (2 small or 1 large).**

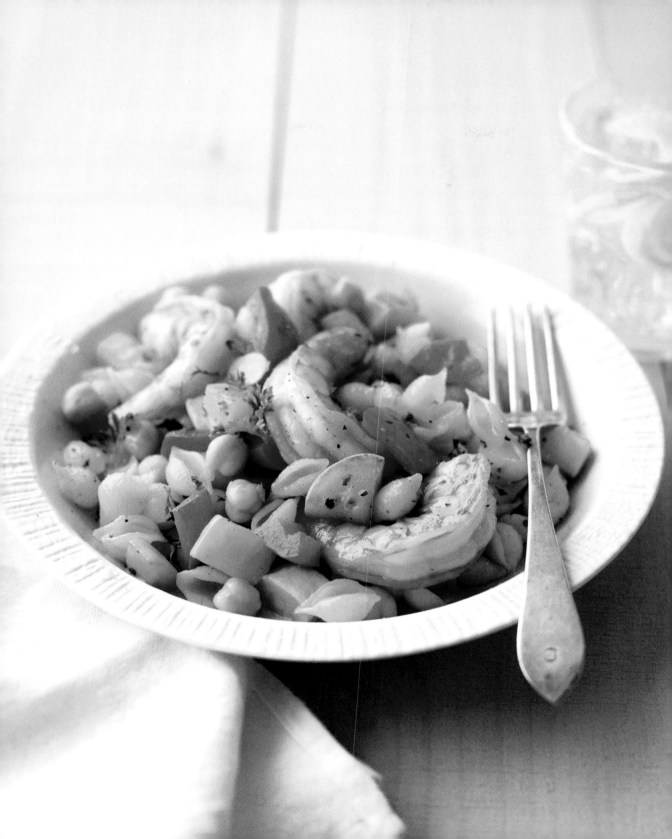

ASPARAGUS, PORTOBELLO, AND TUNA BAKE

HANDS-ON TIME: 20 MINUTES
TOTAL TIME: 1 HOUR 20 MINUTES PLUS STANDING TIME

PHASE
2

PHASE
1

SEE PHASE
SWITCH

Leftovers of this dish hold up really well, making it an ideal lunch to pack and take to work. Divide into single-serving portions, pack into microwave-safe containers, and refrigerate for up to 4 days. When you get to work, it takes just a couple of minutes to reheat on medium power in the microwave.

3 teaspoons extra-virgin olive oil

1 pound asparagus, cut into 1-inch lengths

1 small red onion, slivered

½ pound portobello mushrooms, gills scraped out, cut into ½-inch chunks

1½ cups loosely packed baby spinach

2 cans (5 ounces each) water-packed light tuna, well drained

2 teaspoons grated lemon zest

2 teaspoons fresh lemon juice

½ teaspoon salt

¼ teaspoon freshly ground black pepper

2 tablespoons garbanzo bean flour

1⅓ cups nonfat (0%) plain Greek yogurt

1 large egg

⅓ cup liquid egg whites

½ cup shredded reduced-fat Swiss cheese (2 ounces)

Preheat the oven to 350°F. Coat the bottom and sides of a 7 × 11-inch glass baking dish with 1 teaspoon of the oil.

In a steamer, cook the asparagus until it turns bright green but is still crisp, about 2 minutes.

In a large nonstick skillet, heat the remaining 2 teaspoons oil over medium-high heat. Add the onion and cook until softened, about 3 minutes. Add the portobellos in a single layer on top and cook, without stirring, for 3 minutes. Stir everything together and cook for 1 minute longer.

Scrape the onion and mushrooms into a large bowl and stir in the asparagus, spinach, tuna, lemon juice, salt, and pepper. Toss to combine.

In a small bowl, blend the garbanzo flour with ⅓ cup of the yogurt. Stir in the remaining 1 cup yogurt. Beat in the whole egg and egg whites. Beat in the lemon zest. Stir in the cheese.

Measure out 1 cup of the yogurt mixture and set aside. Add the remainder to the tuna mixture and toss to coat. Scrape the tuna mixture into the baking dish.

Spread the reserved yogurt mixture evenly over the top of the casserole. Bake until the top is nicely browned, about 45 minutes. Let sit for 15 minutes before serving.

MAKES 4 SERVINGS ▶ **Per serving:** 274 calories, 10 g fat, 3 g saturated fat, 33 g protein, 14 g carbohydrate, 3 g fiber, 484 mg sodium

◀ PHASE SWITCH ▶ **To make this a Phase 1 recipe, omit the garbanzo bean flour from the topping.**

TUNA BURGERS WITH CITRUS MAYO

HANDS-ON TIME: 15 MINUTES   TOTAL TIME: 30 MINUTES

Crushed corn tortillas give these burgers some heft, and a bit of olive-oil mayo helps keep the patties moist. Spraying the baking sheet with a little olive oil helps to color the underside of the patties so there's no need to turn them over during cooking.

4 100% corn tortillas (6-inch)

3 cans (5 ounces each) water-packed light tuna, drained

4 tablespoons mayonnaise (made with extra-virgin olive oil)

1 pickled jalapeño (seeded if desired for less heat), finely chopped (1½ teaspoons)

½ teaspoon salt
   Olive oil cooking spray

½ cup nonfat (0%) plain Greek yogurt

2 tablespoons fresh lime juice

1 scallion, thinly sliced

Preheat the oven to 350°F.

Spread the tortillas on a baking sheet and bake until crisp, about 10 minutes. (Leave the oven on.)

When cool enough to handle, crush the tortillas into small bits and transfer to a large bowl. Add the tuna, 3 tablespoons of the mayonnaise, the jalapeño, and the salt to the tortilla crumbs and mix well. Shape into 4 patties.

Spray a large baking sheet with olive oil. Place the patties on the baking sheet and bake until firm and slightly browned, about 5 minutes.

Meanwhile, in a small bowl, stir together the yogurt, lime juice, scallion, and remaining 1 tablespoon mayonnaise.

Serve each burger topped with 3 tablespoons of the citrus mayo.

MAKES 4 SERVINGS ▶ **Per serving:** 247 calories, 7.5 g fat, 0.5 g saturated fat, 27 g protein, 16 g carbohydrate, 1.5 g fiber, 508 mg sodium

◀MAKE AHEAD▶ **The patties can be shaped and individually frozen, wrapped first in wax paper, then foil. They can be cooked straight from frozen; remove their wrappings and increase the baking time by about 10 minutes.**

GRILLED TUNA STEAKS WITH OLD BAY AND ORANGE DRESSING

HANDS-ON TIME: 20 MINUTES   TOTAL TIME: 20 MINUTES

PHASE
2

30
MINUTES
OR
LESS

When you think of Old Bay, you probably think only of crab and shrimp boils. But this classic blend of 18 different spices and herbs is perfect for almost any kind of fish, especially robust types like fresh tuna.

2 navel oranges	⅓ cup finely chopped red onion
4 teaspoons extra-virgin olive oil	4 tuna steaks (5 ounces each)
1¼ teaspoons 30% less sodium Old Bay seasoning	

Using a paring knife, cut a thin slice off one end of each orange so they sit flat on the work surface. Following the curve of the fruit, cut off the peel and the thin white pith underneath. Set a strainer over a small bowl. Working over the bowl to catch the juice, cut in between the membranes to release the orange segments into the strainer. Remove the strainer and squeeze the juice from the membranes into the bowl. Remove all but about 2 tablespoons of the juice and set aside.

Add the orange segments to the 2 tablespoons juice in the bowl along with 2 teaspoons of the oil, ¼ teaspoon of the Old Bay, and the onion. Toss the dressing to combine.

Place the tuna steaks on a plate, rub with the remaining 1 teaspoon Old Bay, and sprinkle with the reserved orange juice.

Heat a grill pan over medium heat and brush with the remaining 2 teaspoons oil. Cook the tuna 1½ minutes per side for medium-rare (or more or less, depending upon your preference). Alternatively, brush the tuna with the 2 teaspoons of oil and broil 4 inches from the heat for 1½ to 2 minutes per side for medium-rare.

Divide the tuna among 4 plates and serve with ⅓ cup of the dressing spooned evenly on top of each steak.

MAKES 4 SERVINGS ❱ **Per serving:** 284 calories, 12 g fat, 2.5 g saturated fat, 34 g protein, 10 g carbohydrate, 2 g fiber, 175 mg sodium

◀ **VARIATION** ▶ **GRILLED TUNA SALAD (to serve 4):** Grill the tuna and make the orange dressing as directed up to a day ahead and refrigerate. When ready to serve, cut the tuna into slices. For each serving, arrange 2 cups of field greens on a plate; top with ½ cup sliced roasted red peppers, 3 olives, and ⅓ cup of the Old Bay orange dressing.

Per serving: 353 calories, 15 g fat, 3 g saturated fat, 35 g protein, 20 g carbohydrate, 4.5 g fiber, 505 mg sodium

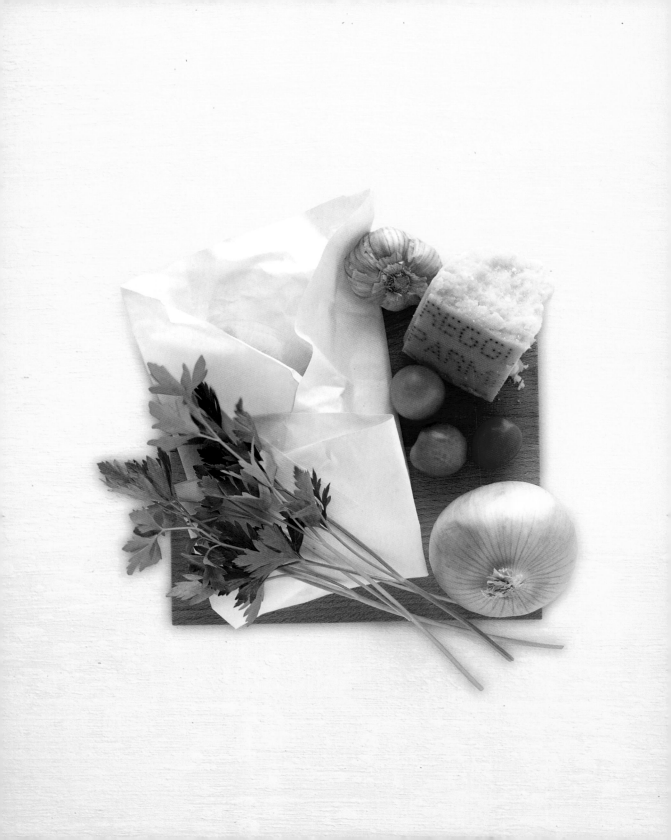

POULTRY

Versatile and easy to prepare, chicken, turkey, and duck breast lend themselves to a wide variety of healthy cooking techniques from grilling and baking to stir-frying and sautéing. This chapter features an international array of dishes, all with gluten-free components (read labels carefully when buying preground turkey and chicken). Many can be made in 30 minutes or less; some, like the Turkey Moussaka and Golden Chicken Cottage Pie, take longer but are well worth the effort for special occasions.

OSSO BUCO–STYLE CHICKEN

HANDS-ON TIME: 15 MINUTES   TOTAL TIME: 30 MINUTES

One of the classic features of osso buco, the popular Italian veal shank dish, is a fresh lemon-parsley-garlic garnish called *gremolata*, which gets sprinkled on just before you serve the dish. It tastes just as good with chicken as it does with veal. We season the sauce with a store-bought herb mixture sold as "Italian season-ing." Since the commercial products can sometimes contain gluten, read labels carefully, or make your own so you know exactly what's in it: Combine equal parts dried basil, rosemary, and oregano.

¼ cup brown rice flour or sorghum flour

4 boneless, skinless chicken breast halves (6 ounces each)

1 tablespoon plus 1 teaspoon extra-virgin olive oil

3 cloves garlic, smashed and peeled

⅔ cup gluten-free low-sodium chicken broth

1 cup coarsely chopped fresh or canned no-salt-added tomatoes

1 tablespoon no-salt-added tomato paste

1½ teaspoons gluten-free Italian herb seasoning

½ teaspoon salt

½ cup chopped fresh flat-leaf parsley

1 teaspoon grated lemon zest

Place the flour in a pie plate or shallow bowl. Dredge the chicken in the flour, shak-ing off any excess.

In a large nonstick skillet, heat the oil over medium-low heat. Add the garlic cloves and cook, turning them as they cook and become golden brown, about 5 minutes. With a slotted spoon, transfer the garlic to a plate and set aside. (Leave the heat on.)

Add the chicken to the pan and brown on both sides, about 2 minutes per side. Add the broth, tomatoes, tomato paste, Italian seasoning, and salt. Bring to a boil, then reduce to a simmer. Cover and cook until the chicken is cooked through but still juicy, about 15 minutes.

Meanwhile, in a small bowl, combine the parsley and lemon zest. Finely chop the garlic and add to the parsley mixture. (This is the gremolata topping.)

Divide the chicken breasts among 4 plates and spoon ⅓ cup of the pan juices around each. Dividing evenly, sprinkle with the gremolata.

MAKES 4 SERVINGS ❱ **Per serving:** 293 calories, 9 g fat, 2 g saturated fat, 40 g protein, 12 g carbohydrate, 1.5 g fiber, 396 mg sodium

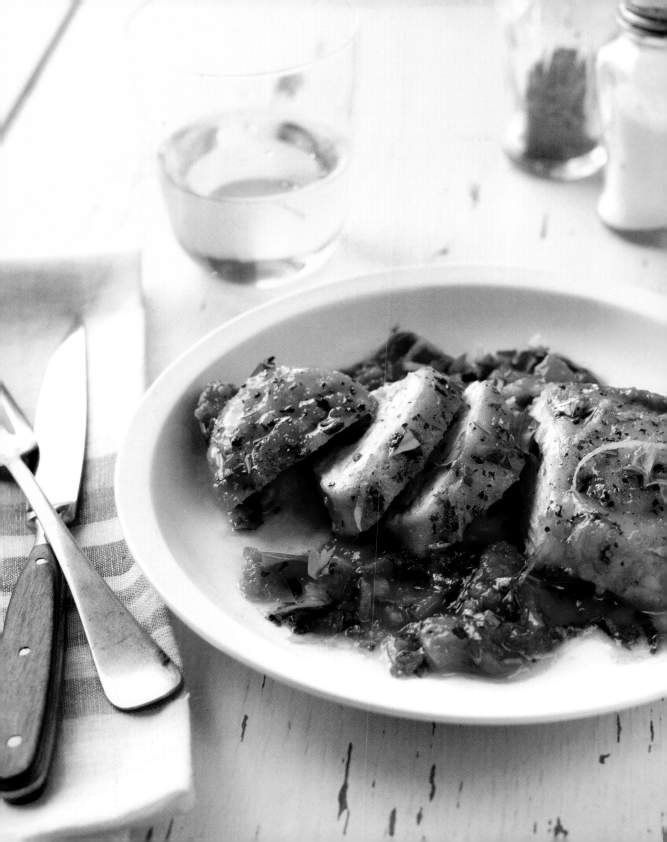

CHICKEN CHILAQUILES

HANDS-ON TIME: 20 MINUTES   TOTAL TIME: 30 MINUTES

Cans of chipotle chiles in adobo sauce can usually be found alongside other condiments and salsas in the grocery store (be sure to look for a gluten-free brand). Both the chiles and the sauce are smoky and hot. Once opened, take the chiles and their sauce out of the can, transfer to an airtight container, and refrigerate for up to a year (or more); they can also be frozen indefinitely.

4   100% corn tortillas (6-inch), each cut into 8 wedges

1   can (14.5 ounces) no-salt-added diced tomatoes

2   tablespoons no-salt-added tomato paste

1   large chipotle chile in adobo sauce, finely chopped (1½ teaspoons)

3   cloves garlic, thinly sliced

½   teaspoon dried oregano

½   teaspoon coarse kosher salt

1¼ pounds boneless, skinless chicken breasts, cut into 1-inch pieces

½   cup nonfat (0%) plain Greek yogurt

Cilantro leaves, for garnish (optional)

Lime wedges, for serving

Preheat the oven to 375°F. Place the tortilla wedges on a baking sheet and bake until crisp, about 10 minutes.

Meanwhile, in a large saucepan, combine the tomatoes, tomato paste, chipotle, garlic, oregano, salt, and ¾ cup water. Bring to a boil over medium heat, then reduce to a simmer. Cover and cook for 5 minutes to blend and intensify the flavors. Add the chicken, cover, and cook until the chicken is cooked through but still juicy, about 7 minutes.

Divide the tortilla wedges among 4 shallow bowls. Dividing evenly, spoon the chicken and its sauce on top. Top each serving with 2 tablespoons of yogurt. Garnish with cilantro (if using) and a lime wedge for squeezing.

MAKES 4 SERVINGS ▶ **Per serving:** 271 calories, 4.5 g fat, 1 g saturated fat, 36 g protein, 21 g carbohydrate, 2.5 g fiber, 489 mg sodium

CHICKEN CHOP SUEY

HANDS-ON TIME: 15 MINUTES   TOTAL TIME: 20 MINUTES

In Chinese, *tsap seui* (chop suey) loosely translates as "bits and pieces" or "a little of this, a little of that." It is a classic American-Chinese restaurant dish with simple, clean flavors. The dish (which may or may not have been invented in this country) was hugely popular in America in the early 1900s, and there were even entire restaurants called "chop suey joints" that specialized in it.

3 tablespoons arrowroot

2 tablespoons gluten-free reduced-sodium tamari soy sauce

1¼ pounds boneless, skinless chicken breasts

1 tablespoon plus 1 teaspoon extra-virgin olive oil

10 ounces white mushrooms, thinly sliced

4 large stalks celery with leaves, thinly sliced on an angle

1 cup slivered red onion (1 medium onion)

1 can (8 ounces) sliced water chestnuts, drained and rinsed

¼ teaspoon freshly ground black pepper

3 cups fresh mung bean sprouts (about 10 ounces)

In a cup, combine the arrowroot, tamari, and 1 tablespoon water. Stir well and set aside.

Halve the chicken breasts lengthwise, then thinly slice crosswise.

In a large nonstick saucepan or Dutch oven, heat the oil over high heat until shimmering. Add the chicken and cook, stirring, until just beginning to brown but still very pink, about 1 minute.

Reduce the heat to medium-high and add the mushrooms, celery, onion, water chestnuts, and pepper. Stir to combine, cover, and cook until the mushrooms have softened, about 5 minutes.

Sprinkle the bean sprouts over the mixture. Re-stir the arrowroot mixture, add to the pan, and stir to combine. Cook, uncovered, until the sauce thickens, 1 to 2 minutes. Divide the chop suey among 4 bowls and serve hot.

MAKES 4 (scant 2-cup) SERVINGS ▶ **Per serving:** 303 calories, 8.5 g fat, 1.5 g saturated fat, 36 g protein, 21 g carbohydrate, 4.5 g fiber, 560 mg sodium

CHICKEN KEBABS
WITH MINTED FETA SAUCE

HANDS-ON TIME: 20 MINUTES   TOTAL TIME: 20 MINUTES

PHASE
1

30
MINUTES
OR
LESS

You can easily make these kebabs on the grill instead of under the broiler. Cook them on a grill topper that you've sprayed lightly with olive oil (away from the grill, of course). And as long as you've got the grill (or broiler) going, make some vegetable kebabs to go along with the chicken: Thread cherry tomatoes, zucchini chunks, and onion pieces on separate skewers and broil or grill them alongside the chicken; they'll take about the same amount of time.

6 teaspoons dried mint	5 teaspoons extra-virgin olive oil
2½ teaspoons garlic powder	¾ cup nonfat plain yogurt
¼ teaspoon coarse kosher salt	⅓ cup crumbled reduced-fat feta cheese
1½ pounds boneless, skinless chicken breasts, cut into 24 pieces	

Preheat the broiler with the rack 4 inches from the heat.

In a medium bowl, combine 4 teaspoons of the mint, the garlic powder, and salt. Add the chicken to the bowl and rub the mixture into it. Drizzle 4 teaspoons of the oil over the chicken and toss to coat.

Thread the chicken onto four 6-inch or larger skewers. Broil, turning the chicken as it cooks, until cooked through but still juicy, 5 to 7 minutes.

Meanwhile, in a small bowl, stir together the yogurt, feta cheese, remaining 2 teaspoons mint, and remaining 1 teaspoon oil.

Divide the skewers among 4 plates and serve each with ¼ cup of the feta sauce on the side.

MAKES 4 SERVINGS ❯ **Per serving:** 298 calories, 12 g fat, 3 g saturated fat, 41 g protein, 5 g carbohydrate, 0.5 g fiber, 513 mg sodium

◀MAKE AHEAD▶ **The minted feta sauce can be made several hours ahead and refrigerated; serve chilled. The mint rub can be made ahead (in even larger amounts) and kept on the spice shelf in an airtight container for up to 2 months. Use it for any grilled meat (it's great on grilled fish, too).**

GARLIC CHICKEN WITH CHIPOTLE-LIME SAUCE

HANDS-ON TIME: 15 MINUTES   TOTAL TIME: 25 MINUTES

The combination of tomato paste, lime juice, agave nectar, and chipotle chile powder mimics a store-bought spicy chile sauce and assures that you aren't inadvertently getting gluten, which is often included as a thickener in this type of prepared product. If you have any leftovers, this would make a great lunch salad: Slice or shred the broiled chicken, steam some broccoli florets, and toss everything together with some of the chilled sauce.

1¼ teaspoons garlic powder

1 teaspoon crumbled dried rosemary

¾ teaspoon coarse kosher salt

4 boneless, skinless chicken breasts (6 ounces each)

1 tablespoon plus 2 teaspoons extra-virgin olive oil

3 tablespoons fresh lime juice

3 tablespoons no-salt-added tomato paste

2 teaspoons agave nectar

1 teaspoon chipotle chile powder

Preheat the broiler with the rack 4 inches from the heat.

In a small bowl, stir together 1 teaspoon of the garlic powder, the rosemary, and ½ teaspoon of the salt. Rub the mixture into both sides of the chicken, then rub the chicken with 1 tablespoon of the oil.

Broil until the chicken is cooked through but still juicy, turning it over midway, about 10 minutes total.

Meanwhile, in a small bowl, whisk together the lime juice, tomato paste, agave nectar, chipotle powder, 2 tablespoons water, and the remaining 2 teaspoons oil, ¼ teaspoon garlic powder, and ¼ teaspoon salt.

Place a chicken breast on each of 4 plates and serve with 2 tablespoons of the chipotle sauce on the side.

MAKES 4 SERVINGS ❭ **Per serving:** 260 calories, 10 g fat, 2 g saturated fat, 35 g protein, 7 g carbohydrate, 1 g fiber, 461 mg sodium

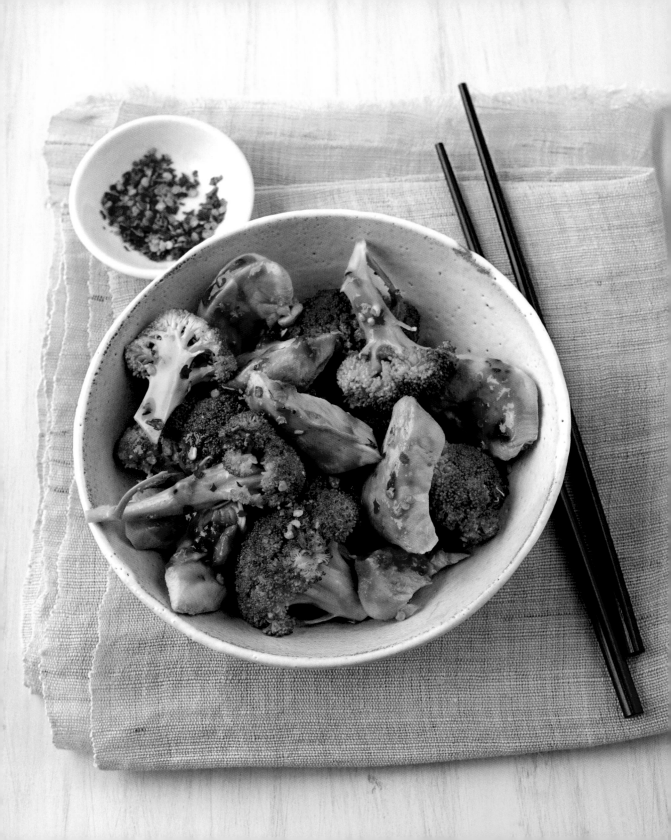

SPICY CHICKEN AND BROCCOLI

HANDS-ON TIME: 20 MINUTES
TOTAL TIME: 20 MINUTES PLUS MARINATING TIME

PHASE 2

To get 4 cups small broccoli florets (if you don't buy them precut), you'll need about 4 medium heads. Don't throw away the stalks. They make a great snack if they are peeled and steamed and served with gluten-free hummus or sugar-free, gluten-free salsa.

1 pound chicken cutlets (thin-cut chicken breast), cut across the grain into ½-inch-wide strips	1 tablespoon garbanzo bean flour
	Pinch coarse kosher salt
¼ cup dry sherry or white wine	1 tablespoon plus 1 teaspoon extra-virgin olive oil
1½ tablespoons gluten-free reduced-sodium tamari soy sauce	1 tablespoon minced fresh ginger
¾ cup gluten-free low-sodium chicken broth	¼ teaspoon red pepper flakes
	4 cups small broccoli florets

In a large bowl, combine the chicken, sherry, and tamari. Toss to coat. Set the chicken aside to marinate at room temperature for 30 minutes (or for several hours in a covered container in the refrigerator).

In a medium bowl, combine ¼ cup of the broth, the garbanzo flour, and salt. Set aside.

In a large nonstick saucepan or Dutch oven, heat the oil, ginger, and pepper flakes over medium heat until the ginger begins to sizzle, about 1 minute. Add the broccoli and toss to coat. Add the remaining ½ cup broth and bring to a boil. Cover and steam until the broccoli is crisp-tender and bright green, 2 to 3 minutes.

Add the chicken (and any marinade) to the pan and cook over medium-high heat, stirring, until the chicken is cooked through but still juicy, 2 to 3 minutes.

Whisk the broth mixture to recombine and stir into the pan. Bring to a boil and cook, stirring, until the sauce is slightly thickened, about 1 minute.

Divide the chicken and broccoli among 4 bowls and serve hot.

MAKES 4 (1-cup) SERVINGS ❱ **Per serving:** 217 calories, 8 g fat, 1.5 g saturated fat, 28 g protein, 6 g carbohydrate, 2.5 g fiber, 461 mg sodium

CHICKEN WITH LEMON-FENNEL COUSCOUS

HANDS-ON TIME: 30 MINUTES   TOTAL TIME: 40 MINUTES

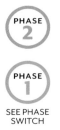

PHASE
2

PHASE
1

SEE PHASE
SWITCH

Moroccan-style dishes—like this couscous—often include sweet-tart apricots. Since fresh apricots make only a brief appearance in our markets (for 3 months in the summer), a nectarine is a more reliable option. But when fresh apricots are in season, use two of them here.

1 tablespoon plus 1 teaspoon extra-virgin olive oil

4 boneless, skinless chicken breast halves (5 ounces each)

½ cup brown rice couscous

½ teaspoon salt

½ teaspoon freshly ground black pepper

1 large yellow onion, finely chopped

5 cloves garlic, minced

1 small fennel bulb, thinly sliced

1 can (15 ounces) gluten-free no-salt-added chickpeas, drained and rinsed

1 can (14.5 ounces) no-salt-added diced tomatoes

1 nectarine, chopped

2 teaspoons grated lemon zest

2 tablespoons fresh lemon juice

1 teaspoon ground fennel seed

In a large nonstick saucepan or Dutch oven, heat the oil over medium heat. Add the chicken and cook until light golden, about 3 minutes per side. Transfer the chicken to a plate.

While the chicken is cooking, in a small saucepan, start the couscous: Cook it according to package directions, adding ¼ teaspoon each of the salt and pepper to the water. Fluff with a fork.

After removing the chicken, add the onion and garlic to the saucepan. Cook over medium heat, stirring frequently, until the onion is just softened, about 4 minutes. Add the fresh fennel, remaining ¼ teaspoon salt, and ¼ cup water. Bring to a boil and cook for 3 minutes.

Stir in the chickpeas, tomatoes, nectarine, lemon zest, lemon juice, ground fennel, another ¼ cup water, and the remaining ¼ teaspoon pepper. Bring to a boil and return the chicken to the pan. Reduce to a simmer, cover, and cook until the chicken is cooked through but still juicy, 8 to 10 minutes.

To serve, mound ½ cup couscous in each of 4 shallow bowls. Top the couscous with 1½ cups vegetables and broth and serve a chicken breast alongside.

MAKES 4 SERVINGS ❱ **Per serving:** 473 calories, 10 g fat, 1.5 g saturated fat, 40 g protein, 56 g carbohydrate, 10 g fiber, 527 mg sodium

❰PHASE SWITCH❱ **For a Phase 1 dish, omit the nectarine and add 1 diced orange bell pepper. Sauté it along with the onion. Skip the couscous and instead ladle the vegetables and broth into a bowl. Slice the chicken and arrange on top of the vegetables.**

CHICKEN-MUSHROOM CROQUETTES

HANDS-ON TIME: 15 MINUTES   TOTAL TIME: 45 MINUTES PLUS CHILLING TIME

Preparing these delicious croquettes is worth the time invested, and you can make the croquette mixture ahead (see Make Ahead, opposite page). Croquettes were invented to use up leftovers, so if you happen to have any leftover cooked chicken or turkey breast, lean pork, or lean beef, use it: You'll need about 3 cups chopped. In that case, since you don't need to cook the chicken, in the first step just simmer the mushrooms with the garlic and salt for about 10 minutes to soften them. The rest of the recipe is the same.

1¼ pounds boneless, skinless chicken breasts, each cut crosswise into 4 pieces

1 ounce dried mushrooms (about 1 cup), preferably porcini

1 clove garlic, grated on a rasp-style citrus zester

½ teaspoon salt

¼ cup black bean flour or garbanzo bean flour

Freshly ground black pepper

1 tablespoon extra-virgin olive oil

¼ cup yellow cornmeal

1 teaspoon dried thyme

Olive oil cooking spray

Lemon wedges, for serving

In a saucepan big enough to hold the chicken snugly in one layer, combine the chicken, dried mushrooms, garlic, ¼ teaspoon of the salt, and 2 cups water. Bring to a low boil, then turn off the heat, cover, and let sit for 10 minutes (this will cook the chicken and soften the mushrooms). Transfer the chicken to a plate to cool, leaving the mushrooms in the broth. When the chicken is cool enough to handle, finely chop and place in a large bowl.

Scoop the mushrooms out of the broth and chop. Strain the broth through a fine-mesh strainer into a 2-cup measuring cup.

In a small saucepan, whisk 1¼ cups of the mushroom broth (add water if you don't have 1¼ cups) with the bean flour. Add the chopped mushrooms and a large pinch of pepper. Cook over medium heat, stirring, until thickened, about 3 minutes.

Add the mushroom sauce to the chicken and stir well. Cover and refrigerate until well chilled, at least 2 hours.

Preheat the broiler. Line a baking sheet with foil (for easier cleanup) and brush the foil with the oil.

In a shallow bowl, combine the cornmeal, thyme, remaining $\frac{1}{4}$ teaspoon salt, and a large pinch of pepper. Pack some chicken mixture into a $\frac{1}{2}$-cup measure, unmold into the cornmeal, and flip to coat both sides. Place the croquette on the baking sheet. Repeat to make 8 croquettes and spray the tops with olive oil.

Broil the croquettes until browned on top, 12 to 15 minutes. Let sit on the pan for 5 minutes before serving with lemon wedges for squeezing.

MAKES 4 (2-croquette) SERVINGS ▶ **Per serving:** 302 calories, 8.5 g fat, 1.5 g saturated fat, 37 g protein, 18 g carbohydrate, 3 g fiber, 364 mg sodium

◀MAKE AHEAD▶ **The croquette mixture can be made at least a day ahead and refrigerated. Form the croquettes while the mixture is still chilled. You can also cook the croquettes, cool, and refrigerate for up to 3 days. Gently reheat in a small covered baking dish in a 325°F oven.**

KNIFE-AND-FORK RATATOUILLE TURKEY BURGERS

HANDS-ON TIME: 35 MINUTES   TOTAL TIME: 45 MINUTES

Pick a long and straight-sided eggplant (instead of a bulbous, squatty one), because you want to get as many hamburger bun–size slices out of it as you can.

1 large eggplant (about 1½ pounds), unpeeled	2 tablespoons no-salt-added tomato paste
¾ teaspoon salt	2 small cloves garlic, grated on a rasp-style citrus zester
1¼ pounds gluten-free ground turkey breast	1 teaspoon extra-virgin olive oil
1 cup finely shredded zucchini (from 1 small)	½ teaspoon ground fennel seed
½ cup chopped grape tomatoes	½ teaspoon dried thyme
	Olive oil cooking spray

Cut the eggplant crosswise into 8 slices about ½ inch thick, cutting from the thickest part of the eggplant because these will be your hamburger "buns." Using ½ teaspoon of the salt, sprinkle both sides of the eggplant slices. Set aside on paper towels to drain a bit while you make the burger mixture.

In a large bowl, combine the turkey, zucchini, tomatoes, tomato paste, garlic, oil, fennel, thyme, and remaining ¼ teaspoon salt. Gently but thoroughly combine. With moistened hands, form the mixture into 4 patties 4 inches across. Make the outer edges of the patties a little higher than the middles (the burgers will plump up as they cook).

Spray a large nonstick skillet with olive oil and heat over medium-high heat. Place the burgers in the skillet and cook for 4 minutes without turning. Flip the burgers, cover the pan, and cook for 4 minutes longer. Add ¼ cup water, re-cover, and cook until the burgers are cooked through but still juicy, 3 to 4 minutes longer. Let stand, covered, for 2 minutes.

While the burgers are cooking, preheat a panini press, hinged electric grill, or large grill pan. (If not nonstick, spray very lightly with olive oil.) Working in batches (depending on how big your press or grill is), cook the eggplant until nicely softened, 5 to 6 minutes (turning once or twice if on a grill pan).

Place each burger on a slice of eggplant and top with another slice of eggplant. If there are pan juices in the skillet, drizzle a little over the tops.

MAKES 4 SERVINGS ❱ **Per serving:** 243 calories, 3.5 g fat, 0.5 g saturated fat, 39 g protein, 17 g carbohydrate, 8.5 g fiber, 373 mg sodium

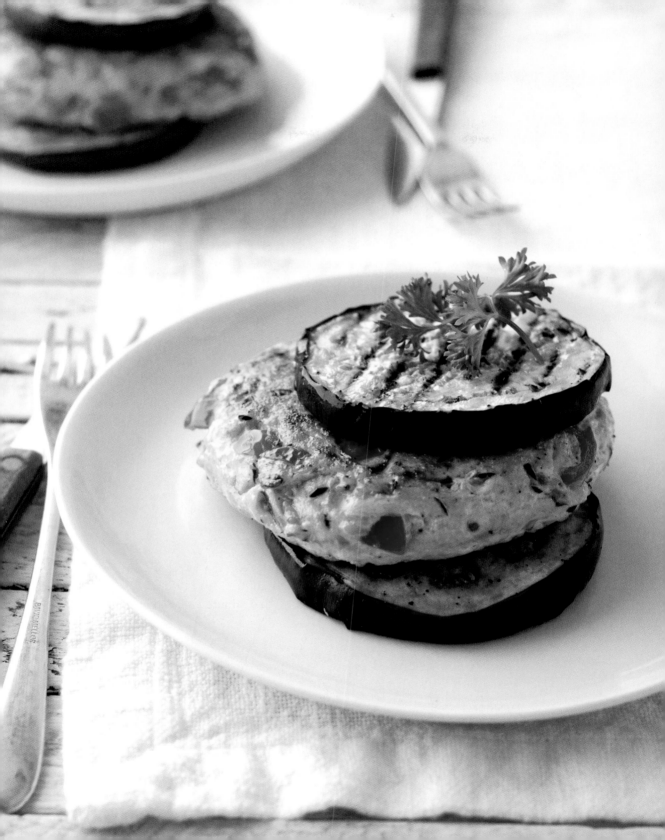

TURKEY MOUSSAKA

HANDS-ON TIME: 25 MINUTES
TOTAL TIME: 1 HOUR 30 MINUTES PLUS RESTING TIME

Like a lasagna, this dish is a multipart affair, but it can definitely be done in stages (see Make Ahead, opposite page). The moussaka also makes great leftovers. Store in the fridge and reheat single portions in the microwave (just 2 or 3 minutes at 50% power).

EGGPLANT

- ⅓ cup liquid egg whites
- ¾ cup almond flour
- ½ cup sorghum flour
- ½ teaspoon salt
- ¼ teaspoon freshly ground black pepper
- 2 pinches ground allspice
- 2 medium eggplants (about 1 pound each), cut crosswise into ½-inch slices

TURKEY SAUCE

- 2 tablespoons extra-virgin olive oil
- 2 cups diced onion (1 large or 2 medium)
- 3 cloves garlic, minced
- 1 can (15 ounces) no-salt-added crushed tomatoes

- ½ cup dry red or white wine
- 3 tablespoons no-salt-added tomato paste
- ¾ teaspoon salt
- ¼ teaspoon ground cinnamon
- 1¼ pounds gluten-free ground turkey breast

TOPPING

- 1½ cups nonfat (0%) plain Greek yogurt
- 2 large eggs
- ⅓ cup liquid egg whites
- ¼ cup grated Parmesan cheese
- 2 tablespoons garbanzo bean flour
- ¼ teaspoon salt

Olive oil cooking spray

For the eggplant: Preheat the oven to 375°F. Line 2 baking sheets with parchment paper.

In a shallow bowl, whisk the egg whites.

In a second shallow bowl, whisk together the almond flour, sorghum flour, salt, pepper, and allspice.

Dip one side of each eggplant slice in the egg whites, then dip the egg-coated side in the almond flour mixture. (Not all of the dredging mixture gets used; discard any remainder.) Place the eggplant slices on the baking sheet, coating-side up, and bake until the eggplant is lightly browned and mostly tender, 25 to 30 minutes (switch the oven racks about halfway through). Remove from the oven and let the eggplant cool on the baking sheet.

Reduce the oven temperature to 350°F.

While the eggplant is baking, make the turkey sauce: In a large nonstick saucepan or Dutch oven, heat the oil over medium-high heat. Add the onion and garlic and cook until the onion is softened, about 5 minutes. Add the tomatoes, wine, tomato paste, salt, cinnamon, and $\frac{1}{3}$ cup water. Bring to a simmer. Add the turkey in small clumps, stirring to incorporate into the sauce. Cook for 2 minutes to partially cook the turkey (it cooks fully in the oven) and blend the flavors. Remove from the heat and set aside.

For the topping: In a medium bowl, whisk together the yogurt, whole eggs, egg whites, Parmesan, garbanzo flour, salt, and $\frac{1}{4}$ cup water.

To assemble the moussaka: Lightly spray the bottom of a 9 × 13-inch baking dish or lasagna pan with olive oil. Saving the larger pieces for the top, layer half the egg-plant, coating-side down, in the bottom of the dish. Spread the turkey sauce over the eggplant, then top with the remaining eggplant, coating-side up. Spread the topping over the eggplant. Bake until the topping is nicely browned and the insides are bub-bling, 45 to 50 minutes. Let the moussaka rest for at least 20 minutes before cutting and serving.

MAKES 8 SERVINGS ❱ **Per serving:** 305 calories, 9.5 g fat, 1.5 g saturated fat, 31 g protein, 23 g carbohydrate, 7 g fiber, 523 mg sodium

◀MAKE AHEAD▶ **You can make both the turkey sauce and the topping ahead and refrigerate for up to 2 days. You can bake the eggplant ahead, too, but it's best done no more than several hours before you're ready to assemble, so you can keep it at room temperature. If you refrigerate it, the coating will get soggy and fall off.**

GOLDEN CHICKEN COTTAGE PIE

HANDS-ON TIME: 20 MINUTES
TOTAL TIME: 1 HOUR 20 MINUTES PLUS STANDING TIME

A cottage pie, another name for shepherd's pie, is inherently gluten-friendly because there is no wheat-based pie crust involved. Instead, the "crust" is made of mashed potatoes. In this version, we give the mashed potato topping a health makeover by opting for sweet potato lightened with cauliflower. And where the filling for a classic cottage or shepherd's pie would be thickened with a little wheat flour, here high-protein bean flour does the job.

- 10 ounces small cauliflower florets (fresh or frozen)
- 1 medium sweet potato (about 10 ounces), peeled and cubed
- ½ teaspoon salt
  Freshly ground black pepper
- 1 cup plus 2 tablespoons gluten-free low-sodium chicken broth
- 1 tablespoon plus 1 teaspoon extra-virgin olive oil

- 1 tablespoon garbanzo–fava bean flour, garbanzo bean flour, or fava bean flour
- ¼ teaspoon turmeric (optional)
- 1 small red onion, diced
- 3 cloves garlic, minced
- 2 stalks celery, diced
- 1 pound gluten-free ground chicken breast
- ½ cup frozen green peas

Preheat the oven to 375°F.

In a medium pot of boiling water, cook the cauliflower for 3 minutes. Add the sweet potato and cook until both vegetables are very tender, about 8 minutes. Drain well and return to the pot. Sprinkle with ¼ teaspoon of the salt and a couple of large pinches of freshly ground black pepper. Add 2 tablespoons of the broth and 1 teaspoon of the oil. Mash until very smooth (an immersion blender does a good job here) and set aside.

Meanwhile, in a small bowl, combine the remaining 1 cup broth and the bean flour. Stir well. Stir in the turmeric (if using).

In a large nonstick skillet, heat the remaining 1 tablespoon oil over medium-high heat. Add the onion and garlic. Cook, stirring, until the onion begins to soften, 3 to 5 minutes. Add the celery and stir for 1 minute. Add the chicken and sprinkle with the remaining ¼ teaspoon salt. Cook, breaking up the chicken with a spoon, until the chicken is still quite pink, 2 to 3 minutes. (It cooks fully in the oven.)

Stir the broth mixture into the skillet and return to a simmer. Cook for 1 minute to thicken. Stir in the peas.

Scoop the chicken filling into a 9- or 10-inch pie plate and spread evenly. Spread the vegetable mash evenly over the top.

Bake until the topping is lightly browned and the filling is gently bubbling, about 1 hour. Let stand at least 15 minutes before serving.

Dividing evenly, scoop the filling and topping into 4 shallow bowls or plates.

MAKES 4 SERVINGS ❯ **Per serving:** 274 calories, 7.5 g fat, 1.5 g saturated fat, 29 g protein, 21 g carbohydrate, 5 g fiber, 509 mg sodium

❮MAKE AHEAD❯ **You can make the sweet potato–cauliflower topping and/or the chicken mixture ahead. Keep at room temperature if baking the pie within 2 hours; otherwise refrigerate, but bring back to room temperature before proceeding. You can also assemble the pie completely about an hour before baking.**

PEKING CHICKEN WRAPS

HANDS-ON TIME: 15 MINUTES   TOTAL TIME: 25 MINUTES

Hoisin sauce—the salty-sweet sauce that traditionally accompanies the Chinese dish called Peking Duck—usually has some wheat flour and sugar added. So here prune butter (which takes the place of the sugar and the wheat in hoisin and gives body to the sauce), gluten-free tamari, rice vinegar, and sesame oil stand in. The Chinese 5-spice powder—a combo of cinnamon, star anise, ground fennel, ground cloves, and Szechuan pepper—is a flavorful addition. Look for it in the spice section of your supermarket.

¼ cup unsweetened prune butter or prune purée

2 tablespoons gluten-free reduced-sodium tamari soy sauce

2 teaspoons rice vinegar or apple cider vinegar

1 teaspoon dark sesame oil

1¼ pounds boneless, skinless chicken breasts

1 teaspoon Chinese 5-spice powder

1 tablespoon extra-virgin olive oil

12 butter lettuce leaves

6 scallions, halved lengthwise

Preheat the broiler with the rack 4 inches from the heat.

In a small bowl, stir together the prune butter, tamari, vinegar, and sesame oil. Set aside.

Rub the chicken with the 5-spice powder and then the olive oil. Broil until the chicken is cooked through but still juicy, turning the chicken over midway, about 10 minutes total.

When cool enough to handle, thinly slice the chicken crosswise. Divide the chicken among the lettuce leaves and top each with a scallion half. Spoon about 2 teaspoons of the sauce over each and roll the leaves up.

MAKES 12 WRAPS (3 per serving) ❱ **Per serving:** 259 calories, 8.5 g fat, 1.5 g saturated fat, 32 g protein, 22 g carbohydrate, 1 g fiber, 520 mg sodium

◀MAKE AHEAD▶ The sauce can be made up to 3 days ahead and refrigerated. It can also be used as a dipping sauce for sliced, cooked pork loin or turkey breast. Bring to room temperature before serving.

QUINOA-STUFFED CHICKEN BREASTS

HANDS-ON TIME: 20 MINUTES   TOTAL TIME: 50 MINUTES

PHASE 2

We opted for creminis (also known as baby bellas) in this dish because they have a slightly more robust mushroom flavor than white button mushrooms. If they aren't available, feel free to use the white mushrooms. And if you don't happen to have poultry seasoning on hand, use ¼ teaspoon each rosemary, sage, and thyme.

1 tablespoon plus 1 teaspoon extra-virgin olive oil

3 ounces cremini mushrooms, coarsely chopped

1¼ cups gluten-free low-sodium chicken broth

¼ cup red quinoa

¾ teaspoon poultry seasoning

½ teaspoon salt

1 cup coarsely chopped arugula (from a 2.5-ounce bunch)

4 boneless, skinless chicken breast halves (6 ounces each)

3 tablespoons brown rice flour

In a small saucepan, heat 1 teaspoon of the oil over medium heat. Add the mushrooms and cook, stirring occasionally, until firm-tender, about 3 minutes. Add ¾ cup of the broth, the quinoa, ½ teaspoon of the poultry seasoning, and ¼ teaspoon of the salt. Bring to a boil, then reduce to a simmer. Cover and cook until the quinoa is tender, about 10 minutes. Stir in the arugula. Cool in the pan to room temperature.

Preheat the oven to 350°F.

With a sharp paring knife, cut a horizontal slit though the thickest portion of each chicken breast to form a deep pocket without cutting through to the other side. Fill each pocket evenly with the quinoa stuffing. Sprinkle the top of each breast evenly with the brown rice flour, patting it on.

In a large nonstick ovenproof skillet, heat the remaining 1 tablespoon of oil over medium heat. Add the chicken and cook until browned on one side, about 2 minutes. Turn the chicken over and add the remaining ½ cup broth, ¼ teaspoon poultry seasoning, and ¼ teaspoon salt. Cover and transfer to the oven. Cook until the chicken is just cooked through and still juicy, about 15 minutes.

Divide the chicken among 4 plates. Spoon any pan juices evenly over the chicken and serve with any of the stuffing mixture that might have slipped out.

MAKES 4 SERVINGS ❫ **Per serving:** 313 calories, 10 g fat, 1.5 g saturated fat, 40 g protein, 15 g carbohydrate, 1 g fiber, 518 mg sodium

SPICE-RUBBED GRILLED DUCK BREAST WITH FRESH PLUM SALSA

HANDS-ON TIME: 15 MINUTES   TOTAL TIME: 20 MINUTES

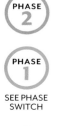

PHASE
2

PHASE
1

SEE PHASE
SWITCH

30
MINUTES
OR
LESS

Although duck has a reputation for being extraordinarily fatty, once you remove the skin and fat below it, duck breasts are actually quite lean. Treat them as you would steak; unlike other poultry, they can be cooked to whatever degree of doneness you prefer, although well-done might be tough. If plums aren't in season, you can make the salsa with any stone fruit you like, even cherries.

1½ teaspoons garam masala

½ teaspoon dried oregano

½ teaspoon coarse kosher salt

4 boneless Long Island (Pekin) duck breast halves (8 ounces each), skinned

4 teaspoons extra-virgin olive oil

1 tablespoon balsamic vinegar

2 teaspoons agave nectar

½ pound plums, halved, pitted, and cut into ½-inch cubes

¼ cup finely chopped red onion

1 fresh jalapeño (seeded if desired for less heat), finely diced

In a small bowl, stir together the garam masala, oregano, and salt. Rub the mixture into both sides of the duck breasts.

Heat a grill pan over medium heat with 2 teaspoons of the oil. Place the duck on the pan and cook for 2 to 3 minutes per side for rare, 1 minute longer per side for medium-rare. Alternatively, in a large nonstick skillet, heat 2 teaspoons of the oil over medium heat. Add the duck and cook as above. Transfer the duck to a cutting board and let sit for 5 minutes before slicing.

While the duck is resting, make the salsa: In a medium bowl, stir together the vinegar, agave nectar, and remaining 2 teaspoons oil. Add the plums, onion, and jalapeño. Toss to combine.

Thinly slice the duck and divide among 4 plates. Spoon ¼ cup of the plum salsa on top of each serving.

MAKES 4 SERVINGS ▶ **Per serving:** 262 calories, 8 g fat, 1.5 g saturated fat, 36 g protein, 11 g carbohydrate, 1 g fiber, 376 mg sodium

◀PHASE SWITCH▶ **For Phase 1, use ½ pound plum tomatoes in the salsa instead of plums.**

MEXICAN TURKEY AND PEPPER STEW

HANDS-ON TIME: 25 MINUTES   TOTAL TIME: 25 MINUTES

PHASE
1

30
MINUTES
OR
LESS

Sesame seeds and chocolate add a richness and incredible depth of flavor to this Mexican-inspired stew. It's mildly spiced, so if you like more heat, use chipotle chile powder instead of a mild chili powder blend and add a minced fresh serrano chile when you cook the bell peppers.

3 tablespoons sesame seeds

2 teaspoons unsweetened cocoa powder

½ teaspoon gluten-free chili powder

½ teaspoon dried oregano

3 teaspoons extra-virgin olive oil

1 pound turkey cutlets or steaks (½ inch thick), cut across the grain into thin strips

1 large sweet onion, chopped

4 cloves garlic, minced

2 medium yellow bell peppers, cut into thin strips 2 inches long

½ teaspoon coarse kosher salt

1 can (15 ounces) no-salt-added crushed tomatoes

1 cup gluten-free low-sodium chicken broth

Chopped fresh cilantro or flat-leaf parsley, for garnish (optional)

In a spice grinder (or coffee grinder), combine the sesame seeds, cocoa powder, chili powder, and oregano. Grind to a fine powder.

In a large nonstick saucepan or Dutch oven, heat 2 teaspoons of the oil over medium-high heat. Add the turkey strips and cook, stirring, until opaque all over (but still pink in the center), about 2 minutes. Transfer to a plate.

Add the onion, garlic, 1 tablespoon water, and the remaining 1 teaspoon oil to the pan. Scrape up any browned bits from the bottom of the pan and cook, stirring, until the onion begins to soften, about 3 minutes. Add the bell peppers, sprinkle with the salt, and cook until they begin to soften, about 3 minutes.

Sprinkle the vegetables with the sesame seed mixture and stir to combine. Add the tomatoes and chicken broth. Bring to a simmer and cook for 5 minutes, stirring occasionally, to develop flavors and thicken the stew.

Return the turkey (and any juices) to the pan and cook for 1 minute to heat through.

Divide the stew among 4 bowls and serve sprinkled with cilantro or parsley, if desired.

MAKES 4 (1¾-cup) SERVINGS ▶ **Per serving:** 293 calories, 8.5 g fat, 1 g saturated fat, 34 g protein, 20 g carbohydrate, 4.5 g fiber, 376 mg sodium

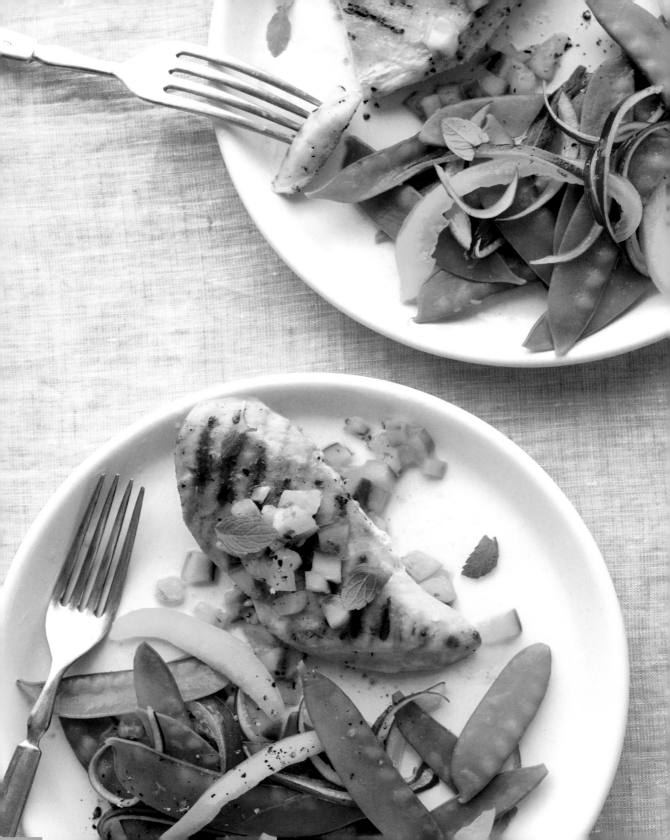

PAN-GRILLED TURKEY CUTLETS WITH THAI RELISH

HANDS-ON TIME: 15 MINUTES   TOTAL TIME: 15 MINUTES

PHASE 1

30 MINUTES OR LESS

If you can find mini cucumbers (also known as Persian cucumbers), use 4 or 5 of them here. You don't have to peel or seed them. Serve this dish with Lemon Snow Peas (page 239), if desired.

1 cucumber, peeled, seeded, and diced

1 teaspoon grated lime zest

2 tablespoons fresh lime juice

2 tablespoons chopped fresh mint

½ teaspoon agave nectar

Coarse kosher salt

4 turkey cutlets or steaks (4 ounces each, ½ to ¾ inch thick)

1 tablespoon extra-virgin olive oil

½ teaspoon ground coriander

Freshly ground black pepper

In a medium bowl, combine the cucumber, lime zest, lime juice, mint, agave nectar, and a pinch of salt. Set the Thai relish aside.

Coat both sides of the turkey with the oil, then sprinkle both sides with the coriander. Season each with a small pinch of salt and pepper on both sides.

Heat a grill pan or cast-iron skillet over medium-high heat. Place the cutlets on or in the pan and cook for 3 minutes. Flip and cook until the cutlets are cooked through but still juicy, about 2 minutes longer.

Place a turkey cutlet on each of 4 plates. Top each with ¼ cup Thai relish.

MAKES 4 SERVINGS ❱ **Per serving:** 168 calories, 4 g fat, 0.5 g saturated fat, 29 g protein, 5 g carbohydrate, 1 g fiber, 223 mg sodium

◀MAKE AHEAD▶ **You can make the Thai relish several hours ahead and refrigerate or leave at room temperature, but any longer than that and the cucumbers will give up too much liquid. Serve chilled or at room temperature.**

CHUNKY TURKEY AND BLACK-EYED PEA STEW

HANDS-ON TIME: 20 MINUTES   TOTAL TIME: 50 MINUTES

PHASE 2

Although we prefer the texture and flavor of black-eyed peas cooked from scratch, you can save a good 40 minutes of cooking time if you use frozen or no-salt-added canned black-eyed peas (you'll need about 2 cups). Cook the frozen or canned peas with the water as directed in the first step, but simmer for only 5 minutes, just to develop flavor. Then continue with the recipe as written.

4 teaspoons extra-virgin olive oil

5 cloves garlic, minced

1 teaspoon dried oregano

½ teaspoon red pepper flakes

1 cup dried black-eyed peas, rinsed and picked over

2½ cups gluten-free low-sodium chicken broth

½ pound red onions, cut into ½-inch chunks

1 pound turkey breast cutlets or steaks (½ to ¾ inch thick), cut into ¾-inch cubes

¾ teaspoon coarse kosher salt

¼ cup almond flour

½ cup unsweetened almond milk

Cilantro leaves, for garnish (optional)

In a large nonstick saucepan or Dutch oven, heat 2 teaspoons of the oil, the garlic, oregano, and pepper flakes over medium heat until fragrant, about 45 seconds. Add the black-eyed peas, broth, and 2 cups water. Bring to a boil, then reduce to a simmer. Cover and cook until the peas are tender, about 45 minutes.

About 20 minutes before the peas are done, in a large nonstick skillet, heat the remaining 2 teaspoons oil over medium-high heat. Add the onions and cook, stirring often, until softened and browned, about 6 minutes.

Add the turkey to the skillet, sprinkle with ¼ teaspoon of the salt, and cook, stirring, until seared all over, about 2 minutes. Remove from the heat and set aside.

In a small bowl, stir together the almond flour and almond milk.

When the peas are done, add the almond milk mixture, the turkey-onion mixture, and the remaining ½ teaspoon salt to the saucepan. Return to a simmer and cook for 3 minutes to cook the turkey through and to thicken the sauce slightly. Divide the stew among 4 bowls and serve hot, garnished with cilantro, if using.

MAKES 4 (1½-cup) SERVINGS ▶ **Per serving:** 384 calories, 9.5 g fat, 1 g saturated fat, 42 g protein, 34 g carbohydrate, 6.5 g fiber, 539 mg sodium

TURKEY TETRAZZINI WITH PORTOBELLOS

HANDS-ON TIME: 20 MINUTES   TOTAL TIME: 55 MINUTES PLUS STANDING TIME

PHASE 2

If you don't happen to have any leftover turkey, poach 1 pound of turkey breast cutlets (or steaks) in a skillet in enough lightly salted water to just cover the turkey. Bring to a gentle boil and cook for 10 minutes. Let cool in the cooking liquid, then remove and chop.

Olive oil cooking spray

Coarse kosher salt

8 ounces gluten-free quinoa radiatore pasta (some brands call them pagodas)

1 tablespoon plus 1 teaspoon extra-virgin olive oil

1 medium green bell pepper, diced

¾ pound portobello mushrooms, gills scraped, caps halved and thinly sliced

3 tablespoons sorghum flour

1½ cups gluten-free low-sodium chicken broth

1½ cups 1% milk

8 tablespoons grated Parmesan cheese

Freshly ground black pepper

2½ cups coarsely chopped cooked turkey breast (about 1 pound)

1 zucchini, diced

Preheat the oven to 375°F. Lightly spray the bottom and sides of a 9 × 13-inch baking dish with olive oil.

Bring a large pot of water to a boil. Add 2 teaspoons salt to the water, then add the pasta and cook according to package directions. Drain well.

While the pasta is cooking, in a large nonstick saucepan, heat the oil over medium-high heat. Add the bell pepper and sprinkle with a pinch of salt. Cook for 1 minute. Add the mushrooms in an even layer and sprinkle with a pinch of salt. Cook without stirring for 2 minutes, then stir and cook until the vegetables are very tender, about 2 minutes longer.

Stir in the flour until well incorporated. Slowly stir in the broth and milk. Bring to a simmer, then cook for 1 minute to lightly thicken. Remove from the heat and stir in 3 tablespoons of the Parmesan, ½ teaspoon salt, and ¼ teaspoon black pepper.

In a large bowl, combine the drained pasta, mushroom sauce, turkey, and zucchini. Transfer the mixture to the baking dish. Sprinkle the remaining 5 tablespoons Parmesan evenly over the top and sprinkle with a little black pepper.

Bake the tetrazzini until the top is browned and the filling is lightly bubbling, 25 to 30 minutes. Let stand 10 minutes before serving.

MAKES 6 SERVINGS ❯ **Per serving:** 364 calories, 7.5 g fat, 2.5 g saturated fat, 33 g protein, 41 g carbohydrate, 4.5 g fiber, 459 mg sodium

TURKEY BREAST STUFFED WITH SPINACH AND RICOTTA

HANDS-ON TIME: 20 MINUTES
TOTAL TIME: 1 HOUR 5 MINUTES PLUS STANDING TIME

PHASE
2

The stuffing for this roasted turkey breast tastes like a rich creamed spinach side dish, but without as much saturated fat—here it's an "inside" dish, since it cooks inside the rolled-up turkey. Although this makes lovely leftovers if you're cooking for fewer than 6 people, it is also a very nice dinner party or buffet dish. Serve it with Smashed Tomatoes (page 232) and a green salad.

4 cloves garlic, minced

1 tablespoon plus 2 teaspoons extra-virgin olive oil

1 package (10 ounces) frozen chopped spinach, thawed and squeezed very dry

⅓ cup part-skim ricotta cheese

3 tablespoons grated Parmesan cheese

1 large egg

1 teaspoon grated orange zest

½ teaspoon freshly ground black pepper

1 boneless, skinless turkey breast half (2 pounds)

1 tablespoon fresh orange juice

½ teaspoon paprika

½ teaspoon salt

Preheat the oven to 375°F.

In a small saucepan, combine the garlic and 1 tablespoon of the oil. Heat over low heat until the garlic is fragrant and is just beginning to sizzle, about 2 minutes. Remove the pan from the heat, add the spinach (shredding it as you do so), and stir to coat with the oil. Let cool slightly.

In a medium bowl, combine the ricotta, Parmesan, egg, orange zest, and pepper. Add the spinach mixture and stir to combine.

With the pointed end of the turkey breast facing you, make a lengthwise and horizontal cut into the thicker side. Slice through the breast, cutting almost to, but not through, the opposite side. Open the turkey up like a book and pound lightly to an even thickness.

Spread the ricotta-spinach mixture over the turkey, leaving a 2-inch border all around. Roll the turkey up as best you can (it will not be an even piece of meat) and tie in several places with kitchen twine. Use small wooden skewers to pin closed any tears or holes (there will definitely be some).

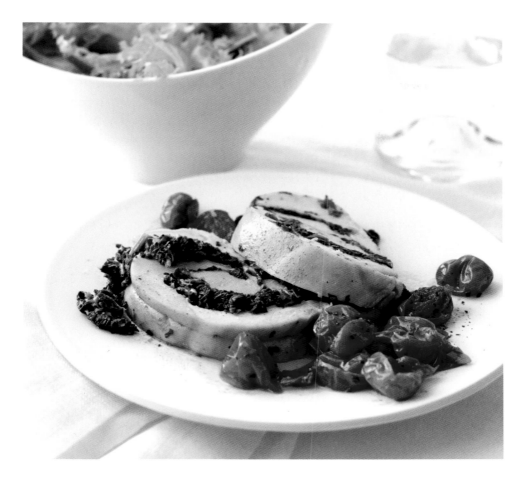

Place the turkey on a rack set over a small roasting pan or baking pan. Pour ½ inch of hot water into the bottom of the pan and cover the pan with foil. Roast the turkey for 30 minutes.

Meanwhile, in a small bowl, combine the orange juice, paprika, salt, and remaining 2 teaspoons oil.

Uncover the turkey, brush with the orange juice mixture, and roast until the turkey is cooked through and an instant-read thermometer inserted in the middle of the stuffing registers 140°F, about 15 minutes longer. Transfer the turkey to a cutting board, tent with foil, and let stand 15 minutes before cutting into 12 slices.

MAKES 6 (2-slice) SERVINGS ▶ **Per serving:** 262 calories, 8.5 g fat, 2.5 g saturated fat, 41 g protein, 4 g carbohydrate, 1.5 g fiber, 359 mg sodium

ITALIAN TAMALES

HANDS-ON TIME: 20 MINUTES   TOTAL TIME: 1 HOUR 10 MINUTES

PHASE 2

A tamale is a sort of steamed dumpling that is common to many parts of Latin America, especially Mexico. A classic Mexican tamale is made with a dough of masa harina (a special type of finely ground corn) and lard that encloses a filling, usually meat. The dough and filling are wrapped in a piece of dried corn husk and steamed for several hours. In this healthy makeover the flavors turn Italian, the lard is replaced by extra-virgin olive oil, and instead of dried corn husks, the wrappers are edible lettuce leaves.

4 teaspoons extra-virgin olive oil

2 cloves garlic, minced

½ teaspoon ground fennel seed

Pinch of red pepper flakes (optional)

10 ounces gluten-free ground turkey breast

¼ cup finely chopped fresh basil

2 tablespoons no-salt-added tomato paste

1 cup masa harina

¼ cup grated Parmesan cheese

½ teaspoon gluten-free baking powder

¼ teaspoon salt

2 heads Bibb lettuce

In a large nonstick skillet, combine 2 teaspoons of the oil, the garlic, fennel, pepper flakes (if using), and 2 tablespoons water. Heat over medium to medium-high heat until the water-oil mixture starts to simmer/sizzle. Add the turkey and cook, breaking it into fine crumbles with a wooden spoon, until opaque throughout, 2 to 3 minutes. Stir in the basil and tomato paste. Remove from the heat and set aside.

In a medium bowl, whisk together the masa harina, Parmesan, baking powder, and salt. Make a well in the center of the dry ingredients and add ⅔ cup water and the remaining 2 teaspoons oil. Mix gently. Adding 1 tablespoon of water at a time, continue to mix, adding enough to create a soft dough. To judge the dough, pinch it: It should stick together and not be crumbly.

Pull off the 8 biggest leaves from each head of lettuce (for a total of 16). Divide the dough into 8 equal portions. Spread a portion of dough all over the top two-thirds of 8 of the leaves. Spoon about 3 tablespoons of turkey down the middle of the dough. Fold one side of the lettuce leaf over the filling and then loosely roll up (leave the ends open). The lettuce leaf will crack, but that's where the second set of leaves comes in. Place the bundle on a second lettuce leaf, making sure that as you roll it up the exposed portion is now covered. Place the bundle, seam-side down, in a steamer basket or insert. Repeat for all 8. (Place the bundles in the steamer a single layer if it is big enough, otherwise in layers.)

Bring the water in the steamer to a boil before adding the basket or insert. Steam the tamales, covered, until firm, 35 to 45 minutes (the longer time for bundles that are stacked). Turn off the heat and let sit in the steamer for 10 minutes before serving.

MAKES 4 TAMALES (2 per serving) ▶ **Per serving:** 255 calories, 8 g fat, 1.5 g saturated fat, 24 g protein, 25 g carbohydrate, 3 g fiber, 333 mg sodium

◀MAKE AHEAD▶ **You can stuff and wrap the tamales ahead of time and refrigerate (but not for longer than a couple of hours). Let them return to room temperature before steaming.**

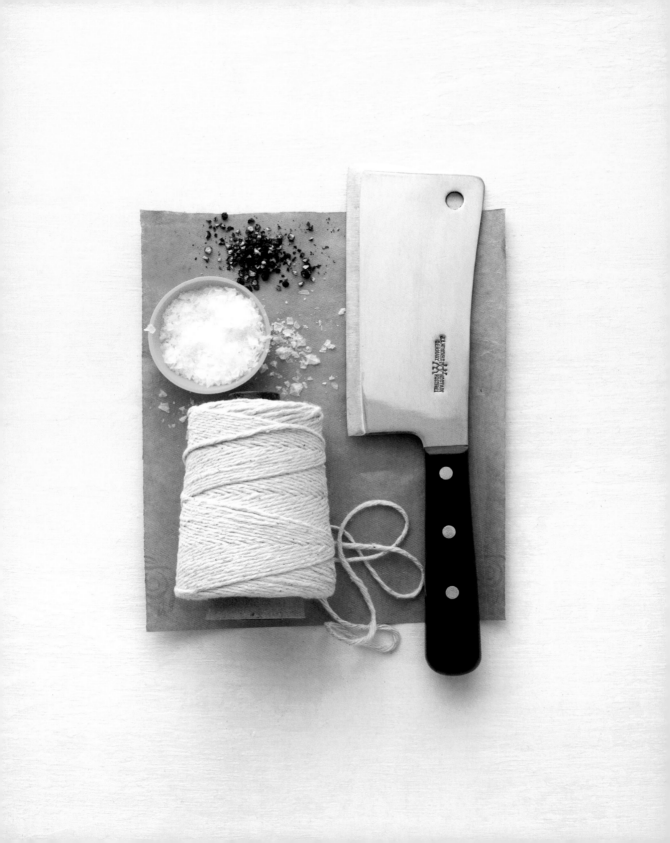

MEATS

This chapter features recipes made with naturally gluten-free lean beef and pork. We have not included lamb, because most cuts are just too high in saturated fat. If your budget allows, try to buy organic grass-fed beef, which provides more heart-healthy omega-3 fatty acids than grain-fed beef. And remember, pork is so lean these days, it only needs to be cooked to 145°F. Try the Pork Meatballs with Broken Spaghetti; there's no bread in the meatballs, and the pasta is gluten free and multigrain.

PAN-SEARED SIRLOIN STEAKS WITH FIERY PEPPER SAUCE

HANDS-ON TIME: 20 MINUTES   TOTAL TIME: 20 MINUTES

PHASE 1

30 MINUTES OR LESS

The fieriness of the sauce will depend on the size of chipotle pepper you use and whether or not you leave the seeds in. Or leave the chipotle out altogether for a nice and tame bell pepper sauce. This dish is delicious served with steamed or sautéed broccoli rabe.

3   scallions, cut into short lengths

¼   cup packed fresh cilantro sprigs (the leafy ends only)

3   cloves garlic, peeled

1   small chipotle chile in adobo (seeded, if desired, for less heat)

1   teaspoon ground cumin

4   thin-cut sirloin steaks (about 5 ounces each)

Freshly ground black pepper

½   teaspoon coarse kosher salt

4   teaspoons extra-virgin olive oil

2   medium bell peppers (any colors), cut into strips

1   can (14.5 ounces) no-salt-added diced tomatoes

In a mini food processor, combine the scallions, cilantro, garlic, chipotle, and cumin. Process to a coarse paste.

Sprinkle the steaks with some black pepper and ¼ teaspoon of the salt.

In a large nonstick skillet, heat 2 teaspoons of the oil over medium heat. Add the steaks and cook until browned on both sides and medium-rare, 3 to 4 minutes total. Transfer the steaks to a plate.

Add the remaining 2 teaspoons oil and the bell peppers to the skillet. Cook, stirring frequently, until the peppers are just slightly softened, about 2 minutes. Add the scallion-chipotle paste, toss to coat the peppers, and cook until quite fragrant and the peppers are crisp-tender, about 2 minutes.

Add the tomatoes and the remaining ¼ teaspoon salt. Cook, stirring occasionally, for 5 minutes to thicken the sauce and develop the flavors.

Place a steak on each of 4 plates. Dividing evenly, top each steak with fiery pepper sauce.

MAKES 4 SERVINGS ▶ **Per serving:** 270 calories, 10 g fat, 2.5 g saturated fat, 33 g protein, 10 g carbohydrate, 2.5 g fiber, 396 mg sodium

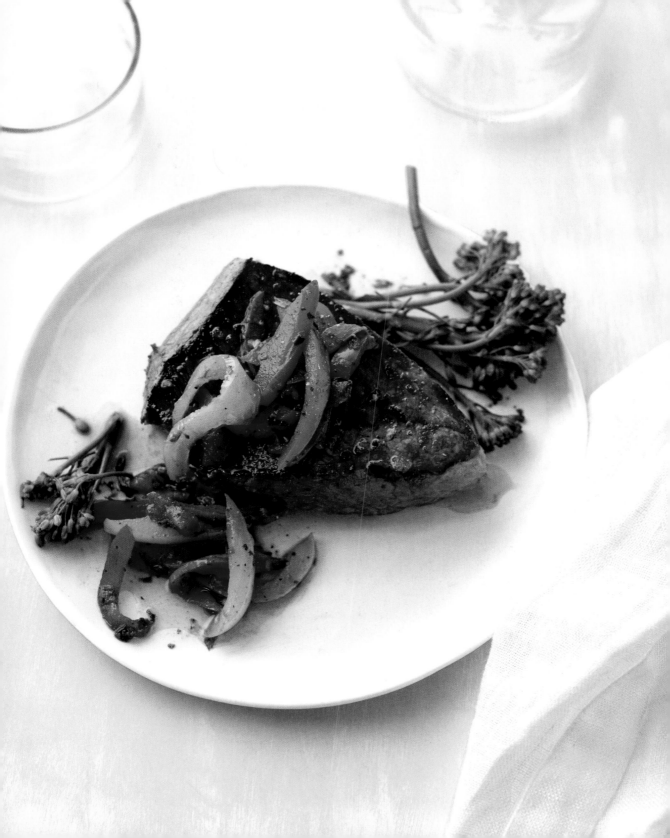

PAN-FRIED FLANK STEAK WITH TOMATO-EGGPLANT SAUCE

HANDS-ON TIME: 20 MINUTES   TOTAL TIME: 20 MINUTES

PHASE 1

30 MINUTES OR LESS

If you plan ahead a bit and pop the flank steak in the freezer for 20 to 30 minutes to firm it up, slicing it will be much easier. If you're having this dish on Phase 2, you can serve it over ½ cup cooked quinoa or brown rice to soak up some of the juices.

1 **pound flank steak**

4 **teaspoons extra-virgin olive oil**

3 **cloves garlic, minced**

½ **teaspoon dried oregano**

¼ **teaspoon red pepper flakes**

1 **small eggplant (about ¾ pound), unpeeled, cut into ½-inch cubes**

¾ **teaspoon coarse kosher salt**

4 **plum tomatoes, halved lengthwise and cut into very thin wedges**

⅓ **cup chopped fresh basil or flat-leaf parsley**

4 **tablespoons grated Parmesan cheese**

Cut the flank steak lengthwise into thirds (following the grain of the meat). Then cut each piece across the grain into very thin slices. In a large nonstick skillet, heat 2 teaspoons of the oil over medium-high heat. Add the steak and cook, stirring, until mostly browned, but still quite pink, 2 to 3 minutes. Transfer to a plate.

Add the garlic, oregano, pepper flakes, and remaining 2 teaspoons oil to the skillet. Cook until fragrant, about 30 seconds. Stir in the eggplant and sprinkle with the salt. Cook, without stirring, for 2 minutes, then stir and cook until the eggplant begins to soften, about 2 minutes. Add the tomatoes, cover, and cook for 3 minutes to break down the tomatoes.

Uncover, return the beef (and the accumulated juices) to the skillet, and cook until the beef is heated through, about 1 minute. Stir in the basil.

Divide the mixture among 4 shallow bowls. Sprinkle each serving with 1 tablespoon Parmesan.

MAKES 4 (1½-cup) SERVINGS ❱ **Per serving:** 264 calories, 13 g fat, 4 g saturated fat, 28 g protein, 10 g carbohydrate, 5 g fiber, 505 mg sodium

JERK FLANK STEAK

HANDS-ON TIME: 5 MINUTES   TOTAL TIME: 15 MINUTES PLUS STANDING TIME

Jerk seasoning, popular in Jamaica, is a combo of hot (red pepper flakes and black pepper), sweet (cinnamon and allspice), and herbal (thyme and scallions). You can find it either as a dry mixture or as a wet mixture, which is what we've made. Here it's used on beef, but it works equally well on poultry.

3 scallions, thinly sliced

1 teaspoon dried thyme

½ teaspoon ground allspice

½ teaspoon ground cinnamon

½ teaspoon coarse kosher salt

¼ teaspoon freshly ground black pepper

¼ teaspoon red pepper flakes

2 tablespoons fresh lime juice

2 teaspoons extra-virgin olive oil

1 teaspoon gluten-free Worcestershire sauce

1¼ pounds flank steak

Preheat the broiler with the rack 6 inches from the heat.

In a food processor, combine the scallions, thyme, allspice, cinnamon, salt, black pepper, pepper flakes, lime juice, oil, and Worcestershire. Process to a coarse paste.

Place the flank steak on a broiler pan and rub the paste over the top. Broil, without turning, until the steak is medium-rare, about 7 minutes. Let stand for 10 minutes before thinly slicing across the grain.

MAKES 4 SERVINGS ▶ **Per serving:** 243 calories, 12 g fat, 4.5 g saturated fat, 29 g protein, 2 g carbohydrate, 0.5 g fiber, 312 mg sodium

◀MAKE AHEAD▶ **The jerk paste can be made up to 3 days ahead and refrigerated.**

CHILI MEATLOAF

HANDS-ON TIME: 15 MINUTES   TOTAL TIME: 1 HOUR 20 MINUTES

PHASE 1

This recipe takes all the components of a bowl of chili (including the garnishes) and combines them in a meatloaf. The beans, in addition to being a chili essential, not only stretch the meat, but add fiber and protein that bread crumbs don't. If you really want to spice things up, make this a 3-Alarm Chili Meatloaf by mixing in a hot chili powder (such as one with chipotle) and adding 2 whole pickled jalapeños, minced. This meatloaf is tasty served hot, room temperature, or even chilled. In fact, there are some people who make meatloaves specifically to have them cold from the fridge the next day—maybe with a spoonful of tomato salsa or a nice dab of Dijon mustard.

1 can (15 ounces) gluten-free no-salt-added pinto beans, drained and rinsed

1 pint grape tomatoes

⅓ cup nonfat (0%) plain Greek yogurt

2½ teaspoons mild to medium gluten-free chili powder

¾ teaspoon salt

1¼ pounds extra-lean ground sirloin

1½ cups finely chopped romaine lettuce

6 scallions, thinly sliced

½ cup shredded reduced-fat Cheddar cheese (2 ounces)

1 large egg

1 large egg white

Preheat the oven to 350°F.

On a cutting board, coarsely chop the beans (don't try to chop in a food processor; the beans need to stay in chunks). Transfer to a large bowl. Coarsely dice the tomatoes and add ¾ cup to the beans. Transfer the remainder to a mini food processor.

To the tomatoes in the mini food processor, add the yogurt, ½ teaspoon of the chili powder, and ¼ teaspoon of the salt. Process to a smooth purée. Measure out ¼ cup and add to the bowl with the beans and tomatoes. Reserve the rest for topping the meatloaf.

To the beans and tomatoes, add the ground sirloin, lettuce, scallions, cheese, whole egg, egg white, and remaining 2 teaspoons chili powder and ½ teaspoon salt. Combine gently but thoroughly.

Pack the meat mixture into a 9 × 5-inch loaf pan, mounding it slightly in the center. Spread the tomato-yogurt mixture over the top of the meatloaf.

Bake until the loaf is firm (and an instant-read thermometer inserted in the center registers 155°F), 50 to 55 minutes. Let stand for 10 minutes for the juices to reabsorb (the internal temperature will also rise by about 10°F).

Cut into twelve ¾-inch-thick slices and serve.

MAKES 6 (2-slice) SERVINGS ❱ **Per serving:** 245 calories, 7 g fat, 3.5 g saturated fat, 28 g protein, 17 g carbohydrate, 5 g fiber, 483 mg sodium

SLOW-COOKER PULLED BEEF

PHASE 2

This recipe makes lots of nice leftovers (freeze in ¾-cup portions). See Variations, opposite, for ideas on how to use them.

1 can (14.5 ounces) no-salt-added diced tomatoes, drained, juices reserved

¾ cup red wine

1 large red onion, sliced

1 medium red bell pepper, sliced

1 apple, peeled and cut into chunks

3 cloves garlic, grated on a rasp-style citrus zester

¾ teaspoon coarse kosher salt

¼ teaspoon freshly ground black pepper

1 bottom round rump roast (3½ pounds)

1 tablespoon plus 1 teaspoon extra-virgin olive oil

1 teaspoon chipotle chile powder

In a 6-quart slow cooker, combine the diced tomatoes (without the juice), wine, onion, bell pepper, apple, garlic, ½ teaspoon of the salt, and the black pepper. Set to high and cook while you brown the meat.

Pat the meat dry. Untie the meat if it was tied as a roast and cut off any external fat. In a large nonstick skillet, heat the oil over medium-high heat until it shimmers. Sprinkle the remaining ¼ teaspoon salt over the bottom of the pan. Add the meat and lightly brown on all sides, including the ends, 5 to 7 minutes total.

Nestle the meat into the tomato mixture in the slow cooker. Add the reserved juice from the tomatoes to the skillet and stir to get up any browned bits. Pour the liquid over the meat. Sprinkle the meat with the chipotle powder. Turn the heat to low and cook for 4 hours. Turn the roast over and cook on low until the beef is tender and you can pull it apart with a fork, 3 to 4 hours longer (check at 3 hours and if it needs more time, turn the roast over again and cook for another hour).

Remove the beef from the cooker and put on a cutting board. When cool enough to handle, use two forks to pull the beef into shreds.

With an immersion blender, purée the sauce in the slow cooker (taste and add more chipotle powder, if desired), then return the beef to the sauce. Serve on its own or spoon over ½ cup cooked quinoa, if you like.

MAKES 12 (¾-cup) SERVINGS ▸ **Per serving:** 230 calories, 8 g fat, 2.5 g saturated fat, 28 g protein, 7 g carbohydrate, 1 g fiber, 162 mg sodium

Per serving (with quinoa): 341 calories, 10 g fat, 2.5 g saturated fat, 32 g protein, 26 g carbohydrate, 3.5 g fiber, 169 mg sodium

Beef Tostadas (to serve 2): Crisp up 4 100% corn tortillas in the oven. Top each with about ⅓ cup warm pulled beef, some chopped scallions and chopped tomatoes, and 2 teaspoons shredded reduced-fat Cheddar per tostada. Serve 2 tostadas per person.

Per serving: 360 calories, 10 g fat, 3.5 g saturated fat, 31 g protein, 34 g carbohydrate, 5 g fiber, 223 mg sodium

Quick Beef Soup (to serve 4): In a medium saucepan, combine 2 portions (1½ cups) pulled beef with 1 (15-ounce) can no-salt-added crushed tomatoes and 2 cups cooked broccoli florets. Reheat (adding water or low-sodium broth to achieve a soupy consistency); add more chipotle powder, if you'd like.

Per serving: 160 calories, 4 g fat, 1 g saturated fat, 17 g protein, 10 g carbohydrate, 3.5 g fiber, 91 mg sodium

Beefy Pasta (to serve 4): Cut 1 portion (¾ cup) pulled beef up a bit to make the pieces less stringy and combine in a saucepan with 1½ cups no-sugar-added bottled marinara sauce. Be sure to add some of the pulled beef sauce, too. Cook 8 ounces gluten-free pasta according to package directions and serve tossed with the marinara and topped with grated Parmesan (1 tablespoon per serving).

Per serving: 336 calories, 4.5 g fat, 1.5 g saturated fat, 15 g protein, 53 g carbohydrate, 3 g fiber, 387 mg sodium

Sloppy Joes (to serve 4): Use in place of the beef mixture in Smoked Portobello Sloppy Joes (page 89). Top each mushroom with a generous ¾ cup of the pulled beef.

Per serving: 281 calories, 10 g fat, 2.5 g saturated fat, 32 g protein, 13 g carbohydrate, 3.5 g fiber, 177 mg sodium

SIRLOIN BURGERS
WITH GRILLED SCALLIONS

HANDS-ON TIME: 20 MINUTES   TOTAL TIME: 20 MINUTES

PHASE
1

30
MINUTES
OR
LESS

Serve the burgers with big slices of beefsteak tomatoes and Green Lentil Salad (page 114). If you're on Phase 2, serve it on a Johnnycake (page 87).

1¼ pounds well-trimmed sirloin, cut into chunks

2 tablespoons gluten-free Worcestershire sauce

16 scallions

2 teaspoons extra-virgin olive oil

1 small yellow bell pepper, diced

¼ cup chopped grape or cherry tomatoes

Olive oil cooking spray

Coarse kosher salt

Place the beef in a food processor and pulse-chop until it is the texture of coarse hamburger meat. Add the Worcestershire sauce and pulse-chop again to combine. Transfer to a medium bowl.

Trim off the scallion roots. Cut off enough of the dark green scallion tops so that 6 inches of the rest remains. Mince the dark scallion greens to get ⅓ cup and add to the beef. Place the whole scallion pieces in a bowl, toss with the oil, and set aside.

Add the bell pepper and tomatoes to the beef. Gently but thoroughly combine. Form the mixture into 4 patties about 1 inch thick.

Preheat a grill pan or cast-iron skillet over medium-high heat. If your pan is big enough, cook the burgers and scallions together, if not, cook the scallions first and set aside. Place the scallions on or in the pan and cook, turning, until nicely browned and softened, 8 to 10 minutes. Spray the burgers on one side with a little olive oil and sprinkle with a pinch of coarse salt. Place the burgers on or in the pan, oiled-side down, and cook for 4 to 5 minutes per side for medium-rare.

Place a burger on each of 4 plates and serve each with 4 grilled scallions on the side.

MAKES 4 SERVINGS ❱ **Per serving:** 247 calories, 8.5 g fat, 2.5 g saturated fat, 32 g protein, 10 g carbohydrate, 2 g fiber, 278 mg sodium

◀MAKE AHEAD▶ **You can grill the scallions several hours ahead of time and serve them at room temperature.**

MOROCCAN-SPICED BEEF BURGERS

HANDS-ON TIME: 20 MINUTES   TOTAL TIME: 25 MINUTES

The seasonings cumin, coriander, ginger, and cinnamon are often found in Moroccan cuisine—a nice blend of sweet, hot, and earthy. Grating the onion for the burger mixture ensures that the onion will not have a raw taste and will cook through along with the burgers. Serve this with Zucchini Ceviche (page 121), if you like.

1 medium onion, peeled

1 pound extra-lean ground beef

⅔ cup plus 2 tablespoons nonfat (0%) plain Greek yogurt

¼ cup no-salt-added tomato paste

1 teaspoon ground coriander

1 teaspoon ground cumin

½ teaspoon ground cinnamon

½ teaspoon ground ginger

½ teaspoon coarse kosher salt

2 ounces reduced-fat goat cheese, crumbled

1 kirby cucumber, peeled, halved lengthwise, and thinly sliced crosswise

On the large holes of a box grater, grate the onion into a large bowl. Add the beef, 2 tablespoons of the yogurt, the tomato paste, coriander, cumin, cinnamon, ginger, and salt and gently combine. Shape the mixture into 4 patties, each about 1 inch thick.

Preheat the broiler with the rack 4 inches from the heat. Broil the burgers until browned on the top, about 3 minutes. Gently turn the burgers over and broil 1 to 2 minutes longer for medium-rare.

Meanwhile, in a medium bowl, stir together the remaining ⅔ cup yogurt, the goat cheese, and cucumber.

Place a burger on each of 4 plates. Dividing evenly, spoon the yogurt mixture on top of each burger.

MAKES 4 SERVINGS ❱ **Per serving:** 217 calories, 7 g fat, 3 g saturated fat, 30 g protein, 12 g carbohydrate, 2 g fiber, 386 mg sodium

◀MAKE AHEAD❱ The burgers can be formed, wrapped individually in foil, and frozen for up to 3 months. Thaw in the refrigerator before cooking.

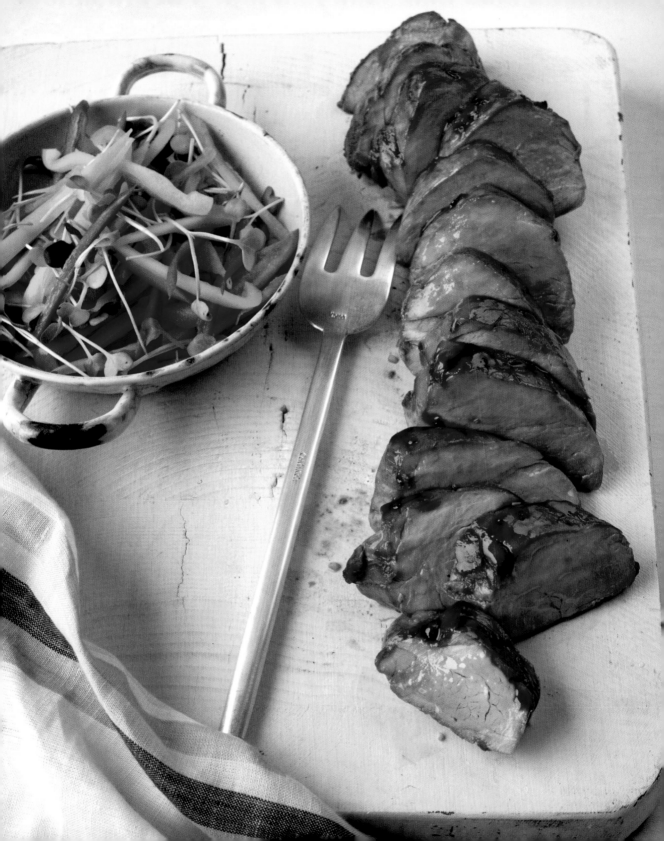

ORANGE-MAPLE PORK TENDERLOIN

HANDS-ON TIME: 10 MINUTES
TOTAL TIME: 45 MINUTES PLUS MARINATING TIME

PHASE 2

The packaged marinated teriyaki tenderloins sold in the supermarket are not gluten free. Here's a simple solution: Make your own marinade. Since the packaged tenderloin from the store usually comes with 2 pieces, you can double the marinade and bake 2 tenderloins at once to have leftovers for other meals. Enjoy the pork with a salad of bell peppers and microgreens.

- 1 navel orange
- 2 cloves garlic, minced
- 2 tablespoons maple-flavored agave nectar
- 2 tablespoons gluten-free reduced-sodium tamari soy sauce
- 1¼ pounds pork tenderloin
- Olive oil cooking spray

Using a vegetable peeler, peel 3 long strips of orange zest from the orange. Squeeze the juice from the orange.

In a small saucepan, combine the juice, zest strips, and garlic. Simmer for 5 minutes to mellow the garlic, infuse the orange juice with flavor, and reduce the liquid a bit.

Meanwhile, in a cup or small bowl, stir together the agave nectar and tamari.

Strain the orange juice mixture into the tamari mixture, pressing on the solids to extract flavor. Let cool slightly, then transfer to a sturdy resealable plastic bag big enough to hold the pork. Add the pork, making sure that it is completely covered by the marinade. Force out the air, seal, and marinate in the refrigerator for at least 30 minutes or preferably for 2 hours (you could also leave it overnight).

Preheat the oven to 375°F. Line a rimmed baking sheet with foil (for easier cleanup).

Reserving the marinade, place the pork (straight from the refrigerator) on the baking sheet and spray very lightly with olive oil. Roast for 20 minutes.

Brush the pork with the reserved marinade (and then discard any unused marinade) and roast until an instant-read thermometer inserted the thickest part of the pork registers 145°F (the meat will be very slightly pink and still juicy), about 10 minutes. Transfer the pork to a cutting board and let stand for 10 minutes. Thinly slice across the grain, divide among 4 plates, and serve.

MAKES 4 SERVINGS ❯ **Per serving:** 189 calories, 4.5 g fat, 1.5 g saturated fat, 27 g protein, 8 g carbohydrate, 0 g fiber, 321 mg sodium

BAKED STUFFED PORK CHOPS

HANDS-ON TIME: 15 MINUTES   TOTAL TIME: 40 MINUTES

PHASE
2

Stuffed pork chops are easy to make and look quite elegant, but if you aren't up for stuffing, simply make the couscous to serve as a side dish (double the amount of couscous and cook with the garlic and salt in 1⅓ cups broth). Keep in mind that unstuffed chops will cook in a shorter amount of time.

¾ cup gluten-free low-sodium chicken broth

¼ cup brown rice couscous

2 cloves garlic, minced

¾ teaspoon coarse kosher salt

3 teaspoons extra-virgin olive oil

½ cup chopped fresh flat-leaf parsley

¼ cup gluten-free dried apricots, coarsely chopped

4 thick-cut boneless pork loin chops (6 ounces each, about 1 inch thick)

½ teaspoon rubbed sage

Preheat the oven to 375°F.

In a small saucepan, combine the broth, couscous, garlic, and ¼ teaspoon of the salt. Bring to a boil over medium heat, then reduce to a simmer. Cover and cook until the couscous is tender and the liquid has been absorbed, 8 to 10 minutes. Add 1 teaspoon of the oil, the parsley, and apricots. Fluff with a fork, then transfer to a bowl to cool to room temperature.

Place the pork on a work surface and, using a sharp paring knife, cut horizontally through the thickest part of each chop to make a deep pocket about 2 inches long (do not cut all the way through). Using a spoon, stuff each chop with one-fourth of the couscous mixture.

Sprinkle both sides of the chops with the remaining ½ teaspoon salt and the sage. Rub with the remaining 2 teaspoons oil. Place the chops on a baking sheet and bake for 10 minutes. Turn the chops over and bake until cooked through but slightly pink, about 5 minutes longer.

MAKES 4 SERVINGS ❱ **Per serving:** 326 calories, 15 g fat, 4.5 g saturated fat, 33 g protein, 15 g carbohydrate, 1.5 g fiber, 448 mg sodium

Per serving (unstuffed with couscous as a side dish): 366 calories, 15 g fat, 4.5 g saturated fat, 34 g protein, 24 g carbohydrate, 2.5 g fiber, 458 mg sodium

❰MAKE AHEAD❱ **The stuffing can be made up to a day ahead and refrigerated. Bring to room temperature before using.**

BRAISED PORK ROLLS

HANDS-ON TIME: 35 MINUTES   TOTAL TIME: 40 MINUTES

PHASE
2

Capers come in different sizes, with nonpareil being the smallest. You'll find them in jars in the condiment aisle in most supermarkets. If these small capers aren't available, buy larger ones and coarsely chop them. Gluten-free sorghum flour is first used to coat the rolls, helping to keep them juicy once cooked, and then used again to lightly thicken the sauce.

½ cup chopped fresh flat-leaf parsley

⅓ cup grated Parmesan cheese

1 tablespoon plus 1 teaspoon nonpareil capers, rinsed

3 cloves garlic, minced

1 teaspoon grated lemon zest

4 boneless center-cut pork loin chops (5 ounces each, about ¾ inch thick)

3 tablespoons sorghum flour

1 tablespoon extra-virgin olive oil

¾ cup gluten-free low-sodium chicken broth

2 tablespoons no-salt-added tomato paste

In a small bowl, combine the parsley, Parmesan, capers, garlic, and lemon zest.

With a sharp knife, slice each chop in half horizontally to make 8 thinner chops. Working with one piece at a time, place between 2 sheets of wax paper or plastic wrap and use a meat mallet or a small skillet to pound each to a ⅛-inch thickness.

Divide the parsley mixture evenly among the 8 cutlets, pressing down and leaving a ¼-inch border all around. Starting at one short end, roll the cutlets up. Press on the rolls to seal. Using 2 tablespoons of the flour, sprinkle the rolls evenly all over.

In a large nonstick skillet, heat the oil over medium heat. Add the pork, seam-side up, and cook until browned, about 2 minutes. Turn the pork, seam-side down, and add the broth and tomato paste to the pan, stirring to combine. Bring to a boil, then reduce to a simmer. Cover and cook until the pork is cooked through but still juicy, about 7 minutes.

With a slotted spoon, transfer 2 pork rolls to each of 4 serving plates, leaving the heat on under the sauce.

In a small bowl, whisk together 2 tablespoons cold water and the remaining 1 tablespoon flour. Whisk the flour mixture into the sauce in the pan and simmer until lightly thickened, about 2 minutes. Spoon 2 tablespoons of the sauce over each serving.

MAKES 4 (2-roll) SERVINGS ❱ **Per serving:** 283 calories, 13 g fat, 4 g saturated fat, 32 g protein, 8 g carbohydrate, 1.5 g fiber, 279 mg sodium

❰MAKE AHEAD❱ **You can stuff and roll the pork early in the day and keep the rolls covered in the refrigerator until ready to make dinner. Bring to room temperature before cooking.**

PIGGY BURGERS

HANDS-ON TIME: 10 MINUTES   TOTAL TIME: 20 MINUTES

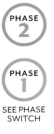

PHASE 2

PHASE 1

SEE PHASE SWITCH

30 MINUTES OR LESS

Grated apple and onion make these burgers juicy. You can grate both on the large holes of a box grater, but if your food processor has a coarse grating disk, grate the apple and onion right over the pork after you've ground it. Just leave the pork in the processor and swap out the metal blade for the grating disk. If you like, top the burgers with your favorite salsa.

1½ pounds pork tenderloin, cut into ½-inch chunks

1 large apple, peeled and grated on the large holes of a box grater

1 medium onion, grated on the large holes of a box grater

2 tablespoons no-salt-added tomato paste

¾ teaspoon coarse kosher salt

½ teaspoon crumbled dried rosemary

½ teaspoon dried thyme

¼ teaspoon freshly ground black pepper

Preheat the broiler with the rack 4 inches from the heat.

In a food processor, pulse the pork until coarsely ground. Add the apple, onion, tomato paste, salt, rosemary, thyme, and pepper. Briefly pulse-chop until just combined.

Shape the mixture into 4 patties, each 1 inch thick. Broil the burgers, turning once, until cooked through and no longer pink, but still juicy, 3 to 4 minutes per side. Serve hot.

MAKES 4 SERVINGS ▶ **Per serving:** 233 calories, 4 g fat, 1 g saturated fat, 37 g protein, 12 g carbohydrate, 2.5 g fiber, 457 mg sodium

◀PHASE SWITCH▶ **For a Phase 1 recipe, omit the apple and add a medium red bell pepper, very finely chopped, to the burger mixture.**

◀MAKE AHEAD▶ **You can form the burgers ahead, wrap individually in foil, and freeze for up to 3 months. Thaw in the refrigerator before cooking.**

PORK AND BUTTERNUT HASH

HANDS-ON TIME: 20 MINUTES   TOTAL TIME: 25 MINUTES

This hash could also be made with 1 pound cut-up turkey cutlets (also called steaks) in place of the pork. The turkey would match very nicely with a tart apple in place of the pear.

- 4 teaspoons extra-virgin olive oil
- 1 pound pork tenderloin, cut into ½-inch cubes
- 1 large yellow onion, diced
- 3 cloves garlic, minced
- 1½ teaspoons gluten-free curry powder
- 1½ cups cubed (⅓-inch) butternut squash
- ½ teaspoon salt
- 1 firm-ripe pear, preferably red-skinned, cut into ⅓-inch cubes
- 4 tablespoons grated Parmesan cheese

In a large nonstick saucepan or Dutch oven, heat 2 teaspoons of the oil over medium-high heat. Add the pork and cook until opaque all over (but still pink in the center), about 2 minutes. Transfer to a plate.

Add the remaining 2 teaspoons oil, the onion, garlic, and curry powder to the pan. Cook until the onion is beginning to soften, about 3 minutes. Stir in the butternut squash, salt, and ¼ cup water. Cover and cook until the squash is firm-tender, about 6 minutes.

Stir in the pear, re-cover, and cook for 1 minute to soften. Return the pork (and any juices) to the pan. Cook, uncovered, stirring occasionally, until the pork is cooked through, about 2 minutes.

Divide the hash among 4 plates. Sprinkle each serving with 1 tablespoon Parmesan.

MAKES 4 (1½-cup) SERVINGS ▶ **Per serving:** 265 calories, 8.5 g fat, 2.5 g saturated fat, 27 g protein, 20 g carbohydrate, 4 g fiber, 433 mg sodium

◀MAKE AHEAD▶ **Make the hash ahead (but cook the pork by 1 minute less than the directions call for) and refrigerate for up to 3 days. Bring back to room temperature and reheat in a covered skillet, with a splash of water or broth, over medium-low heat to get it hot enough to melt the Parmesan that gets sprinkled on at serving time.**

PORK MEATBALLS
WITH BROKEN SPAGHETTI

HANDS-ON TIME: 20 MINUTES   TOTAL TIME: 30 MINUTES

PHASE 2

30 MINUTES OR LESS

If you're making this dish for kids, it might be fun to use one of the gluten-free alphabet pastas now available. For an easy way to cut up the sun-dried tomatoes, use a pair of kitchen scissors and snip the tomatoes right into the bowl with the meatball mixture.

¾ pound boneless center-cut pork loin chops, cut into chunks

8 scallions (including 3 inches of the dark green tops), finely chopped, whites and greens kept separate

¼ cup crumbled reduced-fat feta cheese (1 ounce)

¼ cup minced sun-dried tomatoes

1 tablespoon extra-virgin olive oil

2 medium red bell peppers, diced

¼ teaspoon coarse kosher salt

¼ teaspoon freshly ground black pepper

1 can (14.5 ounces) no-salt-added diced tomatoes

4 ounces gluten-free multigrain spaghetti, broken into 1- to 2-inch pieces (about 1 cup)

5 cups packed baby spinach (about 5 ounces)

In a food processor, pulse-chop the pork until coarsely but evenly ground.

In a medium bowl, combine the pork, scallion whites, feta, and sun-dried tomatoes. Mix until well combined and form into 12 meatballs (about the size of Ping-Pong balls). Set aside.

In a large nonstick skillet, heat the oil over medium-high heat until it shimmers. Add the bell peppers and sprinkle with the salt and pepper. Cook, stirring occasionally, until the peppers are beginning to soften, about 3 minutes.

Stir in the tomatoes and scallion greens. Bring to a boil, cover, and boil for 3 minutes to begin to break down the tomatoes.

Add the meatballs, reduce to a high simmer, cover, and cook for 5 minutes. Turn the meatballs over and cook for 2 minutes longer. With tongs, transfer the meatballs to a bowl and cover to keep warm (the meatballs will cook all the way through from residual heat).

While the meatballs are cooking, bring a medium pot of water to a boil. Add the pasta to the boiling water and cook according to package directions, but undercook by 3 minutes. Drain.

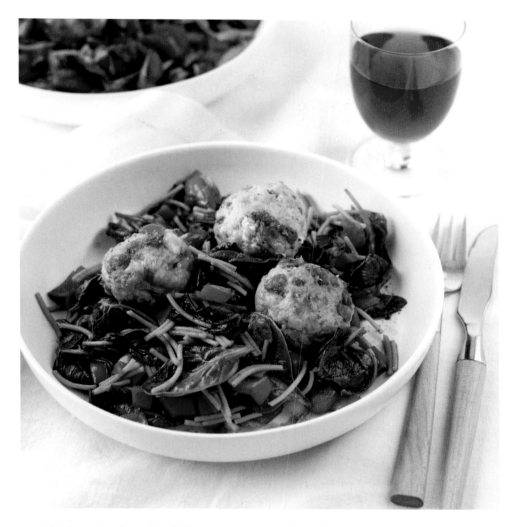

Add the spinach to the skillet, cover, and cook until wilted, about 2 minutes. Stir in the drained pasta and cook, uncovered, until the pasta is al dente, about 3 minutes.

Divide the spaghetti mixture among 4 bowls and top each with 3 meatballs.

MAKES 4 SERVINGS ❯ **Per serving:** 386 calories, 15 g fat, 5 g saturated fat, 24 g protein, 41 g carbohydrate, 7 g fiber, 354 mg sodium

◀MAKE AHEAD▶ **You can freeze the *uncooked* meatballs for up to 3 months. Spread them on a baking sheet and freeze solid, then transfer to a freezer container. Thaw in the refrigerator before using in the recipe.**

PORK AND NAPA STIR-FRY

HANDS-ON TIME: 30 MINUTES   TOTAL TIME: 30 MINUTES

Napa cabbage, a type of Asian cabbage, is softer and more delicate than regular green cabbage. A head of napa is long, rather than round, and its leaves are white with pale green frilly edges. You can find napa in most supermarkets.

1 tablespoon plus 2 teaspoons extra-virgin olive oil

1 head napa cabbage (about 10 ounces), quartered lengthwise and cut crosswise into 1-inch-wide pieces

1 small jícama (about 6 ounces), peeled, thinly sliced, and cut into 1-inch-wide strips

3 quarter-size rounds peeled fresh ginger, slivered

3 cloves garlic, thinly sliced

¾ teaspoon coarse kosher salt

1 pound pork tenderloin, thinly sliced and cut into 1-inch-wide strips

1 tablespoon apple cider vinegar

2 teaspoons dark sesame oil

In a large nonstick skillet, heat 2 teaspoons of the olive oil over medium heat. Add the cabbage, jícama, ginger, garlic, and ¼ teaspoon of the salt. Cook, stirring frequently, until the cabbage is crisp-tender, 3 to 4 minutes. With a slotted spoon, transfer all of the cabbage mixture to a large bowl.

Add the pork and the remaining 1 tablespoon olive oil to the skillet. Sprinkle with the remaining ½ teaspoon salt. Cook, stirring, until the pork pieces are slightly pink inside and still juicy, about 4 minutes.

Return the cabbage mixture to the pan. Add the vinegar and sesame oil and toss to combine. Divide among 4 plates and serve hot.

MAKES 4 (1¼-cup) SERVINGS ▷ **Per serving:** 223 calories, 11 g fat, 2 g saturated fat, 25 g protein, 6 g carbohydrate, 3 g fiber, 429 mg sodium

PORK AND TWO-BEAN STEW

HANDS-ON TIME: 25 MINUTES   TOTAL TIME: 35 MINUTES

PHASE 1

Check the labels on chili powders to make sure they're gluten-free and use your favorite (depending upon how hot you like your chili) in this robust dish.

- 1 pound pork tenderloin, cut into small chunks
- 3 cloves garlic, thinly sliced
- 2 teaspoons gluten-free chili powder
- 2 teaspoons smoked paprika
- 1 tablespoon plus 1 teaspoon extra-virgin olive oil
- 1 large onion, finely chopped

- 1 can (15 ounces) gluten-free no-salt-added red beans, drained and rinsed
- 1 can (14.5 ounces) no-salt-added diced tomatoes
- ½ pound green beans, cut into 1-inch lengths
- ½ teaspoon salt

In a food processor, combine the pork, garlic, chili powder, and paprika. Pulse-chop until the pork is finely ground.

In a large saucepan, heat the oil over medium-low heat. Add the onion and cook, stirring occasionally, until the onion is softened, about 7 minutes. Add the pork mixture and cook, stirring occasionally, until the pork is no longer pink, about 5 minutes.

Add the red beans, tomatoes, green beans, and salt. Bring to a boil, then reduce to a simmer. Cover and cook until the pork is tender and the flavors have blended, about 10 minutes.

Divide among 4 bowls and serve hot.

MAKES 4 (2-cup) SERVINGS ▶ **Per serving:** 318 calories, 8 g fat, 1.5 g saturated fat, 32 g protein, 29 g carbohydrate, 8 g fiber, 413 mg sodium

◀**MAKE AHEAD**▶ **The stew can be made ahead and refrigerated for up to 3 days. Bring back to room temperature before reheating gently over medium-low heat. Add a splash of water or broth if the stew needs to be loosened up a bit.**

SOUTHWESTERN THREE-PEPPER PORK CHILI

HANDS-ON TIME: 25 MINUTES   TOTAL TIME: 30 MINUTES

Not all chilis are red—or made with beef for that matter. In fact many chili-like stews from the Southwest are pork based, and there isn't a tomato in sight.

1 pound boneless center-cut pork loin chops, cut into chunks

1 tablespoon plus 1 teaspoon extra-virgin olive oil

1 medium yellow onion, coarsely chopped

2 medium bell peppers (1 green, 1 yellow), cut into small squares

3 cloves garlic, minced

½ teaspoon salt

2 cups gluten-free low-sodium chicken broth

1 can (15 ounces) gluten-free no-salt-added Great Northern or cannellini beans, drained and rinsed

1 large zucchini, cut into ½-inch dice

1 small to medium (to taste) chipotle chile in adobo, seeded and minced

½ cup nonfat (0%) plain Greek yogurt

3 tablespoons chopped fresh cilantro

2 tablespoons hulled pumpkin seeds (pepitas)

In a food processor, pulse-chop the pork until finely ground but not a paste.

In a large nonstick saucepan or Dutch oven, heat the oil over medium-high heat. Add the onion, bell peppers, garlic, and ¼ teaspoon of the salt. Cook, stirring occasionally, until the peppers are softened, about 5 minutes.

Add the pork, breaking it up with a spoon, then add the broth, beans, zucchini, chipotle pepper, and remaining ¼ teaspoon salt. Bring to a boil, then reduce to a simmer. Cover and cook for 10 minutes to blend the flavors and soften the zucchini.

Meanwhile, in a small bowl, stir together the yogurt and cilantro. In a 350°F oven or in a small dry skillet over medium-low heat, cook the pumpkin seeds (stirring if in a skillet) until they start to puff and turn fragrant, about 3 minutes. Transfer to a plate to stop the cooking.

Divide the chili among 4 bowls and top each serving with 2 tablespoons of the cilantro cream and 1½ teaspoons of the pumpkin seeds.

MAKES 4 (2-cup) SERVINGS ❱ **Per serving:** 364 calories, 11 g fat, 2 g saturated fat, 38 g protein, 29 g carbohydrate, 7 g fiber, 524 mg sodium

❰MAKE AHEAD❱ **The chili can be refrigerated for up to 3 days or frozen for up to 3 months. Freeze in 2-cup portions for easier thawing. Bring back to room temperature before reheating gently over medium heat.**

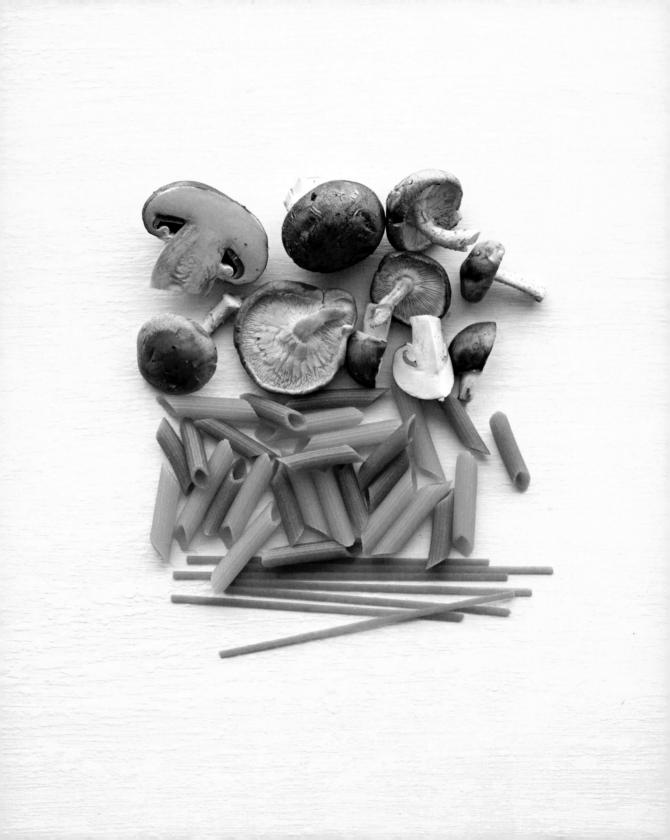

MEATLESS MAINS

Going meatless a few times a week is good for your health and your budget. All too often, though, people rely on pasta, which contains gluten. In this chapter we give you plenty of other options using beans, eggs, and tofu to create dishes like Butternut and Black Bean Stew and Baked Stuffed Tofu that are both wholesome and satisfying. But of course we wouldn't dream of leaving pasta out altogether— we just turn to gluten-free quinoa and brown rice versions that taste delicious.

GREEN AND WHITE PASTA

HANDS-ON TIME: 10 MINUTES   TOTAL TIME: 30 MINUTES

If you happen to have only gluten-free strand pasta (spaghetti, linguine) at home, just break it into 2-inch lengths for this recipe. And for a little added pungency, use half arugula and half spinach.

8 ounces gluten-free brown rice short pasta twists, such as fusilli or rotelle

1¼ teaspoons coarse kosher salt

2 teaspoons extra-virgin olive oil

2 cloves garlic, minced

¼ teaspoon red pepper flakes

1 cup frozen shelled edamame, thawed

2 tablespoons toasted pine nuts or chopped unsalted roasted almonds

4 cups packed baby spinach (4 ounces)

⅓ cup grated Parmesan cheese

In a medium pot of boiling water, cook the pasta according to package directions with 1 teaspoon of the salt.

Meanwhile, in a medium nonstick skillet, heat the oil over medium-high heat. Add the garlic and pepper flakes. Cook until fragrant, about 30 seconds. Stir in the edamame, pine nuts, and remaining ¼ teaspoon salt. Toss to coat. Cook for about 1 minute to heat the edamame through. Remove from the heat and cover to keep warm.

Ladle out 1 cup of the pasta cooking water into a bowl. Drain the pasta and return to the cooking pot. Add the edamame mixture, spinach, Parmesan, and about ½ cup of the reserved pasta cooking water. Toss to coat well and wilt the spinach. Add more cooking water if the mixture looks dry.

Divide the pasta among 4 shallow bowls and serve hot.

MAKES 4 (1-cup) SERVINGS ❯ **Per serving:** 352 calories, 9 g fat, 1.5 g saturated fat, 13 g protein, 50 g carbohydrate, 4.5 g fiber, 317 mg sodium

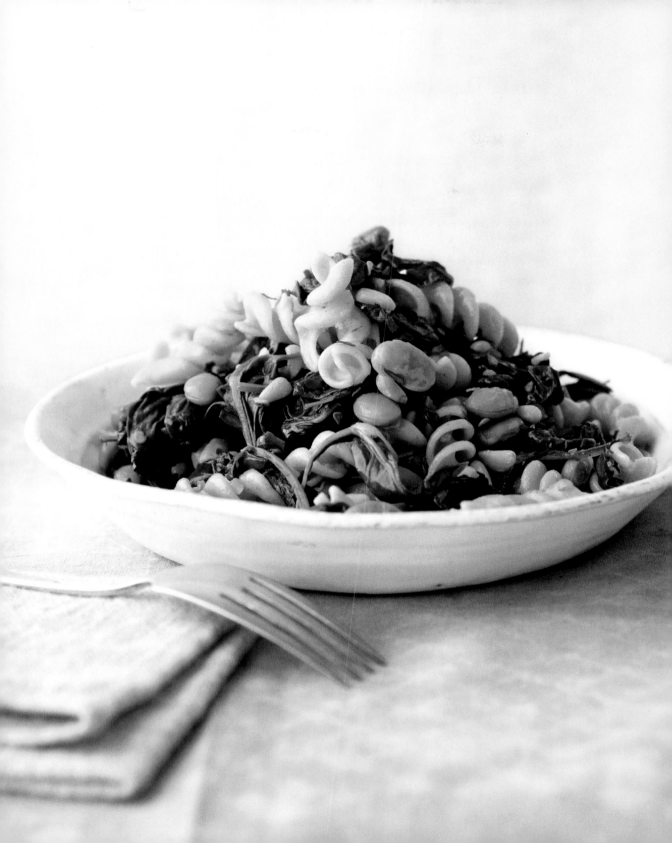

BUTTERNUT AND BLACK BEAN STEW

HANDS-ON TIME: 15 MINUTES   TOTAL TIME: 25 MINUTES

PHASE 2

30 MINUTES OR LESS

Black soybeans have almost twice the protein of regular black beans, so it's definitely worth seeking them out in the natural foods aisle.

1 tablespoon plus 1 teaspoon extra-virgin olive oil

1 large sweet onion, cut into 1-inch chunks

4 cloves garlic, minced

2 medium red bell peppers, cut into ½-inch squares

4 cups cubed (½-inch) peeled butternut squash

1 teaspoon grated lemon zest

1 teaspoon hot paprika

½ teaspoon salt

¼ teaspoon freshly ground black pepper

1 can (15 ounces) gluten-free no-salt-added black soybeans (or regular black beans), drained and rinsed

½ cup chopped fresh cilantro or flat-leaf parsley

2 tablespoons fresh lemon juice, plus more to taste

4 tablespoons shredded reduced-fat Mexican blend cheese (1 ounce)

In a large saucepan or Dutch oven, heat the oil over medium-high heat until it shimmers. Add the onion and garlic, reduce the heat to medium, and cook, stirring frequently, until the onion is softened, about 5 minutes.

Stir in the bell peppers and ¼ cup water, cover, and cook, stirring occasionally, until softened, 5 to 7 minutes.

Add the squash, lemon zest, paprika, salt, and black pepper. Stir to coat. Add 2 cups water, cover, and bring to a boil over high heat. Reduce to a simmer and cook for 5 minutes. Uncover and cook until the squash is tender, about 2 minutes longer. Remove from the heat.

Transfer 2 cups of the vegetable-broth mixture to a food processor and purée until smooth (or purée about one-quarter of the soup right in the pot with an immersion blender). Return the purée to the pan and stir to blend. Stir in the beans, cilantro, and lemon juice. Cook over medium heat to heat through, about 2 minutes. Taste and add more lemon juice, if desired.

Divide the stew among 4 deep serving bowls and sprinkle each with 1 tablespoon cheese.

MAKES 4 (2-cup) SERVINGS ❱ **Per serving:** 283 calories, 12 g fat, 2.5 g saturated fat, 15 g protein, 36 g carbohydrate, 11 g fiber, 383 mg sodium

TOFU FRITTATA WITH ASPARAGUS AND TOMATO

HANDS-ON TIME: 10 MINUTES   TOTAL TIME: 40 MINUTES

PHASE 1

The frittata would be great alongside a tart cabbage slaw or with the Fresh Cucumber-Dill Salad (page 113).

- 1 container (14 ounces) extra-firm tofu, drained
- 3 tablespoons fresh lemon juice
- ½ teaspoon crumbled dried tarragon
- ¼ teaspoon freshly ground black pepper
- ½ pound asparagus
- 5 large eggs
- ½ cup liquid egg whites
- ½ teaspoon salt
- 1 tablespoon plus 1 teaspoon extra-virgin olive oil
- 2 teaspoons gluten-free reduced-sodium tamari soy sauce
- 2 plum tomatoes, seeded and cut into ½-inch chunks

Preheat the oven to 350°F.

Slice the block of tofu in half horizontally. Place the tofu on a double layer of paper towels on a cutting board and top with another double layer of paper towels and a small baking pan with heavy weights in it (like canned goods). Let the tofu drain for at least 10 minutes.

While the tofu is draining, combine the lemon juice, tarragon, and pepper in a container big enough to hold the two slabs of tofu snugly. Let sit to soften the tarragon.

Transfer the tofu to the container and use a knife to cut the tofu into ½-inch cubes right in the container. Spread the cubes out a little so they all are touched by the marinade. Let sit while you prep the remaining ingredients.

In a steamer, cook the asparagus until just tender and bright green, about 2 minutes. When cool enough to handle, cut on an angle into very thin slices.

In a medium bowl, whisk together the whole eggs, egg whites, and salt.

In a large nonstick ovenproof skillet, heat the oil over medium-high heat. Add the tofu and asparagus and distribute evenly in the pan. Drizzle with the tamari. Pour in the egg mixture and dot the tomatoes over the top. Cook until the egg has begun to set around the edges, about 3 minutes. Transfer to the oven and bake until the frittata has puffed and set (it can still be a little wet on top in the center), 13 to 15 minutes. Remove from the oven, cover, and let sit for 5 minutes before slicing into 8 wedges.

MAKES 4 (2-wedge) SERVINGS ❯ **Per serving:** 256 calories, 16 g fat, 3.5 g saturated fat, 22 g protein, 7 g carbohydrate, 2.5 g fiber, 547 mg sodium

CHICKPEA-FENNEL STEW WITH GREENS

HANDS-ON TIME: 15 MINUTES   TOTAL TIME: 20 MINUTES

If you have the time, make a richer broth for the soup: Cut up the fennel stalks that you trim off the bulb and simmer them in the 2 cups chicken broth for at least 30 minutes (partially covered) to add more depth of flavor. Strain the broth and discard the stalks. If a lot of the broth has evaporated, just add water to come up to the original 2 cups, then add it to the stew along with the chickpeas and greens.

1 tablespoon plus 1 teaspoon extra-virgin olive oil

4 cloves garlic, minced

1 large fennel bulb, quartered and thinly sliced

1 medium orange bell pepper, slivered

1 small yellow onion, slivered

¾ teaspoon coarse kosher salt

½ teaspoon gluten-free chili powder

2 cups gluten-free low-sodium vegetable broth

1 can (15 ounces) gluten-free, no-salt-added chickpeas, drained and rinsed

1 package (10 ounces) frozen kale or collard greens, thawed

2 to 4 teaspoons apple cider vinegar (to taste)

½ cup shredded reduced-fat sharp white Cheddar cheese (2 ounces)

In a large nonstick saucepan or Dutch oven, heat the oil over medium-high heat. Add the garlic and cook until fragrant, about 30 seconds. Add the fennel, bell pepper, and onion. Sprinkle with the salt and chili powder. Cook, stirring often, until the fennel is softened, about 5 minutes.

Add the broth, chickpeas, and greens. Cover, bring to a boil, then reduce to a simmer. Cook for 3 minutes to blend the flavors. Remove the pan from the heat and stir in 2 teaspoons of the vinegar. Taste and add 1 to 2 more teaspoons vinegar, if desired. If you'd like a thicker broth, use an immersion blender to purée about one-fourth of the vegetables in the pan and then stir to combine.

Divide the stew among 4 serving bowls. Top each serving with 2 tablespoons of cheese.

MAKES 4 (1½-cup) SERVINGS ❙ **Per serving:** 269 calories, 9 g fat, 2.5 g saturated fat, 13 g protein, 35 g carbohydrate, 8.5 g fiber, 620 mg sodium

❮MAKE AHEAD❯ The stew can be refrigerated for up to 3 days or frozen for up to 3 months. Bring back to room temperature before gently reheating over medium-low heat.

QUINOA MACARONI WITH ASPARAGUS AND ALMONDS

HANDS-ON TIME: 15 MINUTES   TOTAL TIME: 25 MINUTES

Asparagus ranges in thickness from pencil-thin to an almost ¾-inch diameter. If yours are very thick, add them to the pasta water about 30 seconds earlier, so they cook for a total of 2½ minutes. You can change the flavor of this dish by using an onion-flavored light spreadable cheese in place of plain. If you'd like, for slightly richer flavor, you can toast the almonds by placing them on a rimmed baking sheet and toasting at 350°F for about 5 minutes.

- 4 ounces gluten-free quinoa elbow macaroni
- 1 pound asparagus, cut into 2-inch lengths
- 2 cups fat-free milk
- ½ cup almond flour
- 4 wedges (¾ ounce each) light spreadable cheese
- ¼ teaspoon coarse kosher salt
- ¼ teaspoon freshly ground black pepper
- ⅓ cup sliced almonds

In a large pot of boiling water, cook the macaroni according to package directions, adding the asparagus for the last 2 minutes. Drain.

Meanwhile, in a large saucepan, whisk the milk and almond flour until smooth. Cook over medium heat, stirring frequently, until lightly thickened, about 5 minutes. Add the cheese, salt, and pepper. Cook until the cheese has melted. Add the macaroni and asparagus to the sauce and toss well.

Dividing evenly, spoon the pasta onto 4 plates and scatter the almonds over the top.

MAKES 4 (1½-cup) SERVINGS ❱ **Per serving:** 278 calories, 9 g fat, 2 g saturated fat, 23 g protein, 25 g carbohydrate, 4.5 g fiber, 591 mg sodium

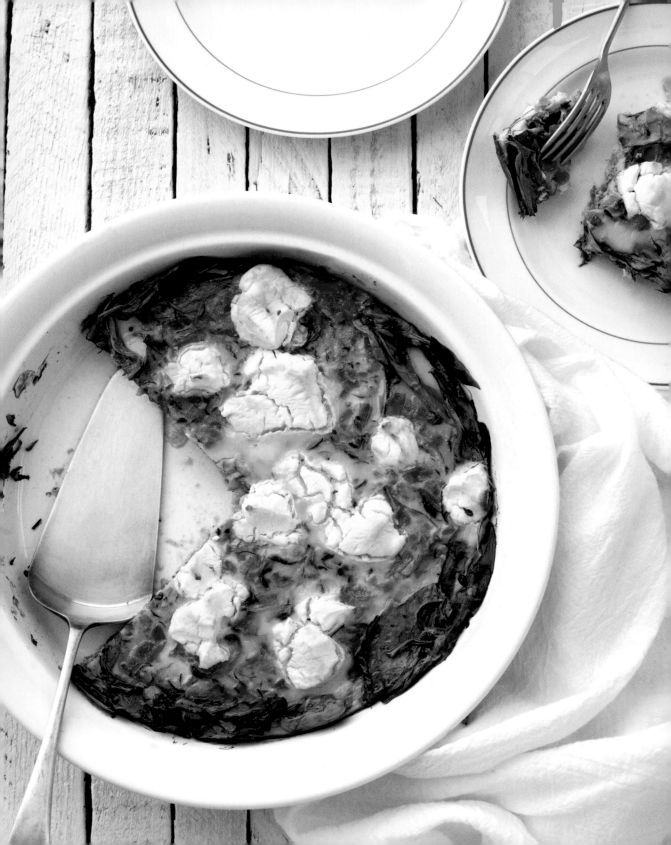

VEGETABLE QUICHE
WITH A SPINACH CRUST

HANDS-ON TIME: 15 MINUTES   TOTAL TIME: 50 MINUTES

PHASE 1

Now you can have the taste of cheesy quiche but without a wheat-based crust. Made from spinach, this "crust" is naturally gluten free—not to mention lower in fat and calories than its traditional counterpart.

4 large eggs	1 cup shredded zucchini
½ cup fat-free milk	½ teaspoon garlic powder
1 teaspoon extra-virgin olive oil	½ teaspoon salt
1 cup white mushrooms, thinly sliced	3 cups baby spinach leaves
1 cup finely diced fresh tomatoes	1 cup crumbled reduced-fat goat cheese

Preheat the oven to 350°F.

In a large bowl, whisk together the eggs and milk.

In a large skillet, heat the oil over medium-high heat. Add the mushrooms, tomatoes, zucchini, garlic powder, and salt. Cook, stirring often, until the vegetables are lightly browned and no liquid remains, 6 to 10 minutes. Remove the pan from the heat to allow the vegetables to cool slightly.

Line the bottom of a 9- to 10-inch quiche pan or glass pie plate with the spinach.

Add the vegetables to the egg mixture and stir to combine. Pour the mixture over the spinach leaves and top evenly with the goat cheese.

Bake until the eggs have fully set and are no longer wobbly (a wooden pick inserted in the center will come out clean), 30 to 35 minutes.

Cut into 4 wedges and serve hot or at room temperature.

MAKES 4 SERVINGS ❯ **Per serving:** 163 calories, 9 g fat, 3.5 g saturated fat, 13 g protein, 8 g carbohydrate, 2 g fiber, 510 mg sodium

THAI EGGPLANT CURRY

HANDS-ON TIME: 15 MINUTES   TOTAL TIME: 20 MINUTES

This recipe is made with two nut milks: store-bought coconut milk and home-made cashew milk. To save some time, you could skip making the cashew milk and use 2 tablespoons of almond butter thinned with water until it's the consistency of sour cream. On Phase 1, serve the curry on its own in a deep soup or chili bowl. On Phase 2, enjoy it with ½ cup of brown basmati rice.

1 ounce raw cashews (about 16)

2 teaspoons extra-virgin olive oil

8 scallions, white and greens kept separate, thinly sliced

½ teaspoon ground cardamom

½ teaspoon ground ginger

½ teaspoon turmeric

Pinch ground cloves

1 small eggplant (about ¾ pound), unpeeled, cut into ¾-inch cubes

¾ teaspoon salt

¾ cup lite coconut milk

1 container (14 ounces) extra-firm tofu, drained and cut into ¾-inch cubes

Sriracha sauce, for serving (optional)

In a mini food processor, pulse-chop the cashews to a paste. Add 2 tablespoons water and process to a smooth mixture (the consistency of thin sour cream).

In a large nonstick saucepan or Dutch oven, heat the oil over medium-high heat. Add the scallion whites and sprinkle with the cardamom, ginger, turmeric, and cloves. Cook, stirring, to toast the spices, about 45 seconds. Add ¼ cup water and stir, then add the eggplant, sprinkle with the salt, and stir to coat well with the spices.

Add the coconut milk and 1 cup water. Bring to a gentle simmer. Cover and cook until the eggplant is almost tender, 3 to 5 minutes. Uncover and stir in the cashew mixture and all but 2 tablespoons of the scallion greens. Cook for 3 minutes to thicken the sauce a bit and finish cooking the eggplant. Stir in the tofu and cook for 1 minute to heat through.

Divide the curry among 4 bowls and serve drizzled with a little Sriracha (if desired) and sprinkled evenly with 2 tablespoons of scallion greens.

MAKES 4 (generous 1-cup) SERVINGS ▶ **Per serving:** 219 calories, 14 g fat, 4 g saturated fat, 13 g protein, 13 g carbohydrate, 5.5 g fiber, 455 mg sodium

TOFU AND EGG MIGAS

HANDS-ON TIME: 25 MINUTES   TOTAL TIME: 35 MINUTES

PHASE 2

Migas is a Tex-Mex breakfast dish of eggs scrambled with torn tortillas (the idea is to use up stale tortillas). This dinnertime version adds lots of bell pepper and some chunks of tofu for more protein.

2   **100% corn tortillas (6-inch)**

4   **teaspoons extra-virgin olive oil**

2   **medium bell peppers (1 green, 1 red), cut into ½-inch squares**

1   **small red onion, cut into ½-inch cubes**

7   **ounces firm tofu, cut into 1-inch cubes**

3   **large eggs**

½   **cup liquid egg whites**

½   **teaspoon chipotle chile powder**

¼   **teaspoon salt**

½   **cup shredded reduced-fat Mexican blend cheese (2 ounces)**

Preheat the oven to 375°F.

Arrange the tortillas on a baking sheet and bake until crisp, about 10 minutes.

In a large nonstick skillet, heat 2 teaspoons of the oil over medium-low heat. Add the bell peppers and onion. Cook, stirring occasionally, until the peppers are tender, about 10 minutes. Add the remaining 2 teaspoons oil and the tofu. Cook until the tofu is heated through, about 3 minutes.

Meanwhile, in a medium bowl, whisk together the whole eggs, egg whites, chipotle powder, and salt.

Break each tortilla into 8 small pieces and add them, along with the egg mixture, to the skillet. Cook, stirring constantly, until the eggs are almost set, about 2 minutes. Add the cheese and cook until the cheese has melted, about 2 minutes longer.

Divide the *migas* among 4 plates and serve hot.

MAKES 4 SERVINGS ❭ **Per serving:** 245 calories, 14 g fat, 3.5 g saturated fat, 18 g protein, 14 g carbohydrate, 3 g fiber, 353 mg sodium

❬MAKE AHEAD❭ **You can toast the tortillas up to 5 days ahead and store in an airtight container at room temperature.**

CRISPY-TOPPED MAC AND CHEESE

HANDS-ON TIME: 15 MINUTES   TOTAL TIME: 35 MINUTES

Quinoa macaroni has a natural al dente–like chewy texture. This baked pasta entrée goes well with steamed vegetables and a simple tossed salad. Or, you could turn it into a one-dish meal by adding vegetables right to the mac and cheese: Before baking, add 2 cups diced roasted bell peppers, chopped cooked broccoli or cauliflower florets, or cut-up cooked green beans.

- 2 100% corn tortillas (6-inch)
- 4 ounces gluten-free quinoa elbow macaroni
- 1 cup fat-free milk
- ½ cup gluten-free low-sodium vegetable broth
- 2 tablespoons white bean flour
- ½ teaspoon coarse kosher salt
- ¼ teaspoon gluten-free mustard powder
- 2 pinches cayenne pepper
- ¾ cup shredded reduced-fat Cheddar cheese (3 ounces)
- ¼ cup plus 3 tablespoons grated Parmesan cheese

Preheat the oven to 375°F.

Arrange the tortillas on a baking sheet and bake until crisp, about 10 minutes.

Meanwhile, in a medium pot of boiling water, cook the macaroni for 1 minute less than the package directions. Drain.

In a medium saucepan, whisk the milk, broth, and bean flour until smooth. Add the salt, mustard powder, and cayenne. Cook over medium heat, stirring constantly, until lightly thickened, about 7 minutes. Remove from the heat and stir in the Cheddar and Parmesan. Stir in the macaroni.

Transfer the mixture to an 8 × 8-inch baking dish and crumble the tortillas evenly over the top. Bake until bubbling, about 20 minutes. Divide among 4 plates and serve hot.

MAKES 4 SERVINGS ▮ **Per serving:** 275 calories, 8 g fat, 4.5 g saturated fat, 14 g protein, 37 g carbohydrate, 4 g fiber, 603 mg sodium

INDIAN SAAG PANEER

HANDS-ON TIME: 10 MINUTES   TOTAL TIME: 30 MINUTES

Saag means spinach and *paneer* is a quickly made fresh cheese, similar in texture to tofu. Here, for added protein, we use tofu as a stand-in for the paneer. Garam masala, available in supermarkets, is a spice blend of both sweet and hot spices. It's great to have on hand, not just for Indian dishes but to use in spice rubs for pork, chicken, and fish.

1 tablespoon plus 1 teaspoon extra-virgin olive oil

1 small onion, finely chopped

3 cloves garlic, thinly sliced

1 piece fresh ginger (1 inch), peeled and finely chopped

2 teaspoons garam masala

½ teaspoon gluten-free curry powder

½ teaspoon salt

2 packages (10 ounces each) frozen chopped spinach, thawed and drained

1 container (14 ounces) firm tofu, drained and cut into ½-inch cubes

¾ cup nonfat (0%) plain Greek yogurt

In a large nonstick skillet, heat the oil over medium heat. Add the onion, garlic, and ginger. Cook, stirring occasionally, until the onion is softened, about 7 minutes. Add the garam masala, curry powder, and salt. Stir to combine.

Add the spinach and cook, stirring occasionally, until the spinach is tender, about 5 minutes. Add the tofu and cook, stirring occasionally, until heated through, about 3 minutes.

Remove the pan from the heat and stir in the yogurt. Return the pan to the heat and cook over low heat, stirring occasionally, just to heat through, about 2 minutes.

Divide among 4 plates and serve hot.

MAKES 4 (1-cup) SERVINGS ❱ **Per serving:** 199 calories, 10 g fat, 1 g saturated fat, 18 g protein, 13 g carbohydrate, 5.5 g fiber, 417 mg sodium

TOFU-MUSHROOM LASAGNA

HANDS-ON TIME: 20 MINUTES   TOTAL TIME: 1 HOUR 10 MINUTES

Extra-firm tofu is a nice alternative to wheat pasta in this meatless lasagna. Look for extra-firm tofu; its low moisture content won't cause the lasagna to become watery. Herbes de Provence is a wonderful herb blend to have on hand, and it goes well with the tomato-mushroom-cheese combination here. However, if you don't have it, just add 1 teaspoon each dried basil, thyme, and rosemary.

- 2 teaspoons extra-virgin olive oil
- ½ cup finely chopped onion
- 2 cloves garlic, thinly sliced
- 6 ounces white or cremini mushrooms, coarsely chopped
- 1 can (15 ounces) no-salt-added crushed tomatoes
- 2 cups 1% cottage cheese

- 6 tablespoons grated Parmesan cheese
- 1 container (14 ounces) extra-firm tofu, drained and cut crosswise into 12 pieces
- 1 tablespoon herbes de Provence
- Fresh basil leaves, for garnish (optional)

Preheat the oven to 350°F.

In a large nonstick skillet, heat the oil over medium heat. Add the onion, garlic, and mushrooms. Cook, stirring occasionally, until the onion is softened, about 7 minutes. Add the tomatoes, bring to a boil, then reduce to a simmer. Cover and cook until the flavors have blended and the sauce is slightly thickened, about 5 minutes longer.

Meanwhile, in a food processor or blender, purée the cottage cheese and Parmesan until smooth. Rub the tofu on all sides with the herbes de Provence.

Spoon about ½ cup of the tomato sauce mixture into the bottom of an 8 × 8-inch baking dish. Top with half the tofu, half of the remaining tomato sauce, and half the cottage cheese mixture.

Repeat with the remaining tofu, tomato sauce, and cottage cheese. Bake until the dish is piping hot and the cheese has set, about 40 minutes. Let stand for 10 minutes before cutting into 4 pieces. Garnish with basil leaves, if desired.

MAKES 4 SERVINGS ❭ **Per serving:** 285 calories, 11 g fat, 3 g saturated fat, 29 g protein, 17 g carbohydrate, 3 g fiber, 581 mg sodium

BAKED STUFFED TOFU

HANDS-ON TIME: 15 MINUTES   TOTAL TIME: 1 HOUR 20 MINUTES

PHASE 1

For more flavor, layer and stuff the tofu several hours ahead and refrigerate. Bring to room temperature before baking.

- 2 containers (14 ounces each) extra-firm tofu, drained
- 1 tablespoon plus 2 teaspoons extra-virgin olive oil
- 2 teaspoons balsamic vinegar
- 4 cloves garlic, grated on a rasp-style citrus zester
- ½ teaspoon freshly ground black pepper
- 1 small red bell pepper, finely diced
- 3 tablespoons minced kalamata olives (about 9 olives)
- 4 cups packed baby spinach (4 ounces), coarsely chopped
- ¾ teaspoon coarse kosher salt

Slice each block of tofu horizontally into thirds. Place the slabs of tofu cut side down on several layers of paper towel on a small baking sheet or cutting board and set aside to drain while you make the filling.

In a medium nonstick skillet, heat the oil, vinegar, garlic, and black pepper over medium-low heat. Cook until fragrant, about 1 minute. Measure out 2 teaspoons of the mixture and set aside.

Increase the heat to medium-high and add the bell pepper and olives to the skillet. Cook until the pepper is beginning to soften, about 2 minutes. Add the spinach and stir. Cook for about 45 seconds to wilt the spinach slightly. Remove from the heat.

Line a rimmed baking sheet with foil (for easier cleanup). Arrange 2 tofu slabs, 1 or 2 inches apart, on the pan. Using ¼ teaspoon of the salt, sprinkle it over both slabs. Top each slab with one-fourth of the spinach filling, spreading it to the edges. Top each with another slab, pressing down lightly. Top the slabs with another ¼ teaspoon salt and the remaining spinach filling. Top with the last 2 slabs of tofu. Let sit while the oven preheats.

Preheat the oven to 325°F.

Drizzle the reserved garlic-vinegar mixture evenly over the tops (spreading it with the back of a spoon) and sprinkle the remaining ¼ teaspoon salt over both stacks. Bake until beginning to turn a golden brown on top, about 1 hour.

Let stand for 10 minutes before slicing each crosswise into 2 pieces.

MAKES 4 SERVINGS ▶ Per serving: 306 calories, 19 g fat, 2.5 g saturated fat, 21 g protein, 12 g carbohydrate, 4.5 g fiber, 553 mg sodium

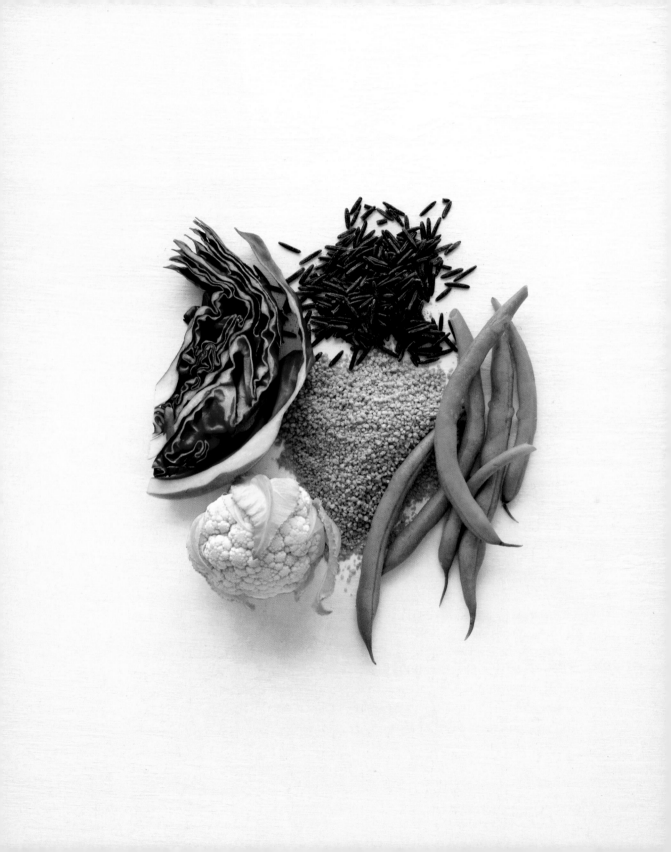

SIDE DISHES

On the South Beach Diet we recommend getting at least ½ cup of vegetables at both lunch and dinner. A great way to do that is with a veggie side dish. Try our healthy Jícama Fries, Lemon Snow Peas, or Sautéed Kale, Bacon, and Sun-Dried Tomatoes, for example. Or, for a heartier side, consider Caramelized Onions and Kasha (buckwheat groats), "Sesame" Noodles (made with gluten-free multigrain spaghetti), or Three Sisters Bread (made from yellow cornmeal, garbanzo–fava bean flour, and winter squash purée).

JÍCAMA FRIES

HANDS-ON TIME: 15 MINUTES   TOTAL TIME: 55 MINUTES

The amount of coating in the recipe is more than you will need; this just makes it easier to dredge the jícama "fries." Be sure to shake off any excess, though—the coating actually browns up better when it's not too thick. Masa harina is the finely ground cornmeal that's used to make tortillas. It has a distinctive flavor (just think of what a corn tortilla tastes like and you'll know the flavor), but you could also use regular yellow cornmeal here.

¼ cup sesame seeds

2 tablespoons masa harina or yellow cornmeal

2 tablespoons grated Parmesan cheese

2 teaspoons ground cumin

2 teaspoons paprika

¼ teaspoon salt

1 large jícama (about 1½ pounds), cut into "steak fries," ½ inch thick and about 3 inches long

2 teaspoons extra-virgin olive oil

Olive oil cooking spray

Hot sauce, for serving

Lime wedges, for squeezing

Preheat the oven to 400°F. Line a large baking sheet with foil (for easier cleanup).

In a mini food processor, grind together the sesame seeds, masa harina, Parmesan, cumin, paprika, and salt. Transfer to a plate or shallow bowl.

Spread the jícama fries on the baking sheet and drizzle with the oil. Use your hands to toss and coat evenly (this might seem messy, but you're oiling the baking sheet in the process).

Working with 2 or 3 at a time, dredge the jícama fries in the sesame seed mixture (tap off the excess) and arrange on the baking sheet.

Lightly spray the tops of the fries with olive oil. Roast until the coating has browned, about 35 minutes. (Note that the jícama will still be crunchy because it does not soften in cooking, the way potatoes do.) Let sit on the baking sheet for 5 minutes before serving.

Serve with hot sauce, for sprinkling, and lime wedges for squeezing.

MAKES 4 SERVINGS ❱ **Per serving:** 138 calories, 6.5 g fat, 1 g saturated fat, 3 g protein, 18 g carbohydrate, 9.5 g fiber, 175 mg sodium

❰MAKE AHEAD❱ **You can make the dredging mixture up to a week ahead of time and refrigerate. Let come back to room temperature before you coat the jícama.**

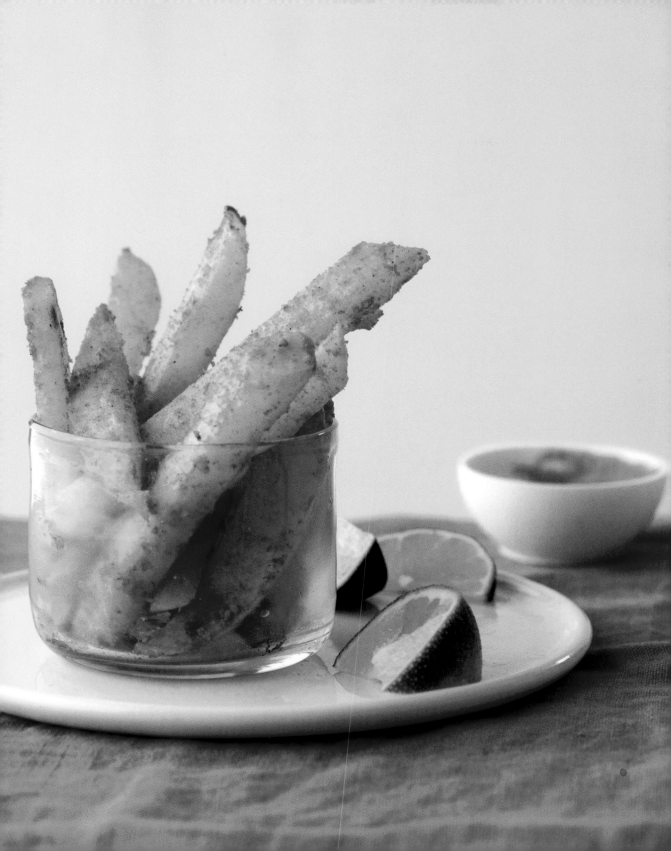

CARAMELIZED ONIONS AND KASHA

HANDS-ON TIME: 20 MINUTES   TOTAL TIME: 30 MINUTES

Despite its name, the buckwheat plant is not at all related to wheat (it's actually in the rhubarb family), making it an ideal choice for the gluten sensitive. Nutty-flavored kasha is simply roasted buckwheat groats—the triangular seeds of the plant. The combo of sweet caramelized onions and kasha is a traditional Eastern European dish.

3 teaspoons extra-virgin olive oil

2 cups chopped onions
   (2 medium onions)

1½ cups gluten-free low-sodium
   chicken broth

⅔ cup medium-granulation kasha
   (roasted buckwheat groats)

1 large egg white

½ teaspoon rubbed sage

½ teaspoon salt

¼ teaspoon freshly ground
   black pepper

In a large nonstick skillet, heat 2 teaspoons of the oil over medium-low heat. Add the onions, stirring to coat. Add ½ cup water, cover, and cook until the onions are softened, about 10 minutes. Uncover and add the remaining 1 teaspoon oil. Cook, stirring frequently, until the onions are golden brown and very soft, about 15 minutes longer.

Meanwhile, in a small saucepan, bring the broth to a simmer over low heat; keep at a simmer while you cook the kasha and egg.

In a small heavy skillet, combine the kasha and egg white. Cook over medium-high heat, stirring frequently, until the kasha is well coated and dry, 2 to 3 minutes.

Transfer the kasha to the pan with the onions. Add the sage, salt, and pepper, stirring to combine. Add the simmering broth, cover, and cook until the liquid has been absorbed, 8 to 10 minutes.

MAKES 4 (⅔-cup) SERVINGS ❱ **Per serving:** 167 calories, 4 g fat, 0.5 g saturated fat, 6 g protein, 29 g carbohydrate, 4 g fiber, 337 mg sodium

HERBED TRICOLOR QUINOA PILAF WITH SHALLOTS

HANDS-ON TIME: 10 MINUTES   TOTAL TIME: 25 MINUTES

PHASE 2

30 MINUTES OR LESS

If you happen to have fresh herbs on hand, use them here. For basil, use about ¼ cup chopped; for tarragon or oregano, you'll need just 1½ teaspoons minced. You could also easily convert this hot side dish to a cold main-course salad (see Variation, below).

1 tablespoon extra-virgin olive oil

3 shallots, thinly sliced

⅔ cup tricolor quinoa (or white quinoa)

1 cup gluten-free low-sodium chicken broth or water

½ teaspoon dried tarragon, basil, or oregano

¼ teaspoon salt

In a medium nonstick saucepan, heat the oil over medium-high heat. Add the shallots and cook until very richly browned, 5 to 7 minutes.

Stir in the quinoa, broth, tarragon, salt, and ¼ cup water. Bring to a boil, then reduce to a simmer. Cover and cook until the quinoa is tender and the liquid has been absorbed, about 15 minutes.

Serve the quinoa warm or at room temperature.

MAKES 4 (½-cup) SERVINGS ▶ **Per serving:** 168 calories, 5 g fat, 0.5 g saturated fat, 6 g protein, 26 g carbohydrate, 2.5 g fiber, 174 mg sodium

◀**VARIATION**▶ **QUINOA AND BEEF SALAD** (for 4 servings): Make the quinoa pilaf and let cool to room temperature. Squeeze a little lemon juice (to taste) into the pilaf and toss with ¾ cup shredded arugula or baby spinach, 1 diced bell pepper (any color), and ¾ cup chopped cooked beef (such as deli roast beef or leftover beef from Slow-Cooker Pulled Beef, page 187). Taste and add more lemon juice, if needed.

Per serving: 231 calories, 7 g fat, 1.5 g saturated fat, 14 g protein, 28 g carbohydrate, 3 g fiber, 199 mg sodium

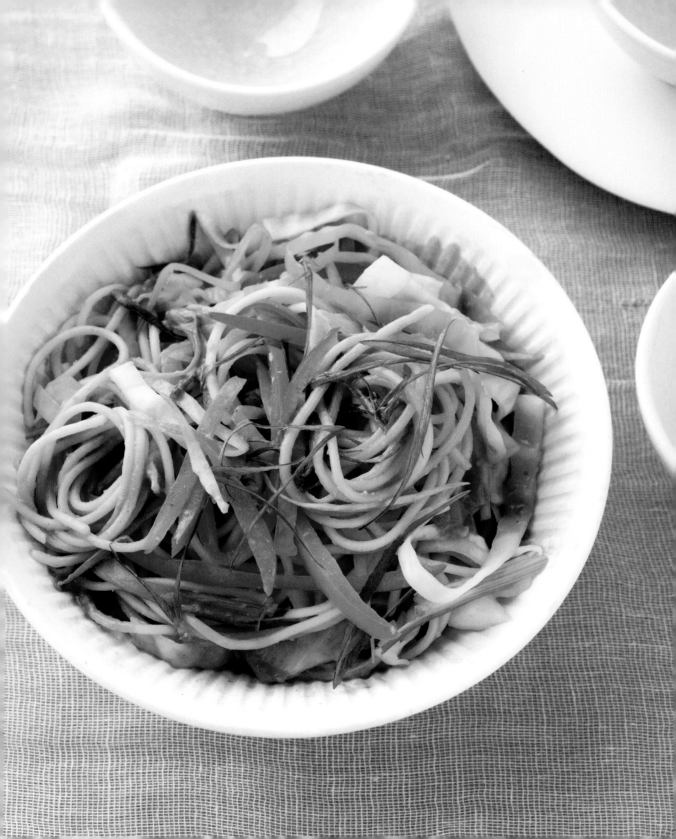

"SESAME" NOODLES

HANDS-ON TIME: 10 MINUTES   TOTAL TIME: 30 MINUTES

PHASE
2

30
MINUTES
OR
LESS

This take-off on the classic Chinese restaurant dish uses gluten-free spaghetti instead of wheat noodles and peanut butter in place of sesame paste for convenience. (You could also try it with almond butter.) The cabbage, which replaces some of the usual noodles, adds fiber.

2 teaspoons salt

2 ounces gluten-free multigrain spaghetti

¼ small head cabbage, cut into long shreds (about 3 cups)

1 medium red bell pepper, finely slivered

4 scallions, halved crosswise and then finely slivered lengthwise

2 tablespoons creamy all-natural peanut butter

1 tablespoon plus 1 teaspoon red wine vinegar

1 tablespoon gluten-free reduced-sodium tamari soy sauce

1 teaspoon agave nectar

2 teaspoons grated fresh ginger

1 small clove garlic, grated on a rasp-style citrus zester

Bring a large saucepan of water to a boil. Add the salt to the water, then add the pasta and stir. About 3 minutes before the pasta should be done (according to the package directions), add the cabbage, bell pepper, and scallions.

While the pasta is cooking, in a large microwave-safe bowl (big enough to hold the cooked noodles and cabbage), combine the peanut butter and 1 tablespoon water. Microwave in 30-second increments, stirring after each, until the peanut butter combines with the water. Stir in the vinegar, tamari, and agave nectar until smooth. Stir in the ginger and garlic.

Drain the pasta and vegetables and add to the peanut butter mixture, tossing well to coat. Serve hot or at room temperature.

MAKES 4 (¾-cup) SERVINGS ▶ **Per serving:** 132 calories, 4.5 g fat, 0.5 g saturated fat, 5 g protein, 18 g carbohydrate, 3.5 g fiber, 304 mg sodium

◀MAKE AHEAD▶ **You can prep the cabbage, bell pepper, and scallions in advance. Just put them all in one bowl, since they go into the pasta water at the same time.**

BRAISED CUCUMBERS

HANDS-ON TIME: 20 MINUTES   TOTAL TIME: 20 MINUTES

Kirby cucumbers, most often eaten in salads or turned into pickles, are meltingly tender and sweet when sautéed; they taste somewhat like summer squash. Unlike other cucumbers, kirbies are not waxed and you don't have to peel them, but occasionally the skin can be a little tough. So to get around that problem, but still get some of the fiber from the skin, the cucumbers here are half-peeled. The striping also adds visual appeal to the dish.

1½ pounds kirby cucumbers	½ teaspoon coarse kosher salt
1 tablespoon extra-virgin olive oil	¼ cup chopped fresh mint
3 scallions, thinly sliced	

With a vegetable peeler, peel the cucumbers in lengthwise stripes, leaving some of the skin on. Halve lengthwise, remove the seeds with a small spoon, and thinly slice crosswise.

In a large nonstick skillet, heat the oil over medium heat. Add the cucumbers and scallions. Cook, stirring frequently, until the cucumbers are heated through, about 3 minutes.

Add 3 tablespoons water, sprinkle with the salt, cover, and cook until the cucumbers are crisp-tender, about 5 minutes. Stir in the mint.

Serve hot, warm, or at room temperature.

MAKES 4 (1-cup) SERVINGS ❯ **Per serving:** 61 calories, 3.5 g fat, 0.5 g saturated fat, 2 g protein, 7 g carbohydrate, 1.5 g fiber, 247 mg sodium

SPICY SWEET POTATO MASH

HANDS-ON TIME: 5 MINUTES   TOTAL TIME: 50 MINUTES

Although baking takes longer than other methods of cooking sweet potatoes (like boiling), it's worth the wait because it brings out the naturally sweet flavors of the vegetable. We've left the skin on for both added texture and fiber, but if you're not a fan, feel free to remove it once the sweet potatoes are done.

- 4 sweet potatoes (about 6 ounces each), well scrubbed
- 1 tablespoon plus 1 teaspoon fresh lime juice
- 1 tablespoon plus 1 teaspoon extra-virgin olive oil
- 1½ teaspoons gluten-free chili powder
- ¼ teaspoon salt
- ¼ teaspoon freshly ground black pepper

Preheat the oven to 400°F. Line a baking sheet with foil (for easier cleanup).

Place the potatoes on the baking sheet and, with a paring knife or a fork, pierce them in several places. Bake until tender, about 45 minutes.

When cool enough to handle, thickly slice and transfer to a serving bowl. Add the lime juice, oil, chili powder, salt, and pepper. Mash with a potato masher or a spoon and serve.

MAKES 4 (¾-cup) SERVINGS ▶ **Per serving:** 145 calories, 5 g fat, 0.5 g saturated fat, 2 g protein, 25 g carbohydrate, 3.5 g fiber, 198 mg sodium

◀MAKE AHEAD▶ **The sweet potatoes can be roasted up to a day ahead and refrigerated. At serving time, mash the potatoes and gently heat with the olive oil, lime juice, seasonings, and 3 tablespoons of water.**

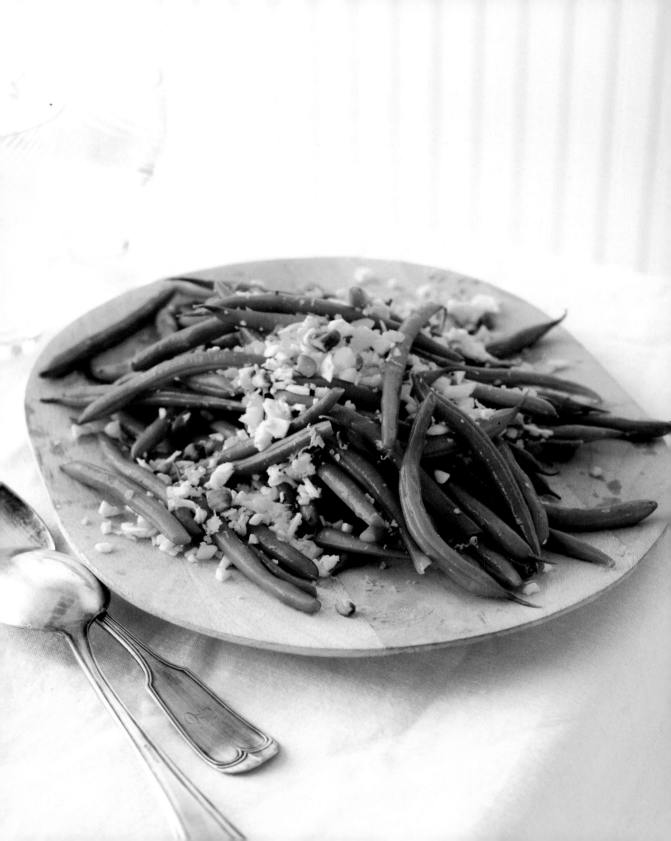

GREEN BEANS MIMOSA

HANDS-ON TIME: 15 MINUTES   TOTAL TIME: 30 MINUTES

In French cooking, the term *mimosa* signifies a dish that is garnished with minced hard-boiled egg because of its resemblance to the tiny yellow flower clusters of the mimosa shrub. In this version, chopped pistachios add a nice hint of green. Try the mimosa mixture to add a little protein and a flavor twist to steamed asparagus or snow peas, too.

1 large egg	2 teaspoons extra-virgin olive oil
1¼ pounds green beans	½ teaspoon coarse kosher salt
2 teaspoons grated lemon zest	3 tablespoons finely chopped unsalted roasted pistachios
2 teaspoons fresh lemon juice	

In a small saucepan, combine the egg and cold water to cover. Bring to a boil over high heat. Remove from the heat, cover, and let stand for 12 minutes, then run under cold water. Peel and very finely chop the egg. Transfer to a small bowl.

While the egg is cooking, in a steamer, cook the beans until crisp-tender, 5 to 9 minutes (depending on the age and size of the beans). Transfer the beans to a medium bowl. Add the lemon juice, oil, and ¼ teaspoon of the salt. Toss to combine. Arrange on a platter.

To the bowl with the chopped egg, add the lemon zest, pistachios, and remaining ¼ teaspoon salt. Stir to combine.

Sprinkle the beans with the egg mixture. (If not serving on a platter, each portion gets about 2 tablespoons of the egg mixture.) Serve hot or warm.

MAKES 4 (1-cup) SERVINGS ▶ **Per serving:** 110 calories, 6.5 g fat, 1 g saturated fat, 5 g protein, 11 g carbohydrate, 4 g fiber, 266 mg sodium

SPICY BROCCOLI PARMESAN

HANDS-ON TIME: 15 MINUTES   TOTAL TIME: 20 MINUTES

The technique of cooking vegetables in a skillet with a small amount of water is called shallow-steaming. Here the shallow-steamed broccoli gets Italian flair from the addition of garlic, red pepper flakes, and a little grated Parmesan.

1 head broccoli (about 1 pound)

1 tablespoon plus 1 teaspoon
   extra-virgin olive oil

2 cloves garlic, thinly sliced

$\frac{1}{2}$ teaspoon red pepper flakes

$\frac{1}{4}$ teaspoon salt

$\frac{1}{2}$ cup grated Parmesan cheese

Separate the broccoli florets from the stalks. With a paring knife, trim off the very bottom of the stalks. Peel the stalks and cut crosswise into $\frac{1}{2}$-inch-thick slices. Cut the florets in half lengthwise.

In a large skillet, heat the oil, garlic, pepper flakes, and salt over medium heat. Add the broccoli florets, stalk slices, and $\frac{1}{4}$ cup water. Bring to a boil, then reduce to a simmer. Cover and cook until the broccoli is tender, 5 to 7 minutes.

Transfer to a serving bowl. Add the Parmesan and toss to coat.

MAKES 4 (1-cup) SERVINGS ❯ **Per serving:** 120 calories, 8 g fat, 2.5 g saturated fat, 7 g protein, 7 g carbohydrate, 2.5 g fiber, 360 mg sodium

ROASTED BABY BOK CHOY AND PEPPERS

HANDS-ON TIME: 5 MINUTES   TOTAL TIME: 35 MINUTES

PHASE
1

Bok choy, a member of the cabbage family, has wide white stems and dark green leaves. It can be found in both large and baby varieties. This recipe calls for baby bok choy, but if you can't find it, sub in regular bok choy and cut it crosswise into 3- to 4-inch lengths.

¾ **pound baby bok choy, left whole**

1 **medium red, orange, or yellow bell pepper, cut into ½-inch-wide strips**

2 **cloves garlic, thinly sliced**

2 **teaspoons extra-virgin olive oil**

1 **teaspoon dark sesame oil**

½ **teaspoon coarse kosher salt**

Preheat the oven to 375°F.

In a 9 × 13-inch baking pan, combine the bok choy, bell pepper, garlic, and olive oil. Roast the vegetables, tossing twice, until both the bok choy and bell pepper are crisp-tender, about 30 minutes.

Transfer to a serving bowl, add the sesame oil and salt, and toss to coat. Serve hot or at room temperature.

MAKES 4 SERVINGS ❯ **Per serving:** 52 calories, 3.5 g fat, 0.5 g saturated fat, 2 g protein, 4 g carbohydrate, 1.5 g fiber, 270 mg sodium

SMASHED TOMATOES

HANDS-ON TIME: 5 MINUTES   TOTAL TIME: 25 MINUTES

Shown pictured with Turkey Breast Stuffed with Spinach and Ricotta on page 175.

Shown pictured with Turkey Breast Stuffed with Spinach and Ricotta on page 175.

PHASE 1

30 MINUTES OR LESS

Grape tomatoes have the most intense flavor, but you can swap in small cherry tomatoes here, or even cut-up plum tomatoes. The needle-like leaves of dried rosemary come in both whole and crumbled form. The crumbled is a much more convenient option, because when you chop whole rosemary leaves, they tend to fly off the cutting board.

4 cups grape tomatoes

1 tablespoon extra-virgin olive oil

2 cloves garlic, thinly sliced

½ teaspoon crumbled dried rosemary

¼ teaspoon freshly ground black pepper

½ teaspoon coarse kosher salt

1 teaspoon anchovy paste (optional)

Preheat the oven to 400°F.

In a 9 × 13-inch baking pan, toss the tomatoes with the oil, garlic, rosemary, and pepper. Sprinkle with the salt and toss to combine.

Roast until the tomatoes start to collapse, about 15 minutes (timing will vary depending on the size of the tomatoes). Gently smash with a fork and continue to roast until the tomatoes are very tender and soft, about 10 minutes longer. Stir in the anchovy paste (if using) and serve.

MAKES 4 (½-cup) SERVINGS ▶ **Per serving:** 78 calories, 3.5 g fat, 0.5 g saturated fat, 2 g protein, 10 g carbohydrate, 1.5 g fiber, 240 mg sodium

◀MAKE AHEAD▶ **The tomatoes can be roasted up to a day ahead and refrigerated. Serve chilled or at room temperature.**

SOUFFLÉED SPINACH

HANDS-ON TIME: 10 MINUTES   TOTAL TIME: 40 MINUTES

PHASE 2

Beaten egg whites are what give this (and every soufflé) its lift. You'll know the whites are beaten to "soft" peaks when you lift up the beaters and the whites lift up into low peaks that droop over. Note that you can't use liquid egg whites here, because they won't whip up properly.

Olive oil cooking spray

1 bag (16 ounces) frozen chopped spinach, thawed

¾ cup fat-free milk

1 tablespoon white bean or garbanzo bean flour

⅓ cup grated Parmesan cheese

¼ teaspoon grated nutmeg

¼ teaspoon salt

¼ teaspoon freshly ground black pepper

1 large egg, separated

2 large egg whites (don't use liquid egg whites here)

Preheat the oven to 350°F. Spray a 6 × 8-inch or 8 × 8-inch baking dish with olive oil.

Place the spinach in a colander and squeeze dry.

In a medium saucepan, whisk the milk and flour until smooth. Cook over medium-low heat, stirring constantly, until the sauce is lightly thickened, about 3 minutes. Stir in the Parmesan, nutmeg, salt, and pepper. Stir in the spinach and egg yolk.

In a bowl, with an electric mixer at high speed, beat the 3 egg whites until soft peaks form. Gently fold the egg whites into the spinach mixture. Transfer the mixture to the baking dish and bake until set and puffed, 25 to 30 minutes.

Cut into 4 pieces and serve warm.

MAKES 4 SERVINGS ❱ **Per serving:** 118 calories, 4.5 g fat, 1.5 g saturated fat, 12 g protein, 9 g carbohydrate, 4 g fiber, 396 mg sodium

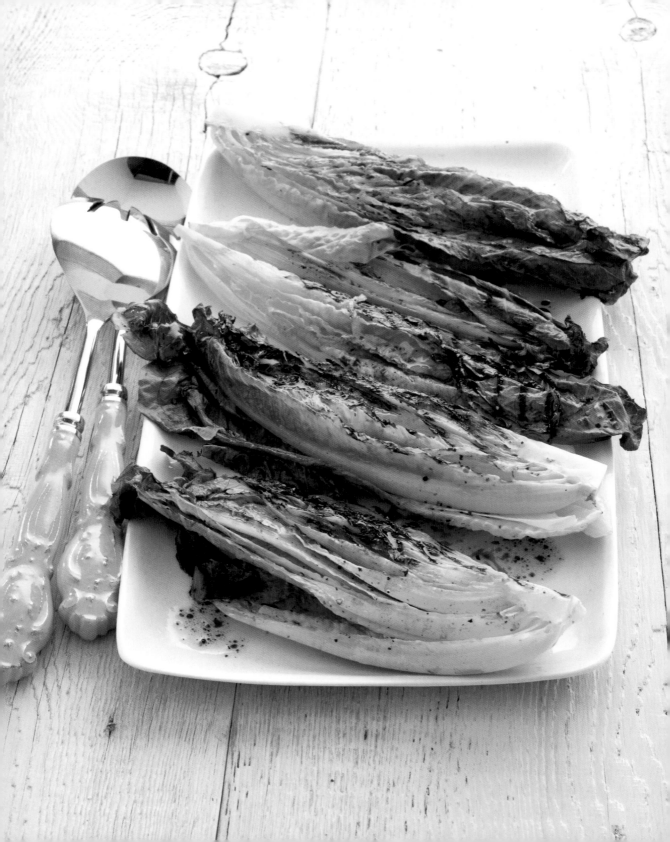

GRILLED ROMAINE LETTUCE

HANDS-ON TIME: 20 MINUTES   TOTAL TIME: 20 MINUTES

Chances are you've never thought about grilling lettuce. Sturdy romaine is the perfect candidate for it and turns soft, tender, and sweet in the process. Don't let its green color fool you; romaine is a good source of the antioxidant beta-carotene. In addition, you'll get vitamin C, folate, and even some iron from the leaves.

Olive oil cooking spray

1 head romaine lettuce, quartered lengthwise and well rinsed

2 tablespoons balsamic vinegar

1 tablespoon plus 1 teaspoon extra-virgin olive oil

½ teaspoon salt

¼ teaspoon freshly ground black pepper

Spray a grill pan or the grates of a grill with olive oil and heat to medium.

Place the romaine quarters, with some water clinging to them, on the grill and cook, turning the romaine as it browns in spots and softens, until crisp-tender, about 10 minutes.

Meanwhile, in a small bowl, whisk together the vinegar, oil, salt, and pepper.

Transfer the grilled lettuce to a platter. Drizzle the dressing over it and serve hot or at room temperature.

MAKES 4 SERVINGS ▶ **Per serving:** 72 calories, 5.5 g fat, 0.5 g saturated fat, 1 g protein, 5 g carbohydrate, 2.5 g fiber, 301 mg sodium

SPICY ROASTED BRUSSELS SPROUTS AND WATER CHESTNUTS

HANDS-ON TIME: 15 MINUTES   TOTAL TIME: 45 MINUTES

PHASE 1

If you have only had boiled Brussels sprouts and think you don't like these little cabbages, then roasted Brussels sprouts will change your mind. Roasting concentrates the flavor and brings out the vegetable's natural sweetness, with no danger of them becoming water-logged. The garlic, ginger, chili powder, and soy combo here was inspired by kimchi, a spicy Korean cabbage condiment.

1 pound Brussels sprouts, halved lengthwise

1 can (8 ounces) sliced water chestnuts, drained

3 cloves garlic, thinly sliced

1 piece fresh ginger (2 inches), peeled and cut into thin matchsticks (¼ cup)

3 scallions, cut into 1-inch lengths

2 teaspoons gluten-free chili powder

1 tablespoon gluten-free reduced-sodium tamari soy sauce

1 tablespoon extra-virgin olive oil

Preheat the oven to 400°F.

In a large bowl, toss together the Brussels sprouts, water chestnuts, garlic, ginger, scallions, chili powder, and tamari until well combined. Drizzle with the oil and toss again until evenly coated.

Transfer the mixture to a rimmed baking sheet and cover with foil. Roast for 20 minutes. Uncover, stir, and roast uncovered until the Brussels sprouts are tender, about 10 minutes longer. (The timing may vary depending upon the size and age of the Brussels sprouts.)

Transfer to a serving bowl and serve hot, warm, or at room temperature.

MAKES 4 (1¼-cup) SERVINGS ▶ **Per serving:** 122 calories, 4 g fat, 0.5 g saturated fat, 5 g protein, 20 g carbohydrate, 6.5 g fiber, 232 mg sodium

SWEET POTATOES BRAVAS

HANDS-ON TIME: 10 MINUTES   TOTAL TIME: 50 MINUTES

Based on a Spanish dish typically made with white potatoes and served with a garlic mayo, the mildly spicy sweet potatoes topped with cool garlicky yogurt is a winning combination of textures and flavors. The yogurt topping would also work well as a dressing in a gluten-free pasta salad.

1 tablespoon plus 1 teaspoon extra-virgin olive oil

1½ teaspoons smoked paprika

½ teaspoon coarse kosher salt

Cayenne pepper

1 pound sweet potatoes, scrubbed and cut into 1-inch chunks

6 cloves garlic, skin on

¾ cup nonfat (0%) plain Greek yogurt

Preheat the oven to 400°F. Line a baking sheet with foil (for easier cleanup).

In a large bowl, whisk together the oil, paprika, ¼ teaspoon of the salt, and 2 large pinches of cayenne (increase the amount if you want more heat). Add the sweet potatoes and toss until well coated.

Wrap the garlic cloves in foil.

Place the potatoes on the baking sheet along with the garlic. Bake the garlic until tender, about 30 minutes. (You'll know the garlic is tender if the packet can easily be pressed and the cloves seem soft.) Bake the potatoes, tossing occasionally, until tender, about 40 minutes.

Once the garlic is soft, remove from the oven and let cool slightly, then remove the skins. Transfer the garlic to a small bowl and mash with a fork. Stir in the yogurt and the remaining ¼ teaspoon salt.

Serve the potatoes hot, each serving with 3 tablespoons of the garlic-yogurt sauce on the side.

MAKES 4 (¾-cup) SERVINGS ❱ **Per serving:** 142 calories, 5 g fat, 0.5 g saturated fat, 4 g protein, 21 g carbohydrate, 2.5 g fiber, 301 mg sodium

◀MAKE AHEAD▶ **You can roast the garlic up to 3 days in advance, mix it with the yogurt, and refrigerate. Bring to room temperature before serving.**

ARTICHOKE GRATIN

HANDS-ON TIME: 5 MINUTES   TOTAL TIME: 15 MINUTES

PHASE 2

30 MINUTES OR LESS

You don't have to serve the gratin piping hot, so it can sit at room temperature while you put together the rest of your meal. If you want a tangier topping for the artichokes, replace half of the Parmesan with grated pecorino cheese.

- 12 ounces quartered frozen artichoke hearts, thawed and halved (i.e., cut into eighths)
- 3 tablespoons minced kalamata olives (about 9 olives)
- 1 teaspoon extra-virgin olive oil
- ¼ teaspoon crumbled dried rosemary
- ¼ teaspoon freshly ground black pepper
- Coarse kosher salt
- 1 cup unsweetened almond milk or fat-free dairy milk
- 2 tablespoons white bean flour
- ¼ cup grated Parmesan cheese

Preheat the broiler with the rack 6 inches from the heat.

In a medium bowl, gently toss together the artichoke hearts, olives, oil, rosemary, pepper, and a large pinch of salt. Spread in an even layer in an 8-inch square baking pan.

In a small saucepan, whisk the milk and bean flour until smooth. Cook over low heat, whisking constantly, until thickened, about 3 minutes. Off the heat, whisk in a large pinch of salt and the Parmesan.

Pour the Parmesan sauce evenly over the artichokes and broil until the topping is golden brown in spots and set, 8 to 10 minutes. Serve hot or warm.

MAKES 4 SERVINGS ▶ **Per serving:** 120 calories, 6 g fat, 1.5 g saturated fat, 5 g protein, 11 g carbohydrate, 6.5 g fiber, 367 mg sodium

◀**MAKE AHEAD**▶ **You can assemble the artichoke portion of the dish 1 or 2 hours ahead and leave at room temperature. Then, before broiling, all you have to do is make the Parmesan sauce.**

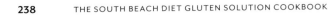

LEMON SNOW PEAS

HANDS-ON TIME: 10 MINUTES   TOTAL TIME: 15 MINUTES

Shown pictured with Pan-Grilled Turkey Cutlets with Thai Relish on page 170.

PHASE 1

30 MINUTES OR LESS

Most snow peas are tender enough that you don't need to pull off the strings that run down both sides of the pod. But if you have fairly large snow peas, they might need stringing. Pull at the stem end of one or two of the larger pods; if a thick string begins to pull away, then the pea needs to be stringed.

½ teaspoon grated lemon zest

2 tablespoons fresh lemon juice

1 tablespoon plus 1 teaspoon extra-virgin olive oil

½ teaspoon agave nectar

½ teaspoon gluten-free curry powder

½ teaspoon salt

1 large yellow bell pepper, slivered

1 small red onion, slivered

1 pound snow peas

In a large serving bowl, combine the lemon zest, lemon juice, oil, agave nectar, curry powder, and salt. Add the bell pepper and onion. Toss to coat.

In a steamer, cook the snow peas until crisp-tender, 4 to 5 minutes. Add to the pepper mixture and toss to coat.

Serve warm or at room temperature.

MAKES 4 (1½-cup) SERVINGS ▶ **Per serving:** 108 calories, 5 g fat, 0.5 g saturated fat, 4 g protein, 14 g carbohydrate, 3.5 g fiber, 297 mg sodium

THREE SISTERS BREAD

HANDS-ON TIME: 5 MINUTES   TOTAL TIME: 30 MINUTES

Three Sisters is a reference to the three crops that Native Americans often planted together: corn, squash, and beans. The corn gave the beans a stalk to climb up, the large leaves of the sprawling squash plant kept the weeds down, and the beans added nitrogen to the soil. The three ingredients find equal harmony in this moist cornbread. If you can't buy a 10-ounce package of frozen winter squash purée, purchase a larger package (it also comes as 12 ounces) and measure out 1 cup of purée.

4 teaspoons extra-virgin olive oil

½ cup yellow cornmeal

½ cup garbanzo–fava bean flour, garbanzo bean flour, or fava bean flour

1 teaspoon gluten-free baking powder

½ teaspoon salt

1 package (10 ounces) frozen winter squash purée, thawed

2 large eggs

Preheat the oven to 375°F. Coat an 8-inch square baking pan with 2 teaspoons of the oil.

In a large bowl, whisk together the cornmeal, flour, baking powder, and salt. Add the squash, eggs, and remaining 2 teaspoons oil. Stir until well combined. Scrape the batter into the pan, smoothing the top.

Bake until golden on top and set, 20 to 23 minutes.

While still hot, cut into 12 pieces and serve.

MAKES 6 (2-piece) SERVINGS ▌ **Per serving:** 163 calories, 5.5 g fat, 1 g saturated fat, 6 g protein, 24 g carbohydrate, 3 g fiber, 312 mg sodium

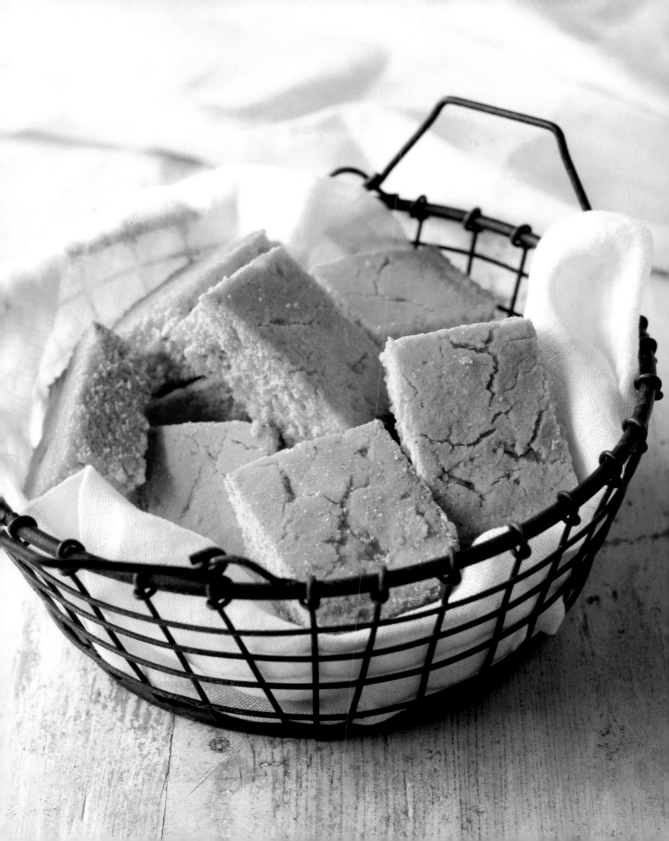

BAKED LENTILS WITH MUSHROOMS AND WALNUTS

HANDS-ON TIME: 30 MINUTES   TOTAL TIME: 1 HOUR 10 MINUTES

PHASE 1

Lentils, mushrooms, and walnuts bring a trifecta of hearty flavors to this dish, each ingredient underscoring the meatiness of the other. Save leftovers to make an excellent main-dish lunch salad (see Variation, below).

2 tablespoons peanut oil

2 medium onions, finely chopped

5 cloves garlic, minced

1½ pounds white or cremini mushrooms, halved and thickly sliced

1 teaspoon salt

¾ teaspoon ground fennel seed or crumbled tarragon

¾ teaspoon freshly ground black pepper

2 cups gluten-free low-sodium chicken broth

1½ cups lentils

30 walnuts (about 2 ounces)

Preheat the oven to 350°F.

In a Dutch oven, heat the oil over medium-high heat. Add the onions and garlic. Cook, stirring frequently, until the onions are softened, about 5 minutes. Add the mushrooms and ½ teaspoon of the salt and cook, stirring occasionally, until the mushrooms are beginning to soften, about 5 minutes.

Stir in the fennel, pepper, and remaining ½ teaspoon salt. Add the broth and lentils. Bring to a boil, cover, transfer to the oven, and bake until the lentils are tender, about 45 minutes.

Meanwhile, in the preheated oven or in a dry medium skillet over medium-low heat, cook the walnuts (stirring if in a skillet) until browned and fragrant, 3 to 5 minutes. Transfer to a cutting board to stop the cooking. Coarsely chop when cool.

Remove the lentils from the oven, transfer to a serving bowl, and stir in the walnuts. Serve hot, warm, or at room temperature.

MAKES 8 (¾-cup) SERVINGS ❯ **Per serving:** 235 calories, 8.5 g fat, 1 g saturated fat, 14 g protein, 29 g carbohydrate, 10 g fiber, 317 mg sodium

◀VARIATION▶ **LENTIL AND CHICKEN SALAD (to serve 1):** Toss ¾ cup of the lentils with a creamy soy dressing made with 1 teaspoon gluten-free reduced-sodium tamari soy sauce, 1 teaspoon of your favorite vinegar, and 2 teaspoons nonfat yogurt. Then add 2 ounces cubed cooked chicken or turkey breast and 2 scallions, chopped.

Per serving: 350 calories, 11 g fat, 1.5 g saturated fat, 33 g protein, 33 g carbohydrate, 11 g fiber, 600 mg sodium

MUSHROOMS AND
SHALLOTS À LA GRECQUE

HANDS-ON TIME: 10 MINUTES   TOTAL TIME: 15 MINUTES PLUS COOLING TIME

PHASE 2

Mushrooms à la Grecque—a cross between a vegetable side and a salad—is a classic French dish. À la Grecque means "in Greek fashion," although there is nothing about the marinated mushrooms that is particularly Greek. Serve alongside simply grilled or roasted chicken breast or flank steak. Although many people use the term *button mushrooms* to mean white mushrooms, its original meaning (in classic French cooking) is a very small mushroom, the size of a man's shirt button. If you can't find small mushrooms for this dish, then just halve or quarter larger ones.

1 tablespoon extra-virgin olive oil

3 shallots, minced

¼ teaspoon coriander seeds

¼ teaspoon dried thyme

1 bay leaf

1 pound button mushrooms

⅔ cup dry white wine

2 tablespoons fresh lemon juice

¼ teaspoon salt

¼ teaspoon freshly ground black pepper

In a large nonstick saucepan or Dutch oven, heat the oil over medium heat. Add the shallots, coriander, thyme, and bay leaf. Cook until the shallots and seasonings are very fragrant, 2 to 3 minutes.

Add the mushrooms, wine, lemon juice, salt, and pepper. Bring to a high simmer and cook until the mushrooms are slightly tender, about 6 minutes.

Remove from the heat and let cool in the cooking liquid. Transfer to a serving bowl and serve at room temperature or chilled (see Make Ahead, below).

MAKES 4 (¾-cup) SERVINGS ❱ **Per serving:** 102 calories, 4 g fat, 0.5 g saturated fat, 4 g protein, 8 g carbohydrate, 2 g fiber, 153 mg sodium

◀MAKE AHEAD▶ The marinated mushrooms and shallots hold up well in the refrigerator and are quite nice served chilled. They will keep for at least 2 weeks.

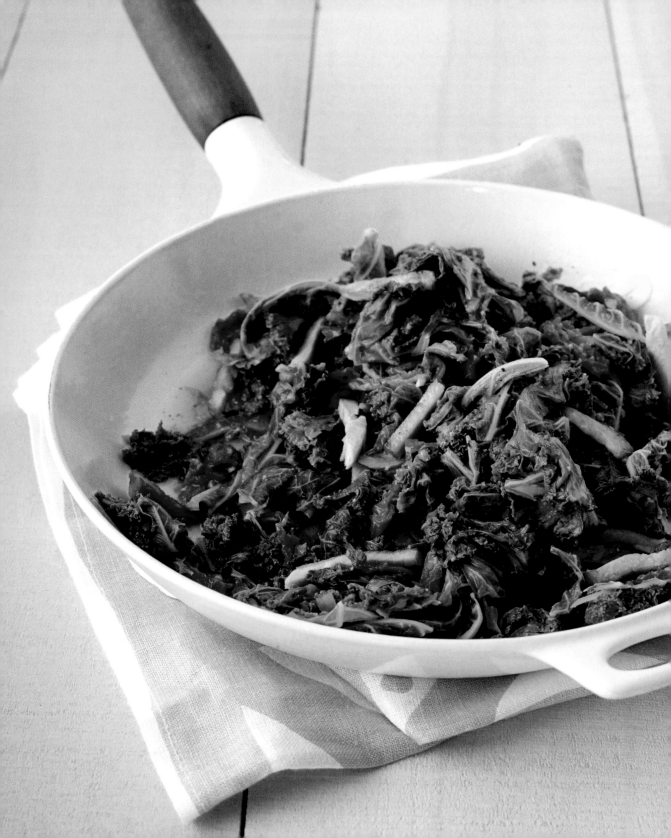

SAUTÉED KALE, BACON, AND SUN-DRIED TOMATOES

HANDS-ON TIME: 15 MINUTES   TOTAL TIME: 20 MINUTES

Kale, a nutritional powerhouse, has thick stems and dark, crinkly green leaves. The stems can be a little tough. You can remove them by cutting them out with a knife, but a good trick for quickly destemming kale is to place the leaf on a cutting board and press down on the stem end with one hand. Then run the fingers of your other hand up both sides of the stem to strip off the leaf.

1 pound kale, stemmed, leaves torn into bite-size pieces

⅓ cup sun-dried tomatoes, cut into thin strips

1 tablespoon extra-virgin olive oil

3 cloves garlic, thinly sliced

2 ounces gluten-free all-natural uncured Canadian bacon, thinly sliced

1 tablespoon red wine vinegar

¼ teaspoon coarse kosher salt

Bring 2 inches water to a boil in a large saucepan. Add the kale, cover, and cook until tender but not mushy, about 5 minutes, adding the sun-dried tomatoes during the last minute of cooking. Drain well.

Meanwhile, in a large skillet, heat the oil over medium-low heat. Add the garlic and Canadian bacon. Cook, stirring occasionally, until the garlic starts to soften, about 1 minute. Add the kale to the skillet, sprinkle with the vinegar and salt, and toss to combine.

Transfer to a serving bowl and serve hot or at room temperature.

MAKES 4 (1-cup) SERVINGS ▶ **Per serving:** 103 calories, 5 g fat, 1 g saturated fat, 6 g protein, 10 g carbohydrate, 2 g fiber, 288 mg sodium

ROASTED CAULIFLOWER AND CELERIAC RÉMOULADE

HANDS-ON TIME: 10 MINUTES   TOTAL TIME: 40 MINUTES

PHASE 1

If you like the flavor of celery, you'll love celery root. This roasted vegetable side dish borrows from the French tradition of pairing celery root with lemon and mustard. If you have any leftovers, they make a great snack, straight from the fridge.

1 celery root (celeriac), about ¾ pound, peeled and cut into ½-inch cubes

3 cups very small cauliflower florets (from a small head)

1 tablespoon plus 1 teaspoon extra-virgin olive oil

¼ teaspoon coarse kosher salt

¼ teaspoon freshly ground black pepper

1 tablespoon fresh lemon juice

2 teaspoons Dijon mustard

Chopped fresh flat-leaf parsley, basil, and/or chives, for garnish (optional)

Preheat the oven to 400°F. Place the celery root and cauliflower in a 9 × 13-inch baking pan.

In a small bowl, stir together the oil and ⅓ cup water. Drizzle the oil-water mixture over the vegetables and toss to coat well. Sprinkle with the salt and pepper.

Cover the pan with foil and roast until the vegetables are beginning to get tender, 12 to 16 minutes. Uncover and stir the vegetables well. Continue roasting, uncovered, until they are fork-tender and a little golden, 10 to 15 minutes longer.

Meanwhile, in a large serving bowl, whisk together the lemon juice and mustard.

Add the hot vegetables to the dressing and toss to coat well. Serve warm or at room temperature, garnished with chopped herbs, if desired.

MAKES 4 (1-cup) SERVINGS ▶ **Per serving:** 94 calories, 5 g fat, 0.5 g saturated fat, 3 g protein, 12 g carbohydrate, 3 g fiber, 277 mg sodium

TRIPLE-GREEN "STIR-FRY" WITH ALMONDS

HANDS-ON TIME: 15 MINUTES   TOTAL TIME: 25 MINUTES

This "stir-fry" is really a "stir-steam-fry." You stir the vegetables with a combination of oil and water, then you steam them in a covered pan. Once the vegetables are almost tender, you uncover the pan to evaporate the water and stir-fry the vegetables in the oil that remains.

2 teaspoons extra-virgin olive oil

½ pound asparagus, cut on an angle into thirds

½ pound green beans, cut on an angle into thirds

8 thin scallions, white and pale-green parts only, cut on an angle into thirds

3 tablespoons slivered almonds

¼ teaspoon coarse kosher salt

¼ teaspoon freshly ground black pepper

In a large nonstick skillet, heat the oil and 3 tablespoons water over medium-high heat until simmering. Add the asparagus, beans, and scallions and stir to coat. Cover and steam until the vegetables are almost crisp-tender, about 6 minutes.

Meanwhile, in a toaster oven at 350°F or in a small dry skillet over medium-low heat, cook the almonds (stirring if in a skillet) until browned and fragrant, 3 to 5 minutes. Transfer to a plate to stop the cooking.

Uncover the large skillet and sprinkle the vegetables with the salt and pepper. Cook, stirring occasionally, to evaporate the liquid and cook the vegetables to your desired degree of doneness, 2 to 3 minutes for crisp-tender.

Transfer to a serving bowl, add the almonds, and toss. Serve hot.

MAKES 4 (½-cup) SERVINGS ▌ **Per serving:** 80 calories, 5 g fat, 0.5 g saturated fat, 3 g protein, 8 g carbohydrate, 3.5 g fiber, 132 mg sodium

◀MAKE AHEAD▶ **The asparagus, beans, scallions, and toasted almonds can all be prepped ahead. If you have all of your ingredients ready to go before starting to cook, this will take only 10 minutes to get on the table.**

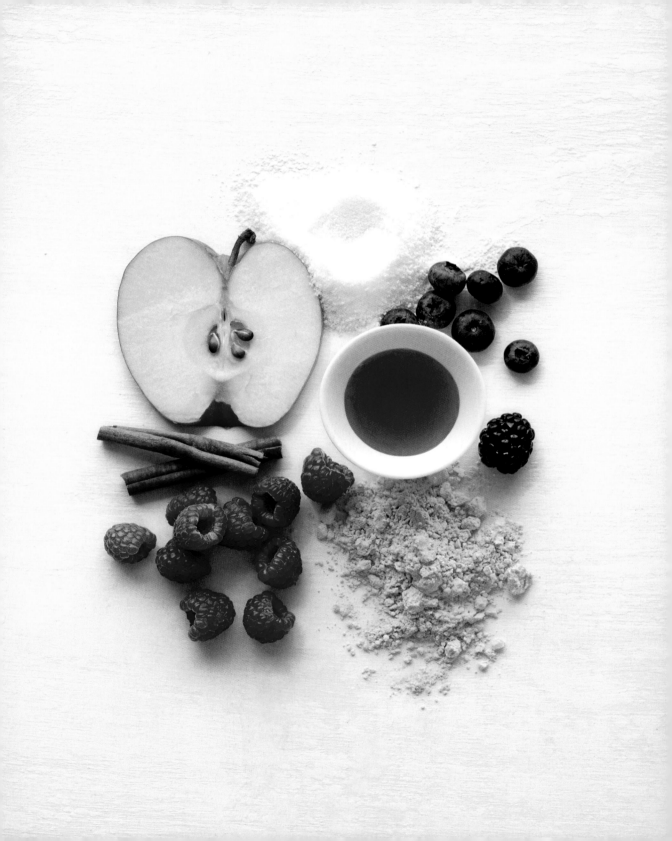

DESSERTS

Yes, you can have dessert on the South Beach Diet, and that includes the occasional piece of cake or pie as well as fruit on Phase 2. As you'll see here, gluten-free desserts like our Caramelized Apple Mini-Shortcakes and Chocolate Walnut Espresso Cake don't have to be flourless or taste like cardboard. And they don't have to be high in saturated fat and sugar, either—often the case in gluten-free baking. For two tasty Phase 1 desserts, see page 6.

POACHED PEARS WITH CARAMELIZED PEAR CREAM

HANDS-ON TIME: 15 MINUTES   TOTAL TIME: 30 MINUTES

PHASE
2

30
MINUTES
OR
LESS

The concentrated pear purée you make here is a delicious, naturally sweet dessert sauce that also happens to boast some fiber.

3 Bartlett pears

3 teaspoons fresh lime juice

¼ teaspoon pure almond extract

Pinch ground allspice

2 tablespoons nonfat (0%) plain Greek yogurt

Cut one of the pears into chunks and place in a small microwave-safe bowl with 1 tablespoon water. Cover the bowl and microwave on high until very soft, 3 to 4 minutes (depending on the ripeness of the pear). Let cool slightly. With a wooden spoon or rubber spatula, push the pear through a fine-mesh strainer back into the same bowl to get a very thin purée (discard the skin and seeds). Add 1 teaspoon of the lime juice, the almond extract, and the allspice to the purée and stir to combine.

Peel, halve, and core the remaining pears. Rub with the remaining 2 teaspoons lime juice to keep them from turning brown.

Place the pears in a medium nonstick skillet, cover with the pear purée, and bring to a simmer over medium-low heat. Cover and simmer (reducing the heat if necessary) until the pears are tender, 10 to 15 minutes (depending on the ripeness of the pears).

With a slotted spatula, lift the pears out of the cooking juices to a plate.

Bring the cooking juices to a high simmer and cook, stirring constantly, until reduced, thickened, and beginning to caramelize, about 5 minutes (there should be about ¼ cup of thickened pear purée).

Scrape the pear mixture into a small bowl and let cool, then stir in the yogurt.

Serve the pears warm, at room temperature, or chilled, dolloped evenly with the pear cream. Sprinkle each with a little allspice, if desired.

MAKES 4 SERVINGS ❯ **Per serving:** 83 calories, 0 g fat, 0 g saturated fat, 1 g protein, 21 g carbohydrate, 4 g fiber, 4 mg sodium

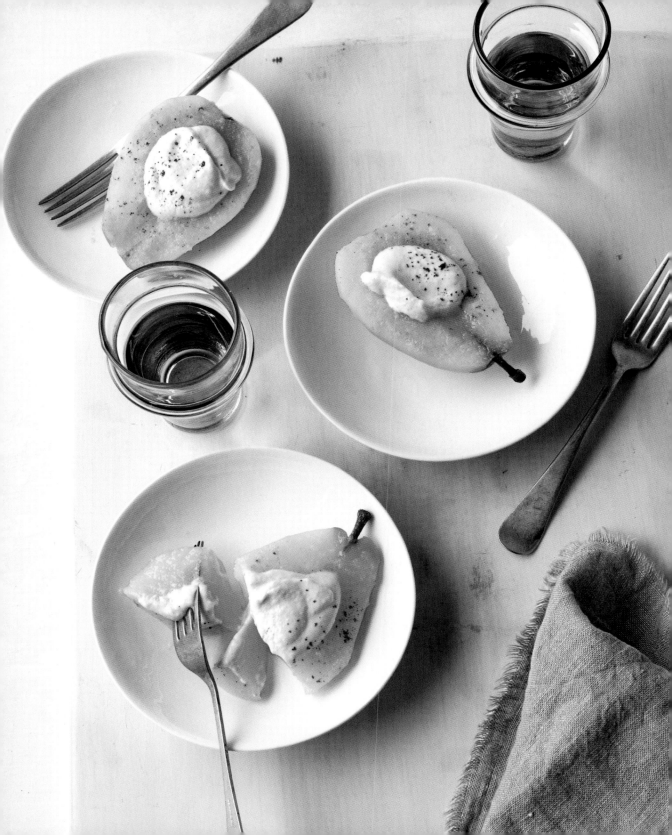

CASHEW BUTTER COOKIES

HANDS-ON TIME: 10 MINUTES   TOTAL TIME: 25 MINUTES

If you like, you can easily make these into peanut butter cookies by swapping in either crunchy or creamy natural peanut butter for the cashew butter. Once you've opened the package of flaxseed meal, be sure to store it in the freezer, where it will keep for up to a year.

⅓ cup all-natural cashew butter

3 tablespoons flaxseed meal

⅓ cup monk fruit natural no-calorie sweetener (baking formula)

2 tablespoons agave nectar

1 large egg white

½ teaspoon baking soda

¼ teaspoon pure vanilla extract

Preheat the oven to 350°F.

In a medium bowl, stir together the cashew butter, flaxseed meal, monk fruit sweetener, agave nectar, egg white, baking soda, and vanilla.

With moistened hands, divide the dough into 12 pieces. Shape into balls and place on an ungreased baking sheet, spacing them 2 inches apart. Flatten each ball to a ½-inch thickness.

Bake until the cookies have puffed and are lightly browned on the bottom, 12 to 15 minutes. Let cool on the baking sheet for 5 minutes, then transfer to a rack to cool completely.

MAKES 12 COOKIES (2 per serving) ▶ **Per cookie:** 64 calories, 4 g fat, 1 g saturated fat, 2 g protein, 5 g carbohydrate, 0.5 g fiber, 58 mg sodium

CHOCOLATE WALNUT ESPRESSO CAKE

HANDS-ON TIME: 15 MINUTES   TOTAL TIME: 35 MINUTES PLUS COOLING TIME

PHASE 2

Flourless chocolate cake is the obvious choice when you're watching your gluten intake. But for those times when you don't want to forgo that typical cakey texture, try this version made with brown rice flour, which also adds a dose of healthy fiber to the cake. The addition of almond milk gives the cake extra richness. You can use pecans or almonds instead of walnuts, if you prefer.

Olive oil cooking spray
1 cup unsweetened almond milk
¼ cup extra-virgin olive oil
1 large egg
2 tablespoons agave nectar
1 teaspoon pure vanilla extract
⅔ cup brown rice flour
½ cup tapioca starch
½ cup monk fruit natural no-calorie sweetener (baking formula)

¼ cup unsweetened cocoa powder
1 tablespoon espresso powder
1 teaspoon gluten-free baking powder
¼ teaspoon salt
⅓ cup walnuts, coarsely chopped
2 ounces gluten-free dark chocolate, coarsely chopped

Preheat the oven to 350°F. Spray a 9 × 9-inch baking pan with olive oil.

In a small bowl, whisk together the almond milk, oil, egg, agave nectar, and vanilla.

In a large bowl, whisk together the brown rice flour, tapioca starch, monk fruit sweetener, cocoa powder, espresso powder, baking powder, and salt. Add the almond milk mixture and stir until smooth. Fold in the walnuts and chopped chocolate.

Scrape the batter into the pan and bake until set and a toothpick inserted in the center comes out clean, 17 to 20 minutes. Let cool in the pan, then invert onto a cake plate.

MAKES 12 SERVINGS ▶ **Per serving:** 157 calories, 9.5 g fat, 2 g saturated fat, 2 g protein, 18 g carbohydrate, 1.5 g fiber, 116 mg sodium

CITRUS YOGURT PIE

HANDS-ON TIME: 25 MINUTES
TOTAL TIME: 1 HOUR 15 MINUTES PLUS CHILLING TIME

This delicious pie will fool you into thinking you are eating a super-rich, super-creamy cheesecake. Bright with citrus flavors—lemon, orange, and lime—the custard filling for the pie is made with thick nonfat Greek yogurt and eggs, so even though it's dessert, you'll actually be getting 6 grams of protein a serving and only a whisper of fat.

CRUST

½ cup sorghum flour

½ cup gluten-free oat flour

⅓ cup coconut flour

¼ teaspoon salt

3 ounces cold light cream cheese, cut into 4 pieces

3 tablespoons extra-virgin olive oil

10 tablespoons ice water

FILLING

1 tablespoon grated lemon zest

1 tablespoon grated orange zest

¾ cup monk fruit natural no-calorie sweetener (baking formula)

2 large eggs

2 large egg whites

½ cup nonfat (0%) plain Greek yogurt

¼ cup fresh lemon juice

¼ cup fresh lime juice

¼ cup fresh orange juice

For the crust: In a food processor, combine the sorghum flour, oat flour, coconut flour, and salt. Pulse a few times to combine. Add the cream cheese and pulse until combined. Add the oil and pulse until the mixture forms coarse crumbs. Add the ice water and pulse 5 to 10 times to combine, or until the dough just holds together when pinched between 2 fingers.

Turn the dough out onto a large piece of plastic wrap. Using the plastic wrap and your hands, guide the dough into a disc, pressing down to fully bring the dough together. Wrap the disc tightly in plastic wrap and refrigerate for 1 hour.

Preheat the oven to 425°F.

Take the dough out of the refrigerator 5 minutes before rolling so that it remains a bit chilled for easier rolling. Place the dough on a sheet of parchment paper that has been lightly dusted with sorghum flour. Flour the top of the dough and place another sheet of parchment on top. Roll out the dough to a 10-inch round (be sure to keep the crust a bit on the thick side since it may shrink when baked). Fit the dough into a 9-inch pie pan, pressing it against the sides and evening the top to make it even with the rim (it does not go over the rim). This dough is fragile but patches together easily, so don't be discouraged if it rips.

Line the pan with foil, leaving an overhang all around. Pour pie weights or dried beans into the foil to weight it down. Place the pan on a baking sheet and bake until the crust is lightly set and golden (lift the foil to see), about 15 minutes. Carefully lift out the foil and pie weights or beans. If the crust has bubbled up, gently press it down. Set the crust aside to cool on a rack. Leave the oven on, but reduce the temperature to 350°F.

For the filling: In a small bowl, combine the lemon zest, orange zest, and monk fruit sweetener.

In a large bowl, whisk together the whole eggs, egg whites, and yogurt. Whisk in the citrus zest mixture, lemon juice, lime juice, and orange juice until well combined.

Pour the custard mixture into the cooled pie crust and bake until lightly set, 30 to 35 minutes. Let cool completely on a rack, then refrigerate until chilled, about 2 hours.

MAKES 10 SERVINGS ❱ **Per serving:** 137 calories, 7 g fat, 2 g saturated fat, 6 g protein, 13 g carbohydrate, 2.5 g fiber, 92 mg sodium

CARAMELIZED APPLE MINI-SHORTCAKES

HANDS-ON TIME: 25 MINUTES   TOTAL TIME: 1 HOUR 15 MINUTES

Shortcakes are sort of like upside-down fruit cobblers, but in perfect individual dessert portions. You can change up the fruits: apples or pears in the fall, peaches or strawberries in the summer (for the soft summer fruits, cook the caramel syrup separately and pour over the cut-up fruit instead of cooking them together). And switch up the flavors in the topping to go with the different fruits: Add a small pinch of allspice for the peaches, a little grated orange zest for the strawberries, and switch the vanilla extract to ¼ teaspoon almond extract for the pears.

SHORTCAKES

Olive oil cooking spray

½ cup coconut flour

2 tablespoons almond flour

¼ teaspoon gluten-free baking powder

½ teaspoon salt

4 large eggs, at room temperature

4 large egg whites (don't use liquid egg whites here), at room temperature

3 tablespoons extra-virgin olive oil

¼ cup monk fruit natural no-calorie sweetener (baking formula)

¼ cup agave nectar

1 teaspoon pure vanilla extract

APPLE TOPPING

1 tablespoon extra-virgin olive oil

2 green apples, unpeeled, coarsely diced

1 red apple, unpeeled, coarsely diced

2 tablespoons agave nectar

1 teaspoon fresh lemon juice

YOGURT TOPPING

1 cup nonfat (0%) plain Greek yogurt

1 teaspoon agave nectar

½ teaspoon pure vanilla extract

For the shortcakes: Preheat the oven to 350°F. Lightly spray a standard 12-cup muffin tin with olive oil.

In a large bowl, whisk together the coconut flour, almond flour, baking powder, and salt.

In a blender, combine the whole eggs, 2 of the egg whites, the oil, monk fruit sweetener, agave nectar, and vanilla. Pulse until thick and fully combined. Add this mixture to the dry ingredients and mix well.

In another bowl, with an electric mixer at high speed, beat the remaining 2 egg whites until stiff peaks form. Gently fold the egg whites into the batter and mix well.

Divide the batter evenly among the muffin cups and bake until golden and a tooth-

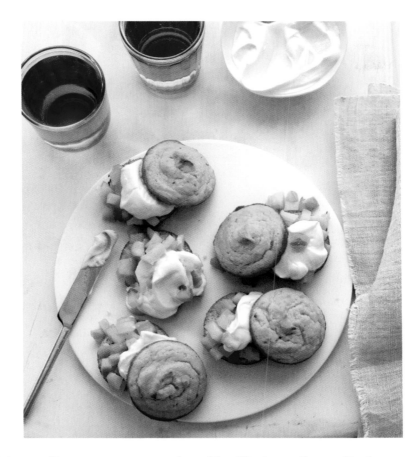

pick inserted in a center comes out clean, 25 to 35 minutes. Let cool in the pan on a rack.

Meanwhile, for the apple topping: In a nonstick skillet, heat the oil over medium heat. Add the apples, agave nectar, and lemon juice. Cook, stirring occasionally, until the apples soften and a caramelized syrup forms around them, 7 to 10 minutes. Remove from the heat.

For the yogurt topping: In a small bowl, mix together the yogurt, agave nectar, and vanilla. Cover and refrigerate until ready to serve.

To assemble the shortcakes, gently slice the shortcakes in half horizontally. Top the bottom halves evenly with caramelized apples. Top each with a dollop of sweetened yogurt, then top with the other half of each shortcake.

MAKES 12 SHORTCAKES (1 per serving) ▶ **Per shortcake:** 159 calories, 7.5 g fat, 2 g saturated fat, 6 g protein, 18 g carbohydrate, 2.5 g fiber, 168 mg sodium

◀MAKE AHEAD▶ The shortcakes are best baked shortly before serving, but you can make both the apple topping and yogurt topping up to 3 days ahead and refrigerate.

LIME CHEESECAKE WITH PECAN-GINGERSNAP CRUST

HANDS-ON TIME: 20 MINUTES
TOTAL TIME: 1 HOUR 15 MINUTES PLUS CHILLING TIME

PHASE 2

Once you taste this rich spiced pecan crust, you'll wonder what you ever saw in the typical gingersnap or graham cracker cheesecake crust. Not only is it gluten free, it's made with healthy fats from the nuts and coconut spread.

CRUST

- 2 cups pecans
- 1 teaspoon monk fruit natural no-calorie sweetener (baking formula)
- ½ teaspoon ground ginger
- 2 tablespoons coconut spread or extra-virgin coconut oil, melted
- Olive oil cooking spray

FILLING

- 10 ounces light cream cheese, at room temperature
- 6 ounces fat-free cream cheese, at room temperature
- ¾ cup fat-free sour cream
- ½ cup monk fruit natural no-calorie sweetener (baking formula)
- 1 large egg
- 2 large egg whites
- Grated zest of 2 limes
- ¼ cup fresh lime juice
- 14 lime slices, for garnish (optional)

Preheat the oven to 350°F.

For the crust: In a food processor, combine the pecans, monk fruit sweetener, ground ginger, and coconut spread. Pulse until finely ground and clumping together.

Lightly spray a 9-inch springform pan with olive oil. Press the pecan-gingersnap mixture into the bottom of the pan and set aside.

For the filling: In a food processor, combine both cream cheeses and the sour cream. With the machine running, slowly add the monk fruit sweetener, whole egg, and egg whites. Process until completely smooth. Add the lime zest and lime juice and pulse until well combined.

Pour the cheesecake mixture over the crust and bake until the center is set, 50 to 55 minutes.

Let the cheesecake cool completely in the pan on a rack, then refrigerate for at least 4 hours, or until well chilled. Garnish each serving with a slice of lime, if using.

MAKES 14 SERVINGS ▶ **Per serving:** 185 calories, 16 g fat, 4 g saturated fat, 6 g protein, 7 g carbohydrate, 1.5 g fiber, 213 mg sodium

STRAWBERRIES WITH RASPBERRY CREAM

HANDS-ON TIME: 15 MINUTES   TOTAL TIME: 1 HOUR 15 MINUTES

When fresh raspberries are in season, you can switch the role the berries play in this dessert. In other words, make a strawberry cream (purée ¾ cup thawed frozen strawberries, the agave nectar, and yogurt) and drizzle it over 2 pints fresh raspberries (don't macerate the raspberries with the agave).

1½ **pounds fresh strawberries, quartered**	¾ **cup frozen unsweetened raspberries, thawed**
1 **tablespoon agave nectar**	3 **tablespoons nonfat (0%) plain Greek yogurt**

In a medium bowl, toss the strawberries with the agave nectar to coat well. Set aside at room temperature to macerate, stirring occasionally, for at least 30 minutes and preferably 1 hour (the longer the berries sit, the more juice they will give off).

Drain the juices from the strawberries into a mini food processor. Add the raspberries and process to a smooth purée. Press through a fine-mesh strainer into a bowl to remove the seeds. Stir in the yogurt.

Divide the strawberries among 4 bowls and drizzle each with 2 tablespoons raspberry cream.

MAKES 4 SERVINGS ▌ **Per serving:** 90 calories, 0 g fat, 0 g saturated fat, 4 g protein, 21 g carbohydrate, 3 g fiber, 4 mg sodium

SUMMER BERRY TART

HANDS-ON TIME: 25 MINUTES   TOTAL TIME: 55 MINUTES PLUS CHILLING TIME

PHASE
2

The crust for this tart is remarkably easy to make and requires no rolling; you simply press it into the pan. The easiest way to do this is to place the dough in the pan, cover it with a sheet of plastic wrap, and then press it out. You can use whatever combo of berries you like (or have on hand); you just need a total of 1½ cups.

TART SHELL

Olive oil cooking spray

1 cup almond flour

½ cup brown rice flour

1 teaspoon grated orange zest

¼ teaspoon baking soda

¼ teaspoon salt

3 tablespoons extra-virgin olive oil

PASTRY CREAM

¼ cup brown rice flour

⅓ cup monk fruit natural no-calorie sweetener (baking formula)

3 tablespoons agave nectar

1 large egg

Pinch salt

2 cups 1% milk

1½ teaspoons pure vanilla extract

TOPPING

¾ cup blackberries plus ¾ cup blueberries; or ¾ cup strawberries (sliced or left whole) plus ¾ cup raspberries

For the tart shell: Preheat the oven to 350°F. Lightly spray a 9-inch tart pan with a removable bottom with olive oil.

In a food processor, pulse the almond flour, brown rice flour, orange zest, baking soda, and salt to combine. Add the oil and 3 tablespoons cold water and let the machine run until the dough almost forms a ball.

Place the dough in the center of the pan and, using your hands, firmly press it into the bottom and up the sides of the pan, making the side walls slightly thicker and then evening the top off. Line the pan with foil, leaving an overhang all around. Pour pie weights or dried beans into the foil to weight it down. Bake for 20 minutes and carefully lift out the foil and pie weights or beans. Return the tart shell to the oven and bake until lightly browned and set, about 10 minutes longer. Transfer the pan to a rack to cool completely.

Meanwhile, for the pastry cream: In a medium saucepan, whisk together the brown rice flour, monk fruit sweetener, agave nectar, egg, and salt until combined.

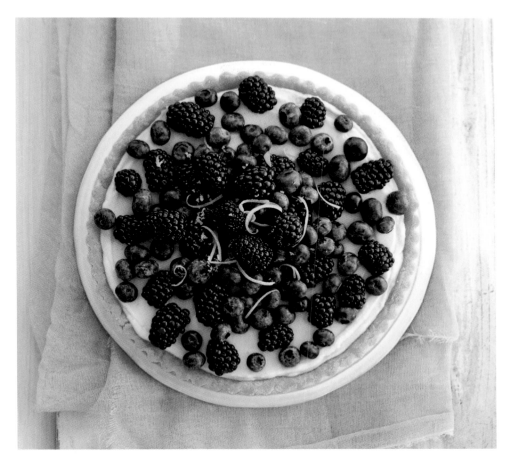

Gradually whisk in the milk until smooth. Cook over medium heat, whisking constantly, until a few big bubbles erupt on the surface and the mixture has thickened, about 10 minutes. Stir in the vanilla. Immediately transfer to a medium bowl to stop the cooking. Let cool to room temperature, then place a sheet of plastic wrap directly on the surface of the pastry cream and refrigerate until chilled, about 2 hours.

To assemble and top the tart: Remove the ring from the tart pan. Run a large metal spatula between the bottom of the pan and the shell and slide the shell onto a cake plate (or leave it on the pan bottom if you'd prefer). Fill with the chilled pastry cream, smoothing the top and spreading the filling to the edge. Top decoratively with the berries.

MAKES 10 SERVINGS ❱ **Per serving:** 200 calories, 11 g fat, 1.5 g saturated fat, 6 g protein, 22 g carbohydrate, 2.5 g fiber, 107 mg sodium

TOASTED OAT AND PEANUT COOKIES

HANDS-ON TIME: 15 MINUTES   TOTAL TIME: 30 MINUTES

Oatmeal cookies are good, but peanut-oatmeal cookies are even better. Grinding roasted peanuts and oats into a flour and including some peanut butter in the mix makes for a cookie with a very peanut-y flavor. Be sure when you buy the oats, you buy the quick-cooking kind (they cook in only 1 minute), not instant oatmeal, which is presweetened.

Olive oil cooking spray

2 cups gluten-free quick-cooking oats

½ cup unsalted dry-roasted peanuts

1½ teaspoons gluten-free baking powder

½ teaspoon salt

½ cup monk fruit natural no-calorie sweetener (baking formula)

¼ cup unsweetened applesauce

2 tablespoons extra-virgin olive oil

2 tablespoons all-natural peanut butter

2 teaspoons pure vanilla extract

1 large egg

Preheat the oven to 375°F. Line a large baking sheet with parchment paper, spray lightly with olive oil, and set aside.

On a second, ungreased baking sheet, spread out the oats and bake until lightly toasted, 5 to 7 minutes. Let the oats cool. Leave the oven on at the same temperature for the cookies.

Measure out ½ cup of the toasted oats and transfer to a mini food processor. Add the peanuts and grind the oats and nuts until they are the texture of coarse flour. Transfer to a medium bowl and stir in the remaining oats, baking powder, and salt.

In a large bowl, with an electric mixer at low speed, beat together the monk fruit sweetener, applesauce, oil, peanut butter, vanilla, and egg until light and fluffy. Slowly add the dry ingredients and mix until well combined.

Drop the dough by generous tablespoons onto the prepared baking sheet for a total of 24 cookies. Press down with a fork to flatten. Bake until lightly golden, 10 to 12 minutes. Let cool on the baking sheet for 5 minutes, then transfer to a rack to cool completely. These cookies are best served fresh from the oven, so for any cookies that won't be eaten right away, store them tightly wrapped in the freezer and reheat for 15 to 30 seconds in the microwave when you want a couple.

MAKES 24 COOKIES (2 per serving) ▌ **Per cookie:** 71 calories, 4 g fat, 0.5 g saturated fat, 3 g protein, 6 g carbohydrate, 1 g fiber, 86 mg sodium

INDIVIDUAL BANANA SOUFFLÉS

HANDS-ON TIME: 10 MINUTES   TOTAL TIME: 25 MINUTES

If you like, you can make these soufflés in a jumbo muffin tin; you'll get 6 slightly smaller soufflés. Line the cups of the muffin tin with paper liners and lightly spray the liners with olive oil. The baking time will be approximately the same. Don't use liquid egg whites in this recipe, because they will not whip up to the volume required to make soufflés.

Olive oil cooking spray

2 medium bananas (not overripe), cut up

1 large egg, separated

1 tablespoon agave nectar (maple flavored if you can find it)

4 large egg whites, at room temperature (don't use liquid egg whites here)

Generous pinch cream of tartar

Position a rack in the lower third of the oven and preheat to 425°F. Generously spray the bottoms and sides of four 8-ounce ramekins with olive oil. Place the ramekins on a baking sheet.

In a mini food processor, process the bananas to a smooth purée. Add the egg yolk and agave nectar and process until smooth. Transfer to a large bowl.

In a bowl, with an electric mixer at high speed, beat the 5 egg whites with the cream of tartar until stiff peaks form. Scoop about one-third of the whites into the banana purée and whisk to lighten the mixture. Add the remaining egg whites to the banana mixture and gently fold until no streaks of egg white remain.

Divide the soufflé mixture among the ramekins and smooth the tops. Bake until puffed and browned on top, 10 to 12 minutes. Serve immediately.

MAKES 4 SERVINGS ❯ **Per serving:** 107 calories, 2 g fat, 0.5 g saturated fat, 6 g protein, 17 g carbohydrate, 1.5 g fiber, 74 mg sodium

DOUBLE PLUM CLAFOUTI

HANDS-ON TIME: 10 MINUTES   TOTAL TIME: 50 MINUTES PLUS COOLING TIME

PHASE 2

Clafouti is a home-style French dessert that's somewhere between a cake and a custard. Don't worry if you can't cut a perfect slice of the "cake"—it's quite moist and full of fruit. If it falls apart, just serve it up in a bowl the way you would cobbler. For a sweeter yogurt topping, add a little monk fruit natural no-calorie sweetener from a packet.

1 teaspoon extra-virgin olive oil

1 pound red or black plums (about 3), cut into ½-inch chunks

6 tablespoons sorghum flour

¼ teaspoon salt

¼ cup unsweetened prune butter or prune purée

3 large eggs

¾ cup unsweetened almond milk

½ teaspoon pure vanilla extract

3 tablespoons sliced almonds

6 tablespoons nonfat (0%) plain Greek yogurt

Preheat the oven to 350°F. Coat the bottom and sides of an 8-inch round cake pan with the oil. Scatter the plums over the bottom of the pan.

In a medium bowl, whisk together the flour and salt.

In a separate medium bowl, beat together the prune butter and 1 of the eggs until evenly combined. Beat in the remaining 2 eggs, the almond milk, and vanilla until well blended. Stir the wet ingredients into the flour until just combined.

Pour the batter over the plums and sprinkle the almonds evenly on top. Bake until risen and set, about 40 minutes.

Let cool to lukewarm or room temperature before cutting into 6 wedges. Dollop each with 1 tablespoon of the yogurt.

MAKES 6 SERVINGS ❯ **Per serving:** 153 calories, 5.5 g fat, 1 g saturated fat, 5 g protein, 22 g carbohydrate, 2.5 g fiber, 155 mg sodium

FRESH PEACH COMPOTE

HANDS-ON TIME: 10 MINUTES   TOTAL TIME: 20 MINUTES PLUS COOLING TIME

PHASE
2

You can peel the peaches if you want, but leaving the skins on makes the compote prettier. Try to get ripe peaches. If they're not, add a little monk fruit sweetener to the cooking syrup. Or opt for 4 cups of unsweetened frozen sliced peaches, but cook them for a shorter amount of time in the first step (you don't want them to get too soft).

1 orange

4 peaches, sliced

   Ground cinnamon

½ cup nonfat (0%) plain Greek yogurt

1 tablespoon agave nectar

   Monk fruit natural no-calorie sweetener from a packet (optional)

4 teaspoons chopped pecans

Grate ½ teaspoon zest from the orange and then juice it. In a medium saucepan, combine the zest, juice, peaches, and a pinch of cinnamon. Bring the mixture to a simmer over medium heat. Stir, cover, and reduce the heat to medium-low. Cook, turning the peaches several times, until softened but not mushy, 5 to 7 minutes (depending on the ripeness of the fruit).

Scrape the peaches and syrup into a serving bowl and set aside to cool to room temperature. Refrigerate if you'd like to serve it chilled.

In a small bowl, whisk together the yogurt, agave nectar, and a pinch of cinnamon. Taste and if you would like the yogurt sweeter, stir in a little monk fruit sweetener. Refrigerate until serving time.

To serve, spoon the peaches and syrup into 4 dessert dishes or goblets. Top each serving with 2 tablespoons of the yogurt mixture and 1 teaspoon of the pecans.

MAKES 4 SERVINGS ▶ **Per serving:** 118 calories, 2 g fat, 0 g saturated fat, 4 g protein, 23 g carbohydrate, 2.5 g fiber, 11 mg sodium

LEMON BARS

HANDS-ON TIME: 20 MINUTES
TOTAL TIME: 1 HOUR 15 MINUTES PLUS COOLING TIME

PHASE 2

Almond flour and coconut flour add just the right amount of richness to the short-bread base in this gluten-free version of the classic lemon bars recipe. Be sure when you make the lemon topping that you go for fresh lemon juice; bottled or frozen just won't have the right zing, plus you need to use some grated lemon zest here to really notch up the lemon flavor. In a typical lemon bar, the thickener for the lemon topping could include wheat flour; here garbanzo flour is used instead to add a little protein plus a mildly buttery flavor.

CRUST

- 1 cup almond flour
- ½ cup coconut flour
- ½ cup gluten-free quinoa flour
- ¼ cup monk fruit natural no-calorie sweetener (baking formula)
- ¼ cup extra-virgin olive oil

TOPPING

- 1 cup monk fruit natural no-calorie sweetener (baking formula)
- ½ cup agave nectar
- 2 large eggs, beaten
- 2 large egg whites
- 1 tablespoon grated lemon zest
- ⅔ cup fresh lemon juice (3 or 4 lemons)
- 1½ tablespoons garbanzo bean flour
- 1 teaspoon gluten-free baking powder
- ¼ teaspoon salt

Preheat the oven to 300°F.

For the crust: In a food processor, pulse together the almond flour, coconut flour, quinoa flour, and monk fruit sweetener. Add the oil and pulse until well blended and the dough comes together.

Press the dough into the bottom of an 8 x 8-inch glass baking dish. Bake for 25 minutes to set the crust. Remove from the oven and let the crust cool on a rack for 10 minutes. Leave the oven on but increase the temperature to 350°F.

Meanwhile, for the topping: In a medium bowl, whisk together the monk fruit sweetener, agave nectar, whole eggs, egg whites, lemon zest, and lemon juice.

In a small bowl, whisk together the garbanzo flour, baking powder, and salt.

Add the flour mixture to the lemon mixture and stir well to combine. Pour the topping over the cooled crust.

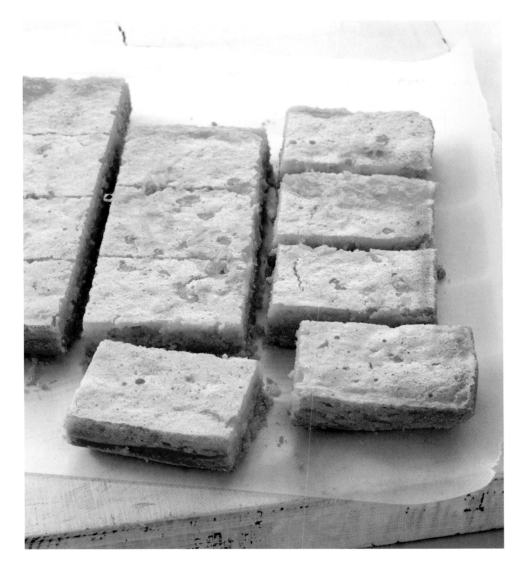

Bake until the topping sets, 35 to 40 minutes.

To serve warm, let cool in the pan on a rack for at least 20 minutes before cutting into 12 bars. To serve chilled, let cool to room temperature, then refrigerate for at least 3 hours before cutting into bars.

MAKES 12 BARS (1 per serving) ❯ **Per bar:** 195 calories, 11 g fat, 2 g saturated fat, 5 g protein, 21 g carbohydrate, 3.5 g fiber, 131 mg sodium

CHOCOLATE PANNA COTTA

HANDS-ON TIME: 10 MINUTES   TOTAL TIME: 10 MINUTES PLUS CHILLING TIME

Panna cotta popped up on the dessert scene in upscale restaurants several years ago and has stayed there because it's so good. While *panna cotta* means "cooked cream" in Italian, we've swapped in 1% milk for the cream and used unsweetened cocoa powder for a deep chocolate flavor. This version is certainly not as decadent as the original, but definitely delicious—and easy to make.

2 cups 1% milk	1 teaspoon pure vanilla extract
¼ cup unsweetened cocoa powder	1 envelope (¼ ounce) unflavored gelatin
3 tablespoons agave nectar	
2 tablespoons monk fruit natural no-calorie sweetener (from packets)	

In a medium saucepan, gradually whisk 1½ cups of the milk into the cocoa powder until smooth. Whisk in the agave nectar, monk fruit sweetener, and vanilla. Bring to a simmer over medium-low heat.

Meanwhile, in a small bowl, sprinkle the gelatin over the remaining ½ cup milk. Gently swirl the bowl to moisten all the gelatin. Let stand until the gelatin is softened and swollen, about 5 minutes.

Stir the gelatin mixture into the saucepan of simmering milk, stirring until the gelatin has dissolved.

Divide the mixture among four 6-ounce custard cups or ramekins. Refrigerate, covered, until set, at least 2 hours or up to 3 days.

MAKES 4 SERVINGS ▶ **Per serving:** 115 calories, 1.5 g fat, 1 g saturated fat, 7 g protein, 21 g carbohydrate, 2 g fiber, 57 mg sodium

COCONUT CUSTARD PUDDING

HANDS-ON TIME: 5 MINUTES   TOTAL TIME: 30 MINUTES PLUS CHILLING TIME

PHASE 2

You won't need a whole can of coconut milk for this pudding, so pour the remainder into an ice cube tray and freeze. Once frozen, pop the coconut cubes out of the ice cube tray and transfer to resealable plastic bags. Each cube (if you used a standard ice cube tray) is 2 tablespoons of coconut milk. Try adding some to a salad dressing or pan sauce.

1 very ripe banana, cut up

¾ cup lite coconut milk

¾ cup 1% milk

1 large egg

1 large egg white

1 tablespoon plus 2 teaspoons monk fruit natural no-calorie sweetener (from packets)

Pinch of salt

2 tablespoons unsweetened coconut flakes

Preheat the oven to 350°F.

In a blender, combine the banana, coconut milk, 1% milk, whole egg, egg white, monk fruit sweetener, and salt. Purée until very smooth.

Pour the mixture into four 6-ounce custard cups or ramekins. Place the cups in a baking dish large enough to hold them snugly. Pour boiling water to come halfway up the sides of the custard cups. Bake until the pudding is just set, 25 to 30 minutes.

Place the coconut flakes on a baking sheet and bake alongside the puddings until lightly browned, about 7 minutes. Transfer the toasted coconut to a small bowl or plate.

Carefully remove the puddings from the water bath, transfer them to a rack to cool, then refrigerate until chilled, about 2 hours. Serve topped evenly with the toasted coconut flakes.

MAKES 4 SERVINGS ▶ **Per serving:** 129 calories, 6.5 g fat, 5 g saturated fat, 5 g protein, 14 g carbohydrate, 1.5 g fiber, 95 mg sodium

GLOSSARY OF INGREDIENTS

Following the South Beach Diet Gluten Solution Program isn't just about replacing wheat with other whole grains. Plenty of nutritious, waistline-friendly foods are naturally gluten free, and we take advantage of many of them in the healthy and delicious recipes in this book. Use this selected list as a guide for more information on how to buy and cook with this wide variety of ingredients. Though the majority of these items are supermarket staples, some of the more uncommon flours and spices may be easier to find online (see page 295). With the exception of gluten-free grains, gluten-free pasta, alcohol, starchy vegetables, and fruit (which are not allowed on Phase 1 of the Gluten Solution Program but are reintroduced on Gluten Solution Phase 2), most of these ingredients are fine for any phase. Where useful, we have provided page references to various recipes using particular ingredients.

AGAVE NECTAR: Agave nectar, which has a consistency similar to honey, is a natural sweetener made from a plant indigenous to Mexico called the blue agave. It is 1½ times sweeter than sugar, so you don't need to use a lot of it. It can be enjoyed in moderation on all phases of the South Beach Diet Gluten Solution Program. Agave nectar comes in light, dark, and flavored varieties, such as maple and hazelnut. Light agave imparts sweetness, while dark agave has a richer, caramel taste, but they are interchangeable in recipes. We've used agave nectar in the Amaranth, Almond, and Apricot Breakfast Cereal (page 30) and the Caramelized Apple Mini-Shortcakes (page 256), and we call for maple-flavored agave nectar in the Orange-Maple Pork Tenderloin (page 191).

ALCOHOL: Starting on Gluten Solution (GS) Phase 2, you can enjoy certain types of alcohol, in moderation, with a meal. Women should stick to 1 alcoholic beverage a day, and men to 1 or 2 a day. We recommend you opt for dry red or white wine, dry sherry, ouzo, extra-brut champagne, extra-brut cava, or extra-brut prosecco, which are all gluten free and have no or very little residual sugar. Currently there are no brands of gluten-free light beer on the market. Most people with gluten sensitivity can also enjoy distilled alcoholic beverages, even those that are made from gluten-containing grains, such as scotch, whiskey, and gin. If you are highly gluten sensitive, however, you may be able to consume only potato-based vodka (avoid flavored varieties, which may contain gluten) and rum (made from sugar cane) or tequila (made from agave), which are sure to be gluten free. See also Wine (page 293).

ALMOND FLOUR: See Nut Flours (page 285).

ALMOND MILK, UNSWEETENED: Unsweetened almond milk is a flavorful (and vegan) alternative to dairy milk. It is allowed on all phases of the Gluten Solution Program. We use it in our Mexican Rolled Omelet (page 39) and Chocolate Walnut Espresso Cake (page 253).

AMARANTH: An ancient food that was a staple crop of the Aztecs, tiny round amaranth seed is not a true cereal like rice or wheat, though it's used like one and is generally lumped into the grain category. Gluten free and high in protein, fiber, and iron, sweet, slightly nutty-tasting amaranth cooks quickly and is a good substitute for oatmeal in the morning. We use it in our Amaranth, Almond, and Apricot Breakfast Cereal (page 30). You can also use amaranth flour in baked goods, although we do not call for it in this book.

BACON: Gluten-free Canadian bacon and turkey bacon can be enjoyed on all phases of the South Beach Diet Gluten Solution Program (check labels carefully). They're a great substitute for regular bacon because they have the same smoky flavor without all the saturated fat. We add a slice of gluten-free Canadian bacon to each of our Baked Breakfast Stacks (page 33) for extra protein and use it for flavoring the Sautéed Kale, Bacon, and Sun-Dried Tomatoes side dish (page 245).

BAKING POWDER: Baking powder is a leavener typically consisting of baking soda (an alkali), acids, and starch (sometimes made from wheat) to keep it from sticking together. Because gluten-free flours aren't as elastic as those with gluten, adding baking powder helps to lighten gluten-free baked goods like the scones, biscuits, muffins, and breads in this book. Check labels carefully to make sure the baking powder is wheat free and gluten free.

BEAN FLOURS: High in protein, fiber, and iron, so-called bean flours are made by grinding dried beans and other legumes like lentils, chickpeas, and green peas into a fine powder. Bean flours are typically combined with other gluten-free flours in baking (using them alone produces too heavy a result). You can also use them instead of white flour for thickening soups, stews, and sauces and for making dips. The flour generally tastes like the bean it's ground from (see Beans and Other Legumes on page 272) and some, like black bean flour, produce a darker product. To keep your bean flour in the best possible condition, store it airtight in the freezer for up to 6 months. Bean flours that have been stored for too long at room temperature can develop a bitter flavor. We use the following bean flours in a variety of ways in this book:

- **Black bean flour:** See Chicken-Mushroom Croquettes (page 158).
- **Fava bean flour:** See Cheddar-Arugula Pinwheels (page 53).
- **Garbanzo bean (or chickpea) flour:** See Creamy Hot Broccoli Dip (page 48), Lemon Zucchini Bread (page 44), and Asparagus, Portobello, and Tuna Bake (page 142).
- **Garbanzo–fava bean (Garfava) flour:** See Golden Chicken Cottage Pie (page 164) and Three Sisters Bread (page 240).
- **White bean flour:** See Crispy-Topped Mac and Cheese (page 214), Souffléed Spinach (page 233), and Artichoke Gratin (page 238).

BEANS AND OTHER LEGUMES: A good source of protein and fiber, beans such as black, white, fava, and kidney, and other legumes like lentils, green peas, and chickpeas, also contain iron, folate, potassium, and antioxidants (darker beans like black beans, black soybeans, pinto, and kidney beans are particularly high in the antioxidants called anthocyanins, which have been shown to help prevent diseases related to inflammation). All legumes can be eaten on all phases of the South Beach Diet Gluten Solution Program. Most come dried and canned and, in the case of edamame, fresh and frozen. Look for canned beans that are gluten free with no salt added and avoid those that contain brown sugar, lard, or molasses. If you are highly gluten sensitive, avoid dried legumes stored in bulk bins because cross-contamination from wheat, barley, and rye stored in nearby bins is possible. The following beans and other legumes are called for in this book (see also Bean Flours, above.):

- **Black beans:** Also known as Mexican, Spanish, or black turtle beans, black beans have a slightly mushroomy flavor and are a staple throughout South and Central America and the Caribbean. They are typically used in black bean soup and as a side dish. Try them in our Chunky Tomato and Black Bean Chipotle Dip (page 46), Faux Caviar (page 49), and Gluten Solution SuperSalad (page 108).
- **Black soybeans:** This type of soybean, which tastes more like black beans than yellow soybeans, has almost twice the protein of regular black beans. Look for them in the natural foods aisle of large supermarkets or in health-food stores. You can use them in any recipe that calls for black beans. We use the canned variety in Butternut and Black Bean Stew (page 206).

- **Cannellini beans:** These white, kidney-shaped Italian beans (also called white kidney beans) have a slightly nutty flavor and creamy texture that suits our Italian White Bean and Artichoke Dip (page 47), Spinach-Stuffed Mushrooms (page 63), and Kale and Smoked Turkey Soup (page 75). You can use them interchangeably with Great Northern beans (below).

- **Chickpeas:** Also called garbanzo or ceci beans, these delicious legumes have a mild, nutty flavor and a firm yet creamy texture. They're delicious in a wide range of dishes including Chickpea Breakfast Hash (page 41), Spicy Chickpea "Nuts" (page 58), Chickpea and Sweet Potato Bisque (page 76), and Chickpea-Fennel Stew with Greens (page 208).

- **Edamame:** Immature soybeans that are eaten when they are still green, edamame, like all soybeans, are a source of complete protein, which means they provide all of the essential amino acids. Like all soybeans, they are relatively high in fat, but nearly all of the fat is unsaturated. Edamame are available fresh in the pod, frozen in the pod, or frozen shelled. We use frozen shelled edamame in Mockamole (page 52), Artichoke, Edamame, and Walnut Salad (page 106), and Green and White Pasta (page 204).

- **Great Northern beans:** Smaller than cannellini beans and oval in shape, Great Northern beans have a dense, nutty flavor and a slightly grainy texture. They can be used in any recipe calling for white beans. We use canned Great Northern beans in Faux Caviar (page 49) and Southwestern Three-Pepper Pork Chili (page 200).

- **Kidney beans:** This dark red bean is kidney shaped (thus its name). Its full-bodied flavor makes it a particularly good choice for chilis and hearty soups and stews. We use kidney beans in Pasta e Fagioli ("pasta and beans" in Italian), page 81.

- **Lentils:** Lentils have an earthy flavor and come in a wide variety of colors. The most common and least expensive are brown lentils, which are available both dried and canned, but dried green, red, orange, black, and white lentils are also available, mainly in Middle Eastern or East Indian markets. Dried lentils do not need presoaking. In this book we use dried French green lentils (sometimes sold as petite or Puy lentils) in the Green Lentil Salad (page 114) and dried brown lentils in the Greek-Style Turkey and Lentil Soup (page 74) and Baked Lentils with Mushrooms and Walnuts (page 242). In recipes where the type of lentil is not indicated, you can use whichever type you prefer, but cooking times will vary.

- **Pinto beans:** Also known as red Mexican beans, pintos are a type of kidney bean, but oval in shape. They are named for their pinkish-brown streaks (*pinto* is Spanish for painted), which disappear when the beans are cooked. We use them in Mexican Bean and Cheese Salad (page 107) and Chili Meatloaf (page 184).
- **Soybeans:** See Edamame; Black soybeans (above).
- **Split peas:** Once peas are dried and the skins removed, they split naturally. Even in their dried state, split peas (which come in both green and yellow varieties) do not require soaking, and they cook quickly. All varieties have an earthy flavor that's different from that of fresh peas. We use green split peas in Creamy Asparagus-Pea Soup with Deviled Shrimp (page 79).
- **White beans:** See Cannellini beans; Great Northern beans (page 273).

BEEF: A good source of protein, iron, zinc, and vitamin B_{12}, beef is delicious and easy to cook. But not all cuts are equal when it comes to fat. Look for lean cuts like flank steak, London broil, tenderloin (filet mignon), T-bone, top round, bottom round, eye of round, sirloin, and top loin; veal chops and cutlets are also fine. Trim any visible fat before cooking. When choosing ground beef, look for extra lean, lean, or sirloin. Purchase range-fed (grass-fed) beef when possible because it contains more omega-3s than grain-fed beef. Among the recipes calling for beef in this book are Pan-Fried Flank Steak with Tomato-Eggplant Sauce (page 182), Jerk Flank Steak (page 183), Pan-Seared Sirloin Steaks with Fiery Pepper Sauce (page 180), and Sirloin Burgers with Grilled Scallions (page 188).

BLACK BEAN FLOUR: See Bean Flours (page 271).

BREAD: Avoid all types of bread on Phase 1 of the Gluten Solution Program. Gluten-free whole-grain breads, such as multigrain (brown rice with millet, for example), and those made with amaranth, corn, and/or quinoa flour, can be enjoyed when you gradually reintroduce gluten-free grains starting on GS Phase 2. Choose varieties that have 2 grams or more of fiber per serving. Try our "Everything" Oat Bread (page 86) made with gluten-free oat flour, flaxseed meal, almond flour, and coconut flour, or our Three Sisters Bread (page 240), a type of cornbread created by our Native American ancestors.

BROTH: All of the recipes calling for beef, chicken, or vegetable broth in this book were developed with low-sodium broth. Look for brands that contain no more than 140 milligrams per cup; some brands have as little as 80 milligrams. Watch out for chicken, beef, and vegetable broths containing wheat flour or hydrolyzed wheat protein; they will contain gluten. Broth can be used on all phases of the Gluten Solution Program. It's obviously a key component in soups, but you can also try cooking beans, vegetables, and, on GS Phase 2, gluten-free grains in broth instead of water to enhance the flavor.

BROWN RICE: Because it has its germ intact, gluten-free brown rice is a good source of fiber and other nutrients, including thiamin, iron, and some vitamin E. You can enjoy a ½-cup serving, cooked, as a side dish beginning on GS Phase 2 (avoid flavored brown rice products, since the flavorings may contain gluten). We recommend serving regular brown rice with Pan-Fried Flank Steak with Tomato-Eggplant Sauce (page 182) and brown basmati rice with Thai Eggplant Curry (page 212). See also Brown Rice Couscous (below); Brown rice flour (page 282); Brown rice pasta (page 288).

BROWN RICE COUSCOUS: You can enjoy a ½-cup serving of cooked brown rice couscous as a side dish beginning on GS Phase 2. It's a finer-textured alternative to regular brown rice and cooks more quickly. Unlike wheat-based couscous, which is prepared by soaking in boiling water for just 5 minutes off the heat, gluten-free brown rice couscous takes about double that to become tender. We use it in Baked Salmon with Spinach and Couscous (page 135), Chicken with Lemon-Fennel Couscous (page 156), and Baked Stuffed Pork Chops (page 192).

BUCKWHEAT: Not wheat at all but a relative of rhubarb, buckwheat is naturally gluten free. It is sold as a whole grain, as kasha (roasted buckwheat groats), and as a flour (see Buckwheat flour, page 282). Look for products made with 100% buckwheat, since it is sometimes blended with wheat flour. We use medium-granulation kasha in the Caramelized Onions and Kasha recipe (page 222).

BUCKWHEAT FLOUR: See Flours, Gluten-Free (page 281).

BUTTERMILK: Low-fat (1.5%) or light (1% or 1.5%) buttermilk can be enjoyed on all phases of the South Beach Diet Gluten Solution Program. Buttermilk makes dishes extra creamy without the added fat. We use it in the dressing for Artichoke, Edamame, and Walnut Salad (page 106) and Mexican Bean and Cheese Salad (page 107).

CANADIAN BACON: See Bacon (page 271).

CASHEW BUTTER: See Nuts/Nut Butters (page 286).

CHEESE: You can enjoy cheese on all phases of the South Beach Diet Gluten Solution Program. We recommend choosing low- or reduced-fat varieties that contain no more than 6 grams of fat per serving, as regular cheese can be high in saturated fat and calories. Low- and reduced-fat cheeses are just as rich in protein and calcium. A note of caution: Cheeses that have been presliced in the deli department rather than by the manufacturer may be cross-contaminated with gluten from deli meats sliced on the same machine. Watch out for canned and tube cheese spreads, as well as beer-washed cheeses, and for certain types of blue cheese that may have been made with mold cultured on gluten. The following types of cheese are used in this book:

- **Cheddar:** This firm cow's-milk cheese is available in a range of flavors from mild to sharp. Use the reduced-fat variety and buy it preshredded to save time. We use it in Cheddar-Arugula Pinwheels (page 53), Crispy-Topped Mac and Cheese (page 214), and Chili Meatloaf (page 184).

- **Cottage cheese:** Choose 1%, 2%, or fat-free cottage cheese. In this book we use 1% cottage cheese in the Tofu-Mushroom Lasagna (page 216).

- **Cream cheese:** Both light cream cheese and fat-free cream cheese take the place of full-fat cream cheese in our Lime Cheesecake with Pecan-Gingersnap Crust (page 258). We also use light cream cheese in the Citrus Yogurt Pie (page 254).

- **Feta:** Crumble this tangy Greek cheese over salads like our Asparagus Salad with Feta and Toasted Nuts (page 111) or use it in a sauce, as we do for Chicken Kebabs with Minted Feta Sauce (page 152). Be sure to buy the reduced-fat variety, which can be purchased precrumbled.

- **Goat cheese:** Also called *chèvre*, goat cheese has a creamy texture and tart flavor that complements a wide variety of dishes. In this book we use reduced-fat goat cheese in the filling for Vegetable Quiche with a Spinach Crust (page 211), and we combine it with Greek yogurt as a topping for Moroccan-Spiced Beef Burgers (page 189).

- **Mexican blend cheese:** This mix of preshredded sharp Cheddar, Colby, Monterey Jack, and sometimes queso blanco and/or asadera cheese as well, is good for south-of-the-border–inspired dishes such as our Tofu and Egg Migas (page 213), Mexican Bean and Cheese Salad (page 107), and Oat Cake Quesadillas (page 90). Be sure to buy the reduced-fat variety.

- **Parmesan:** This nutty-tasting hard cheese doesn't come in low-fat or reduced-fat versions, but due to its powerful flavor it is used in small quantities and therefore allowed on all phases of the South Beach Diet Gluten Solution Program. It's at its best when freshly grated. Since Parmesan is so versatile, we use it often in this book in recipes like Green and White Pasta (page 204), Crispy-Topped Mac and Cheese (page 214), Italian Tamales (page 176), Spicy Broccoli Parmesan (page 230), and Artichoke Gratin (page 238). You can use a box grater, rasp-style citrus zester, or hand-cranked mill grater to get the texture you prefer. Or you can buy Parmesan pregrated (but avoid the canned varieties).

- **Provolone:** This Italian cow's-milk cheese has a mild, smoky flavor and is ideal for melting or grating. We use it in our Jícama Cheese Toasties (page 83). Be sure to buy the reduced-fat variety.

- **Spreadable cheese:** Buy this light, creamy cow's-milk cheese (which comes in ¾-ounce wedges) in a variety of flavors and experiment. We use French onion in Creamy 'n' Cheesy Scrambled Eggs (page 36) and the chipotle flavor in the Mexican Rolled Omelet (page 39).

- **Ricotta:** This smooth cheese resembles cottage cheese but is sweeter and has four times more calcium. Look for part-skim ricotta, which has all the flavor of the whole-milk version but 40 percent less fat. It's a key component in the stuffing for Turkey Breast Stuffed with Spinach and Ricotta (page 174).

- **Swiss cheese:** This favorite holey cheese is great for sandwiches or for melting. We use reduced-fat Swiss in our Asparagus in a Blanket (page 51) and Spinach-Stuffed Mushrooms (page 63).

CHIA SEEDS: See Seeds (page 291).

CHICKEN: See Poultry (page 289).

CHICKPEAS: See Bean Flours (page 271); Beans and Other Legumes (page 272).

CHIPOTLES IN ADOBO: These smoked, dried jalapeño chiles come canned and packed in a dark red sauce made from vinegar and seasonings. Both the peppers and the sauce add punch to chilis and other stews. We use them to flavor Pan-Seared Sirloin Steaks with Fiery Pepper Sauce (page 180), in Chicken Chilaquiles (page 150), and in our delicious Southwestern Three-Pepper Pork Chili (page 200).

CHOCOLATE: Dark chocolate, including semisweet, is allowed in moderation beginning on Phase 2 of the Gluten Solution Program. For this book, pick a brand that contains at least 70% cacao, since it has more of the antioxidant flavonoids that are thought to be heart protective. Whether you're cooking with chocolate or enjoying a piece as a special treat, read labels carefully, because certain brands have gluten additives. Look for chocolate that does not contain unspecified modified food starch, barley malt, unspecified natural flavors, or artificial colors, which can all be indicators of the presence of gluten. We use gluten-free dark chocolate in our Chocolate Walnut Espresso Cake (page 253). See also Cocoa Powder (below).

COCOA POWDER: Imparting a deep chocolate flavor to both sweet and savory dishes, cocoa powder is simply dried and ground cocoa beans. Be sure to look for sugar-free and gluten-free brands labeled 100% cacao. We use unsweetened cocoa powder in the Chocolate Walnut Espresso Cake (page 253), Chocolate Panna Cotta (page 268), and Mexican Turkey and Pepper Stew (page 169).

COCONUT: Shredded or flaked unsweetened coconut can be used in moderation on all phases of the Gluten Solution Program to add sweetness to baked goods, fruit salads, toppings for gluten-free puddings, and coatings for poultry and shrimp. We use shredded coconut in our Coconut-Apple Muffins (page 25) and mix it with almond flour for the coating for Coconut-Almond Chicken Strips (page 56). Unsweetened coconut flakes flavor the Coconut Custard Pudding (page 269).

COCONUT FLOUR: See Nut Flours (page 285).

COCONUT MILK, LITE: Coconut milk is made from coconut and water steeped together to produce a coconut-flavored liquid. Canned lite coconut milk can be used occasionally and in moderation in cooking on all phases of the Gluten Solution Program. It adds creaminess to the Thai Eggplant Curry (page 212) and Coconut Custard Pudding (page 269). Avoid full-fat varieties.

COCONUT OIL/COCONUT SPREAD: While coconut oil is predominantly a saturated fat, we do allow it in moderation on the South Beach Diet Gluten Solution Program because natural, nonhydrogenated extra-virgin coconut oil has been shown to actually increase HDL and improve the cholesterol profile. You can use coconut oil, or the new coconut spread product, in the crust for our Lime Cheesecake with Pecan-Gingersnap Crust (page 258).

COOKING SPRAY: We recommend using a little olive oil cooking spray to keep foods from sticking to skillets and baking pans. Avoid butter-flavored sprays. You can buy a commercial product or use your own sprayer filled with extra-virgin olive oil.

CORNMEAL: Cornmeal, which is simply ground dried corn, can be enjoyed beginning on GS Phase 2. Available in white, yellow, and blue, it is a good gluten-free option for baked goods such as our Three Sisters Bread (page 240) and in the johnnycakes used for our Johnnycake Chicken Sandwiches (page 87). It's also the primary ingredient in the Italian dish polenta (a medium-ground cornmeal is usually used), but before ordering it at a restaurant, ask if the dish is gluten free: Polenta is sometimes made with wheat semolina. Because of its oil content ground cornmeal can become rancid quickly, so keep it refrigerated in a tightly covered container. See also Masa Harina (page 284); Tortillas, Corn (page 292).

COUSCOUS: See Brown Rice Couscous (page 275).

DELI MEATS: All-natural, lower-sodium and nitrite- and nitrate-free cold cuts and other deli meats are always preferred. Avoid those that are honey or maple flavored. Watch out for deli meats that have modified food starches, which are used to bind water. We use deli-sliced gluten-free all-natural uncured smoked ham for our Green Eggs and Ham recipe (page 40) and deli-sliced all-natural uncured mesquite smoked turkey breast for our Kale and Smoked Turkey Soup (page 75).

DRIED FRUITS: Dried fruits, such as dried cherries (page 29) and dried apricots may be enjoyed in moderation beginning on GS Phase 2. Be aware that certain dried fruits may have a dusting of flour to prevent clumping (look for packages that say 100% pure fruit).

DUCK: See Poultry (page 289).

EDAMAME: See Beans and Other Legumes (page 272).

EGGS: An economical source of protein, eggs are also packed with vitamin B_{12}, riboflavin, and selenium. They are not limited on any GS phase, unless otherwise directed by your doctor. All of the recipes in this book use large eggs. In some of the recipes we have used liquid egg whites for convenience. Never use liquid egg whites in recipes that call for beating eggs to peaks, because pasteurization prevents them from whipping up properly. You can experiment with using liquid egg whites in recipes where we call for whole eggs, but they don't always work the same way, particularly in baking.

ESPRESSO POWDER: Made from ground espresso coffee beans, instant espresso powder adds a complex coffee flavor to baked goods. You can find it at specialty-food stores or make your own by drying leftover espresso grounds (from the cups of espresso you've made) on a baking sheet in a low oven for about an hour, then grinding them to a fine texture using a coffee grinder or mini food processor.

Espresso powder is a key ingredient in our Chocolate Walnut Espresso Cake (page 253) because it enhances the flavor of the dark chocolate.

EVAPORATED MILK: We use fat-free canned evaporated milk, also known as dehydrated milk, to add creaminess to the Chickpea and Sweet Potato Bisque (page 76).

EXTRACTS: Flavored extracts like pure almond, vanilla, lemon, peppermint, and black walnut can be enjoyed on all phases of the South Beach Diet Gluten Solution Program. Use them in baked goods and to flavor smoothies and yogurt desserts. Be sure to choose pure extracts, made without barley malt, which contains gluten.

FISH AND SHELLFISH: Fish and shellfish are a good source of protein. Fattier types, such as salmon, sardines, and lake trout, are high in heart-healthy omega-3 fatty acids. Since there are so many types available, we can't provide information on all of them here—but we do cover those that are used in this book. Some fish, such as canned albacore tuna, swordfish, tilefish, king mackerel, orange roughy, and shark, should be limited because of their high mercury content.

- **Bay scallops:** Harvested from bays along the East Coast from New England to North Carolina, bay scallops (once removed from the shell) are only about ½ inch in diameter. They have a firm texture and a very sweet delicate flavor. Try them in Green Curry with Scallops and Peppers (page 138).

- **Clams:** You can buy live, fresh clams in the shell, as well as shucked and frozen or canned. We call for tiny, sweet fresh Manila clams, which we serve in the shell for "Spaghetti" with Red Clam Sauce (page 124). Look for them at large supermarkets and fish markets.

- **Cod:** This very tasty, lean white fish has a firm texture and a mild flavor. Enjoy it in Batter-Baked Cod with Homemade Mango Chutney (page 126) or as part of our Fish Cakes with Pepper Salsa (page 131).

- **Grouper:** Firm-textured grouper has a mild flavor that's a cross between bass and halibut. Red grouper is sweeter and milder than black grouper. You can use either in California Fish Tacos (page 128).

- **Mahi mahi:** This mild-tasting, meaty fish is the perfect complement to the Asian-inspired oil we make for the Broiled Mahi Mahi with Sizzling Scallion Oil recipe (page 127).

- **Salmon:** Thiamin, niacin, omega-3 fatty acids, potassium, and the vitamins

B_6, $B_{12,}$ and D are just a few of the healthful nutrients salmon offers. Salmon is available fresh, smoked, and canned; we use fresh salmon fillets in the Salmon Salade Niçoise (page 105), Sesame Salmon Fingers with Lemon-Dill Cream (page 132), and Baked Salmon with Spinach and Couscous (page 135), and canned pink or sockeye salmon in our Mini Salmon Loaves (page 136).

- **Shrimp:** This popular shellfish is widely available both fresh and frozen (and also peeled and deveined). Shrimp lend themselves to a variety of cooking techniques: sauté, grill, steam, or bake them. Remember, shrimp cook up in mere minutes, so don't overcook them or they'll become tough and flavorless. We use shrimp in Shrimp and Chicken Pad Thai (page 139), Quinoa Pasta Salad with Shrimp (page 140), and Creamy Asparagus-Pea Soup with Deviled Shrimp (page 79).

- **Striped bass:** We use this firm, well-flavored fish in Manhattan Fish Stew (page 130) and Fish Cakes with Pepper Salsa (page 131).

- **Tilapia:** Also known as St. Peter's fish, tilapia is a firm-fleshed, mild-tasting, farm-raised fish that is widely available in many supermarkets. We broil it coated with miso paste for Miso-Glazed Tilapia (page 137).

- **Trout:** These freshwater fish have a mild, sweet flavor and are good broiled, grilled, or baked. We bake brook trout for Lemon-Baked Trout with Green Goddess Sauce (page 129).

- **Tuna:** An excellent source of B vitamins, tuna is rich in omega-3 fatty acids and the mineral selenium. Buy it fresh for Grilled Tuna Steaks with Old Bay and Orange Dressing (page 145) and Pepper Tuna Rolls (page 59) and use light, water-packed tuna for Asparagus, Portobello, and Tuna Bake (page 142) and Tuna Burgers with Citrus Mayo (page 144). Avoid canned albacore tuna, which can be high in mercury.

FLOURS, GLUTEN-FREE: Avoid all flours, gluten free or not, on Gluten Solution Phase 1. You can cook or bake with gluten-free flours beginning on GS Phase 2. The following flours are used in this book, usually in combination for enhanced flavor and lighter texture. As you become more confident with gluten-free baking, you can experiment with your own combinations in recipes. Most of these flours can be purchased at major supermarkets; you can also find them at health-food stores and online (see page 295 for online sources). See also Bean Flours (page 271); Nut Flours (page 285).

- **Brown rice flour:** Because it contains the bran, brown rice flour is higher in fiber and contains more protein than white rice flour (which we do not recommend using on any phase of the Gluten Solution Program). Brown rice flour adds a slightly nutty flavor to baked goods such as our Bacon-Pecan Breakfast Biscuits (page 22), Summer Berry Tart (page 260), and Chocolate Walnut Espresso Cake (page 253). It can also be used to thicken sauces and make coatings for baked fish and poultry. Brown rice flour should be stored in the freezer to keep it from becoming rancid.

- **Buckwheat flour:** Made from ground buckwheat, 100% buckwheat flour is a good gluten-free option to whole-wheat flour in pancakes, muffins, and other baked goods. It is typically ground with the outer bran, which is high in fiber and other nutrients. It's the bran that turns the resulting flour a rich brown color, with dark flecks. Because it is strongly flavored, we combine buckwheat flour with other gluten-free flours in our Belgian Waffles (page 24), Gingerbread Muffins (page 26), and Peanut Butter–Banana Pancakes (page 27).

- **Flaxseed meal (flour):** Nutty-tasting flaxseeds are extremely nutritious: They contain both soluble and insoluble fiber, plant-based omega-3s in the form of ALA, and a good amount of protein. Using a little ground flaxseed (flaxseed meal) with other gluten-free flours lends suppleness to gluten-free baked goods. Buy preground flaxseed meal or grind whole flaxseeds in a coffee grinder or blender, since grinding the seeds allows your body to absorb their nutrients (whole seeds pass through your system undigested). Because of its oil content, store flaxseed meal in the freezer. (Whole flaxseeds keep at room temperature for at least a year.) We use flaxseed meal in our Coconut-Apple Muffins (page 25), Gingerbread Muffins (page 26), Oatmeal Breakfast Wedges (page 31), and Cashew Butter Cookies (page 252).

- **Oat flour:** Oat flour has the subtle, sweet flavor of whole oats and is best combined with other gluten-free flours in baked goods to produce a lighter texture. High in protein, calcium, and fiber, oat flour does not contain gluten, but like other oat products is subject to potential cross-contamination by other grains in the field, or in facilities that also handle wheat. Look for certified gluten-free oat flour or make your own by grinding certified gluten-free rolled oats or oatmeal flakes in a clean coffee grinder or blender. We combine it with flaxseed meal, almond flour, and coconut flour in "Everything" Oat Bread (page 86).

- **Quinoa flour:** Made by grinding quinoa, this earthy-tasting, high-protein flour is generally used in small quantities in combination with other gluten-free flours (using it alone can make baked goods heavy) to add moisture and a good crumb. We combine it with almond and coconut flours in the crust for our Lemon Bars (page 266).
- **Sorghum flour:** High in protein and fiber, sorghum flour has a slightly sweet taste similar to wheat and a darker color than many other gluten-free flours. We use it in combination with other gluten-free flours in our Gingerbread Muffins (page 26), to coat the fish for our California Fish Tacos (page 128), and in the dumplings for Chicken Soup with Dumplings (page 82).
- **Tapioca flour:** See Tapioca Starch (page 292).
- **Teff flour:** Made from the tiny, khaki-colored gluten-free grain called teff, which is similar to millet, this nutty-tasting flour has twice the iron and three times the calcium of the flour made from many other grains. It is commonly used to make injera (Ethiopian flatbread). We combine it with buckwheat flour in our Belgian Waffles (page 24).

GUAR GUM: This powder, made from a beanlike plant, is often used, like Xanthan Gum (page 294), to keep gluten-free baked goods from becoming too dry and crumbly. Guar gum is less expensive than xanthan gum. We do not use guar gum or xanthan gum in this book, but have included information on it for your interest.

HAM: See Deli Meats (page 279).

HERBS: Adding herbs to your dishes not only enhances flavor but also allows you to use less salt in cooking. In the summer, fresh herbs are particularly plentiful, but you can use dried as a substitute. A rule of thumb: Because fresh herbs are generally less potent and not as concentrated as dried herbs, you'll need more (three times the amount of fresh herbs as dried). For example, if a recipe calls for 1 teaspoon of dried thyme, you'll need 1 tablespoon of fresh thyme to achieve the same level of flavor. Check labels on herb blends, such as Italian seasoning, for gluten additives.

HORSERADISH: You can enhance sauces, spreads, dressings, and sandwiches with prepared horseradish, which can be found jarred in the refrigerated section of the supermarket. You can also purchase this spicy member of the cabbage family fresh in the produce section and grate it yourself. It gives the yogurt sauce for Pepper Tuna Rolls (page 59) a nice kick.

JÍCAMA: Also known as yam bean or Mexican turnip, jícama is a large, bulbous root vegetable native to Central America. High in fiber and vitamin C, it has a sweet, nutty flavor that resembles a water chestnut. It's delicious raw in salads and on crudité platters, and it can also be cooked. We bake it for our Jícama Fries (page 220) and Jícama Cheese Toasties (page 83). Be sure to peel off the thin outer skin before using.

KASHA: See Buckwheat (page 275).

LENTILS: See Beans and Other Legumes (page 272).

MASA HARINA: Made from hominy that has been soaked in lime (calcium oxide, not lime juice), this finely ground cornmeal flour is typically used to make corn tortillas. It's the basis for the dough for our Italian Tamales (page 176), and we use it to coat Jícama Fries (page 220). If you don't have masa harina on hand, you can use yellow cornmeal instead.

MAYONNAISE: Used sparingly, mayonnaise makes a delicious addition to sandwiches, salad dressings, dips, and sauces. You can use regular mayonnaise, low-fat mayo, or light mayo. Avoid fat-free varieties, because they often contain added sugar, such as high-fructose corn syrup. In this book we use regular mayonnaise made with extra-virgin olive oil in our Creamy Hot Broccoli Dip (page 48), Tuna Burgers with Citrus Mayo (page 144), and other recipes.

MILK: Milk is an important source of protein, calcium, and vitamins A, D, and B_{12} on all phases of the Gluten Solution Program and is used in a wide variety of recipes in this book. Choose fat-free or 1% milk, which contain the same nutrients as whole milk but without the high amount of saturated fat. See also Almond Milk, Unsweetened (page 271); Buttermilk (page 275); Coconut Milk, Lite (page 278); Evaporated Milk (page 280).

MILK POWDER, NONFAT DRY: Nonfat dry milk is the most concentrated form of milk. With all of the water removed, dry milk powder has about 27 percent protein, versus dairy milk with about 3.25 percent . We use it to add richness and extra protein to our Bacon-Pecan Breakfast Biscuits (page 22), Banana Cream Pie Breakfast Shake (page 32), and Amaranth, Almond, and Apricot Breakfast Cereal (page 30).

MISO PASTE: Miso is a fermented soybean paste generally sold in resealable packages or plastic or glass containers in Japanese groceries, as well as in most health-food stores and many larger supermarkets. In general, the lighter in color the miso, the less salty it is. "White" miso is actually golden yellow in color and has a sweet flavor. Read the label carefully, because some misos can contain barley or wheat, and thus gluten. We use white miso paste for Miso-Glazed Tilapia (page 137).

MONK FRUIT NATURAL NO-CALORIE SWEETENER: Monk fruit got its name from the Buddhist monks who cultivated the fruit centuries ago in southern China. Today the fruit is available as a natural, calorie-free sweetener that comes as a very sweet white powder (in packets) or in bulk (called baking formula). In this book we developed our recipes using all-natural Monk Fruit In The Raw baking formula (if we used the packets, it is indicated in the recipe). If you buy another brand of monk fruit baking formula, you will have to experiment, since sweetness can vary. We use the sweetener, sometimes in tandem with a little agave nectar, in our breads, muffins, and desserts. See also Agave Nectar (page 270); Sugar Substitutes (page 292).

MUSTARD: Most types of mustard are gluten free, including Dijon, which we use in this book. Certain brands of yellow mustard and mustard powder may have gluten additives, however, so check labels carefully. Also avoid honey mustard and honey-mustard dressing, which contain high amounts of added sugar, on all GS phases. Dijon flavors our Roasted Cauliflower and Celeriac Rémoulade (page 246) and Mustard-Roasted Pork and Apple Salad (page 101).

NUT FLOURS: Nut flours are made from ground nuts and work best in combination with other gluten-free flours. Because of their high oil content, nut flours can go rancid quickly. Store them airtight in the freezer for up to 6 months. The following nut flours are used in this book:

- **Almond flour:** Also sold under the name almond meal, this off-white, high-protein flour is usually ground from blanched almonds and can be used in any number of ways. We put it in the coating for Coconut-Almond Chicken Strips (page 56) and in the cheese sauce for Quinoa Macaroni with Asparagus and Almonds (page 209), and we mix it with other gluten-free flours for our Cinnamon Cherry Scones (page 29), Lemon Zucchini Bread (page 44), and Lemon Bars (page 266). You can make your own almond flour by grinding blanched almonds in a blender or food processor. Take care not to overprocess or you will have almond butter.
- **Coconut flour:** Ground from defatted coconut meat, this fragrant, slightly sweet high-fiber flour (just 2 tablespoons has 5 grams of fiber!) is typically

found mixed with other flours in baked goods (your desserts will fall apart if coconut flour is used alone). We use it in our Gingerbread Muffins (page 26), Peanut Butter–Banana Pancakes (page 27), and Caramelized Apple Mini-Shortcakes (page 256).

NUTS/NUT BUTTERS: Nuts and nut butters, such as peanut butter and cashew butter, can be enjoyed on all phases of the South Beach Diet Gluten Solution. High in plant protein and fiber, they make a great snack and add a wonderful crunch to a wide variety of dishes. Because nuts are calorie-dense, they should be enjoyed in moderation. Be aware that if you buy seasoned nuts that have been coated with a flavoring agent, they may be processed on equipment that also processes wheat. Check labels on dry-roasted nuts; some may have flavorings with added gluten. Also avoid those with sugary coatings. Many varieties of nuts, such as almonds and pistachios, come pretoasted or roasted.

- **Almonds:** Rich in vitamin E, these heart-healthy nuts also contain riboflavin, iron, and magnesium and are higher in fiber and calcium than most other nuts. We use almonds in the Quinoa Macaroni with Asparagus and Almonds (page 209), Grilled Duck and Pear Salad with Almonds (page 99), and Triple-Green "Stir-Fry" with Almonds (page 247).
- **Cashew butter:** Made from raw or roasted cashews, cashew butter can be used in smoothies, sauces, and desserts, or as a substitute for peanut butter. We use it in our Cashew Butter Cookies (page 252). Choose all-natural cashew butter with 1 gram of sugar or less per 2 tablespoons.
- **Cashews:** These nuts are always sold shelled and come raw (unroasted), roasted, or dry roasted. We grind cashews to a paste to add depth to the sauce for Thai Eggplant Curry (page 212).
- **Peanut butter:** High in monounsaturated fat, folate, and resveratrol (the phytochemical also found in red wine that helps protect against heart disease and cancer), peanut butter is wonderful in Peanut Butter–Banana Pancakes (page 27), Spiced Peanut Wafers (page 62), Chicken and Sweet Potato Salad with Spicy Peanut Dressing (page 96), and "Sesame" Noodles (page 225). It also makes a satisfying, high-protein snack spread onto celery or endive on GS Phase 1 or onto gluten-free crackers or fruit slices on GS Phase 2. Choose all-natural peanut butter with 1 gram of sugar or less per 2 tablespoons.
- **Peanuts:** Though used and thought of as nuts, peanuts are actually legumes.

Sold raw, roasted, or dry roasted, they contain good amounts of vitamin E, folate, niacin, and magnesium. We use unsalted dry-roasted peanuts in the Toasted Oat and Peanut Cookies (page 262).

- **Pecans:** Rich in thiamin, zinc, and fiber, pecans are available shelled and unshelled. We grind them for the batter for our Bacon-Pecan Breakfast Biscuits (page 22), use them in Lime Cheesecake with Pecan-Gingersnap Crust (page 258), and sprinkle them atop Fresh Peach Compote (page 265).

- **Pine nuts:** Also known as pignoli or *piñon,* pine nuts are the seeds of certain pinecones, in particular those from the Mexican and Colorado piñon pine. Delicious in salads, pastas, and baked goods, they come toasted and untoasted. Because of their high oil content, it's best to keep pine nuts in the refrigerator or freezer. Enjoy them in Green and White Pasta (page 204) and Baked Salmon with Spinach and Couscous (page 135).

- **Pistachios:** Pistachios provide vitamin E, iron, thiamin, and magnesium. Sprinkle them over salads, vegetable dishes, and desserts. We combine them with chopped hard-boiled eggs for the topping for Green Beans Mimosa (page 229).

- **Walnuts:** Walnuts are unique in the nut world in that they are the only nut that contains alpha-linolenic acid (ALA), a polyunsaturated fatty acid related to the heart-protective omega-3s. We use them in our Artichoke, Edamame, and Walnut Salad (page 106), Asparagus Salad with Feta and Toasted Nuts (page 111), Baked Lentils with Mushrooms and Walnuts (page 242), and Chocolate Walnut Espresso Cake (page 253).

OATS: Oats are impressively high in fiber and also a good source of thiamin, iron, selenium, magnesium, and zinc. Be aware that oats and oat products (such as oat flour and oatmeal, as well as gluten-free breads made with oats and oat bran) may be cross-contaminated with wheat during processing; look for oat products labeled certified gluten-free. We use certified gluten-free quick-cooking oats in the Oatmeal Breakfast Wedges (page 31) and Toasted Oat and Peanut Cookies (page 262) and rolled oats and oat bran in the Oat Cake Quesadillas (page 90). See also Oat flour (page 282).

OILS: Healthy unsaturated oils are extremely important ingredients on all phases of the Gluten Solution Program. You'll use them for sautéing, for making salad dressings, and for drizzling over grilled vegetables, for example. They're also an important component in baked goods. You'll want to store most oils in a cool, dark place (except for nut oils, which belong in the refrigerator). We use the following oils in this book:

- **Canola oil:** This bland-tasting oil comes from the seeds of the same plant that gives us the vegetable broccoli rabe. The oil is rich in alpha-linolenic acid (ALA), a heart-protective polyunsaturated fatty acid. Although canola oil is not used in this book, we include it here because it can be used in place of extra-virgin olive oil in some recipes, if you prefer.

- **Extra-virgin olive oil:** Made from the first pressing of olives, this primarily monounsaturated oil has a low acid content and a delicate flavor. Research now shows that many of olive oil's health benefits may actually come from the more than 30 plant compounds it contains that have antioxidant and anti-inflammatory effects.

- **Peanut oil:** A combination of mono- and polyunsaturated fats, mildly nutty-tasting peanut oil (which also contains the antioxidant resveratrol) is a good alternative to canola oil for sautéing because of its high smoke point (use the unroasted oil for cooking).

- **Sesame oil:** Dark-brown roasted sesame oil is used in many recipes in this book. Look for it in the Asian section of larger supermarkets and be sure to store it in the refrigerator.

PASTA, GLUTEN-FREE: You can enjoy nutritious, fiber-rich gluten-free pasta beginning on GS Phase 2. Choose varieties with 2.5 to 4 grams or more of fiber per ½-cup cooked serving if you're enjoying it as a side dish. While many types of gluten-free pastas are available, including some made from bean flours and soy, as well as 100% buckwheat soba noodles, we use the following gluten-free pastas in this book:

- **Brown rice pasta:** Brown rice pasta is made from ground brown rice. It comes in a variety of shapes. You can use either fusilli or rotelle in Green and White Pasta (page 204) and brown rice spaghetti or linguine in Shrimp and Chicken Pad Thai (page 139).

- **Multigrain pasta:** This pasta is typically made from a combination of rice bran, quinoa, and amaranth flours. We use multigrain penne pasta in the Gluten Solution SuperSalad (page 108) and multigrain spaghetti in Pork Meatballs with Broken Spaghetti (page 196) and in "Sesame" Noodles (page 225).

• **Quinoa pasta/elbow macaroni:** Quinoa pasta is made from ground quinoa and is often combined with corn flour. We use quinoa elbow macaroni in Quinoa Macaroni with Asparagus and Almonds (page 209) and Pasta e Fagioli (page 81); quinoa shells in Quinoa Penne Salad with Shrimp (page 140); and quinoa radiatore in Turkey Tetrazzini with Portobellos (page 173).

PEPPERONCINI: Also known as Tuscan peppers or sweet Italian peppers, these pickled chile peppers are widely available jarred and range from medium to medium-hot. We use them in our Jícama Cheese Toasties (page 83).

PEPPERONI, TURKEY: Low in saturated fat, turkey pepperoni is a good alternative to fatty beef pepperoni on all phases of the Gluten Solution Program. Make sure to look at labels and buy brands that are gluten free. We use it in the Spicy Sausage, Black Bean, and Pepper Soup (page 73).

PORK: Pork chops, cutlets, loin, and tenderloin are all excellent sources of lean protein as well as vitamin B_{12} and niacin. Among the delicious pork recipes you'll find in this book are Garlicky Roast Pork and Tomato Salad (page 102), Mustard-Roasted Pork and Apple Salad (page 101), Baked Stuffed Pork Chops (page 192), Braised Pork Rolls (page 193), and Orange-Maple Pork Tenderloin (page 191). See also Bacon (page 271); Deli Meats (page 279).

POULTRY: You can enjoy skinless chicken, turkey, and duck breast, as well as ground turkey and chicken breast, on all phases of the Gluten Solution Program. You can also have gluten-free turkey bacon, turkey pepperoni, and gluten-free low-fat turkey or chicken sausages (with 3 to 6 grams fat per 60-gram serving). If you are buying sliced deli chicken or turkey breast, watch out for brands that have modified food starches, which contain gluten and are used to bind water. Also choose deli meats that are all-natural, lower-sodium, and nitrite and nitrate free. Avoid dark meat chicken and turkey (legs and wings), as well as goose, which contain more saturated fat. Also avoid processed poultry nuggets and patties, which often contain gluten. Purchase natural, free-range chicken and turkey when possible. We use poultry in soups, salads, and main dishes, including Chicken Soup with Dumplings (page 82), Grilled Duck and Pear Salad with Almonds (page 99), Salsa Grilled Turkey and Macaroni Salad (page 110), Chicken Chop Suey (page 151), and Spanish-Spiced Turkey Meatballs (page 57), among other recipes.

PRUNE BUTTER/PURÉE: Prune butter (also called prune purée) refers to a spread that is made from pitted prunes (dried plums) and water or fruit juice. Look for unsweetened varieties. You can use prune butter as a healthy spread or in recipes for gluten-free baked goods. If you like, make your own by puréeing prunes in a mini food processor with a little hot water until smooth. We add it to Peking Chicken Wraps (page 166), and it's the second "plum" in the Double Plum Clafouti (page 264).

QUINOA: Botanically a relative of Swiss chard and beets, quinoa is often referred to as a "super grain" because it is high in protein and fiber. While many brands of quinoa are sold prerinsed, some recommend rinsing to remove the naturally occurring residue of bitter saponins, the plant's defense against insects (follow package directions). Quinoa comes in a variety of colors, including white, red, and tricolor; the darker the quinoa the more antioxidant-rich beta-carotene it has. We use tricolor quinoa in Herbed Tricolor Quinoa Pilaf with Shallots (page 223) and red quinoa in Chicken, Butternut, and Quinoa Soup (page 66), but you can use whatever you have on hand. See also Quinoa flour (page 283); Quinoa pasta/elbow macaroni (page 289).

RICE: See Brown Rice (page 275).

RICE VINEGAR: See Vinegar (page 293).

SALAD DRESSING: In this book, we offer many easy, healthy salad dressings within recipes for the various salads (not in a separate dressing and condiment section). If you find a few you love, you can always make them to dress a simple mixed green salad or even to drizzle over a side of vegetables. If you do purchase a prepared salad dressing, look for a low-sugar variety that contains no more than 3 grams of sugar per serving. Remember to steer clear of low-fat salad dressings, which are often high in sugars and may have gluten additives.

SALSA: Typically containing chopped tomatoes, onions, chiles, and cilantro, salsa comes canned, jarred, and fresh (in the refrigerated section of many supermarkets). Check labels carefully for added gluten. We use medium-hot gluten-free jarred salsa for Salsa Grilled Turkey and Macaroni Salad (page 110) and make our own for Fish Cakes with Pepper Salsa (page 131) and Spice-Rubbed Grilled Duck Breast with Fresh Plum Salsa (page 168).

SALT: Using a small amount of salt in cooking helps to enhance the flavors of food. Table salt is the most common type of salt used for cooking, but in this book we also use coarse kosher salt (which has less sodium by volume than table salt). Do not substitute equivalent amounts of table salt for kosher salt in recipes because your recipe will be far too salty.

SEEDS: All seeds are high in fiber, and many are excellent sources of plant protein. They add a wonderful crunch to salads, baked goods, smoothies, and more, and can be enjoyed on all phases of the Gluten Solution Program. Seeds are also used to make oils. Because of their high oil content, seeds can become rancid quickly and should therefore be stored airtight in the refrigerator, where they will keep for up to 6 months. We use the following seeds in recipes in this book:

- **Chia seeds:** These tiny seeds are an excellent source of fiber and heart-healthy omega-3 fatty acids. They come in both black and white varieties (though there is virtually no difference in the nutrients between the two). They can be used as a natural thickener in smoothies, soups, salad dressings, and sauces, and can be ground and used instead of whole-wheat bread crumbs as a binder for meatballs and burgers. We add chia seeds to our Bacon-Pecan Breakfast Biscuits (page 22) and Banana Cream Pie Breakfast Shake (page 32).

- **Poppy seeds:** The small dried seeds of the poppy plant, these crunchy black seeds are most often used in baking. They add texture and an almost nutty flavor to baked goods such as our Lemon Zucchini Bread (page 44) and "Everything" Oat Bread (page 86).

- **Pumpkin seeds:** Pumpkin seeds, also known as pepitas, are an excellent source of zinc, and also provide essential and nonessential fatty acids. They are sold in the shell, shelled, roasted, and raw in health-food stores and better supermarkets. We sprinkle them over Southwestern Three-Pepper Pork Chili (page 200) and Mexican Bean and Cheese Salad (page 107).

- **Sesame seeds:** These tiny oval seeds come hulled and unhulled. The unhulled type, which are darker in color, have the bran intact and are a source of iron and phosphorus. You can use either type in the coatings for Sesame Salmon Fingers with Lemon-Dill Cream (page 132) and Jícama Fries (page 220), and in the dressing for Rainbow Chard Salad with Sesame-Carrot Dressing (page 115).

SHELLFISH: See Fish and Shellfish (page 280).
SORGHUM FLOUR: See Flours, Gluten-Free (page 281).
SOY SAUCE: Many brands of soy sauce are made with wheat (and therefore gluten) and are also high in sodium. In this book we use gluten-free reduced-sodium tamari soy sauce to flavor Ginger-Garlic Eggplant Skewers (page 61), Grilled Duck

and Pear Salad with Almonds (page 99), Shrimp and Chicken Pad Thai (page 139), Chicken Chop Suey (page 151), and Spicy Chicken and Broccoli (page 155).

SPICES: These aromatic seasonings come from the bark, buds, fruit, roots, seeds, or stems of plants and trees. In general spices do not contain gluten, but check labels on spice blends and chili powder in particular. Using spices in your cooking is an easy—and quick—way to add more flavor to food. Buy spices ground or whole and store them in a cool, dark place for up to 6 months.

SPLIT PEAS: See Beans and Other Legumes (page 272).

SUGAR SUBSTITUTES: While there are many types of sugar substitutes available, including sucralose (Splenda), stevia, stevia and erythritol (Truvía), aspartame (Equal, NutraSweet), and saccharin (Sweet'N Low), we chose to go all-natural in this book, using agave nectar and monk fruit for our baked goods and other recipes. See Agave Nectar (page 270); Monk Fruit Natural No-Calorie Sweetener (page 285).

TAMARI: See Soy Sauce (page 291).

TAPIOCA STARCH: Tapioca starch (also called tapioca flour) is ground from the starchy, tuberous root of the cassava plant, and thus it's gluten free. Tapioca adds body and a chewy texture to gluten-free baked goods. We combine it with brown rice flour in our Chocolate Walnut Espresso Cake (page 253).

TEFF FLOUR: See Flours, Gluten-Free (page 281).

TOFU: Made from soymilk curd, which is pressed into small blocks (similar to the way that cheese is made), tofu is rich in iron and is also a good source of protein. Tofu comes in silken and regular varieties, which in turn are divided into soft, firm, and extra-firm. Silken tofu is smoother and generally better for baking or smoothies; regular is more granular in texture and works better for the recipes in this book. We use firm tofu in the Indian Saag Paneer (page 215) and Tofu and Egg Migas (page 213) and extra-firm in the Tofu Frittata with Asparagus and Tomato (page 207), Baked Stuffed Tofu (page 217), and Tofu-Mushroom Lasagna (page 216). Be aware that some preseasoned types of tofu may contain gluten additives.

TORTILLAS, CORN: You can use 100% corn tortillas in cooking beginning on GS Phase 2. Check labels carefully, because some brands that are not 100% corn may include wheat and/or gluten additives. Also choose varieties that have 3 grams or more fiber per serving and no trans fats. We use corn tortillas in our Spanish-Spiced Turkey Meatballs (page 57), Tofu and Egg Migas (page 213), California Fish Tacos (page 128), Chicken Chilaquiles (page 150), and Crispy-Topped Mac and Cheese (page 214).

TURKEY: See Poultry (page 289).

VINEGAR: Vinegar adds a bright, jazzy flavor to marinades and salad dressings. Among the most popular varieties are balsamic vinegar, champagne vinegar, apple cider vinegar, rice vinegar, sherry vinegar, and red and white wine vinegar. Here's a quick rundown on those we use in a wide variety of recipes this book:

- **Apple cider vinegar:** Made from the fermented juice of pressed apples, this is a pungent, acidic vinegar that's a good addition to salad dressings, stews, vegetable side dishes, and more. We use it in Hot and Sour Cabbage Soup with Pork (page 71), Chickpea-Fennel Stew with Greens (page 208), and other recipes.

- **Balsamic vinegar:** This flavorful, slightly sweet fruit vinegar is made in Modena, Italy, from highly concentrated grape juice that never becomes wine. It's reduced by cooking, then aged in wooden barrels. Long-aged balsamics are too intensely sweet for the recipes in this book. We use the supermarket variety in Asparagus Salad with Feta and Toasted Nuts (page 111), Grilled Romaine Lettuce (page 235), and other recipes.

- **Rice vinegar:** Made from fermented rice, this mild, slightly sweet vinegar is often used in Asian cooking. Look for rice vinegar, made from fermented rice, in the Asian section of large supermarkets or, for the highest quality, in Asian liquor stores. It's used to flavor our Peking Chicken Wraps (page 166).

- **Wine vinegar:** Made from a variety of wines, these acidic vinegars include red wine vinegar, white wine vinegar, and sherry vinegar. We use red wine vinegar in Warm Beef and Broccoli Romesco Salad (page 100) and other recipes, and sherry vinegar or white wine vinegar in Grilled Duck and Pear Salad with Almonds (page 99).

WHITE BEAN FLOUR: See Bean Flours (page 271).

WINE: Red or white wine can be enjoyed as a beverage starting on GS Phase 2. Drink a glass of wine with a meal or right after, because wine contains natural sugar that can raise blood sugar and cause cravings. It can also be used in cooking on all GS phases, because the alcohol evaporates. In this book we use dry sherry or white wine in the Spicy Chicken and Broccoli (page 155), dry red or white wine in the Turkey Moussaka (page 162), and red wine to flavor Slow-Cooker Pulled Beef (page 186), for example.

WORCESTERSHIRE SAUCE: This piquant condiment typically contains anchovies, tamarind, and vinegar and may contain gluten in the form of soy sauce.

Look for gluten-free Worcestershire sauce, now widely available. We use it in the beef mixture for Smoked Portobello Sloppy Joes (page 89) and in the jerk paste for Jerk Flank Steak (page 183).

XANTHAN GUM: A white powder typically produced by fermenting corn sugar, xanthan gum is often used to prevent gluten-free breads and other baked goods from becoming dry and crumbly. It can be used interchangeably with guar gum. Some xanthan gum products may be derived from other sources such as wheat or soy, so reading labels is essential. We do not use xanthan gum or guar gum in this book but we have included information here for your interest.

YOGURT: High in calcium, yogurt also provides protein, B vitamins, and minerals. It's a versatile ingredient that can be enjoyed in a wide variety of dishes from breakfasts to desserts. Plain nonfat or low-fat yogurt is fine on all Gluten Solution phases. We use regular nonfat plain yogurt for Oatmeal Breakfast Wedges (page 31) and Banana Cream Pie Breakfast Shake (page 32). We also use nonfat (0%) plain Greek yogurt (which is strained more than regular yogurt and has a thicker texture and considerably more protein than regular yogurt) in a wide variety of recipes in this book, including Sesame Salmon Fingers with Lemon-Dill Cream (page 132), Turkey Moussaka (page 162), Sweet Potatoes Bravas (page 237), Citrus Yogurt Pie (page 254), and Strawberry-Apple Breakfast Fool (page 34).

ZEST: Many recipes in this book call for the grated zest of a lemon or lime—the flavorful, colorful part of the peel. To zest a fruit, wash the fruit, then use a rasp-style citrus grater or the fine side of a box grater to remove the zest, being careful to avoid the white pith underneath (which has a bitter taste). Lemon zest adds zing to our Lemon Zucchini Bread (page 44) and lime zest enhances the flavor of Lime Cheesecake with Pecan-Gingersnap Crust (page 258). You can have lemon, lime, and even orange zest (but not the orange fruit itself) on all phases of the South Beach Diet Gluten Solution Program.

RESOURCES

ONLINE SHOPPING

Always check nutrition labels carefully, if possible, when shopping online to make sure you get the healthiest products.

BEFREEFORME
befreeforme.com
Offers free coupons and samples to consumers with celiac disease, gluten intolerance, or food allergies.

THE GLUTEN-FREE MALL
glutenfreemall.com
You can shop for more than 1,000 gluten-free products from 130-plus leading brands.

GLUTEN-FREE TRADING COMPANY
gluten-free.net
Gluten-free groceries from suppliers around the world.

GLUTEN SOLUTIONS
glutensolutions.com
Offers a wide variety of gluten-free foods.

Online Suppliers of Gluten-Free Flours, Grains, and More

AMAZON
amazon.com
Check out their prices for gluten-free pastas, grains, and more from many purveyors.

BARRY FARM FOODS
barryfarm.com/flours.htm
Offers a large selection of gluten-free flours, including amaranth, sorghum, green pea, cashew, pistachio, and almond, to name just a few.

THE BIRKETT MILLS
thebirkettmills.com
The world's largest manufacturer of buckwheat products, established in 1797 in Penn Yan, NY, sells groats, kasha (whole, coarse, fine, and medium granulation), buckwheat flour, buckwheat cereal, and more.

BOB'S RED MILL
bobsredmill.com
The online source for an expansive line of gluten-free whole grains and flours, cereals, and other products, which you might not be able to find in your local supermarket. Excellent product descriptions help in ordering.

DEBOLES
deboles.com
Shop online for this company's delicious gluten-free rice and corn pastas in all shapes.

GF HARVEST
glutenfreeoats.com
Shop here for a variety of gluten-free oats and oat products.

KALUSTYAN'S
kalustyans.com
A New York City–based purveyor of specialty foods with a wide range of spices, herbs, and spice blends. Check blends carefully for gluten.

MEXGROCER
mexgrocer.com
This site offers more than 3,000 specialty Mexican and Latin products, including masa harina, chile peppers, spices, and more from imported and national leading brands.

MONK FRUIT IN THE RAW
intheraw.com
To find a retailer or order the Monk Fruit In The Raw Bakers Bag (the monk fruit baking formula we used for testing the recipes in this book), check out their website. This natural, zero-calorie sweetener measures cup for cup like sugar.

NORTHERN QUINOA CORPORATION
quinoa.com
This Canadian supplier offers a wide variety of quinoa products.

NUTS.COM
nuts.com
Offers a large selection of nuts (including many organic varieties), seeds, sugar-free dried fruits, and other gluten-free products. Certified by the Gluten-Free Certification Organization.

PENZEYS SPICES

penzeys.com

Great prices on a wide range of spices.

TRADER JOE'S

traderjoes.com/fearless-flyer/article.asp?article_id=412

This chain has its own brand of tricolor organic quinoa. You can't buy it online, but you can get it at one of their stores. Check out the article and the store finder.

VITACOST

vitacost.com

This discount supplier of nutritional supplements also sells a wide variety of gluten-free grain products, including Ancient Harvest quinoa pasta, Eden Foods red quinoa, and Arrowhead Mills organic quinoa, at great prices.

Other Useful Sites

CELIAC.COM

celiac.com

A comprehensive, well-written online resource dedicated to the support of those who have celiac disease and gluten sensitivity.

GLUTEN FREE GIRL AND THE CHEF

glutenfreegirl.com

Excellent food blog from celiac sufferer Shauna James Ahern and her chef husband, with recipes, videos, articles, and links.

NO GLUTEN, NO PROBLEM

Noglutennoproblem.blogspot.com

Musings on the gluten-free life, with recipes, product reviews, sports commentary, and more from runner and author Pete Bronski and his wife, Kelli. Great index of past articles.

GLUTEN-FREE DIET

glutenfreediet.ca

Resource center for information about celiac disease, gluten intolerance, and a gluten-free diet from respected nutritionist and author Shelley Case.

SIMPLY . . . GLUTEN-FREE

simplygluten-free.com

Television chef, freelance writer, and cookbook author Carol Kicinski's gluten-free blog. Recipes, recommendations for gluten-free products, and lots more.

GLUTEN-FREE DIETITIAN

glutenfreedietitian.com

How to follow a nutritious, gluten-free diet from respected nutritionist, dietitian, and author Tricia Thompson.

PUBLICATIONS FOR THE GLUTEN AWARE

DELICIOUS LIVING

deliciousliving.com

A complimentary publication distributed by natural-food stores. It began as a food magazine for the natural-foods industry but now covers a wide range of natural health topics. Search on "gluten" or "gluten-free" for recipes and articles.

DELIGHT GLUTEN-FREE MAGAZINE

delightglutenfree.com

A bimonthly international food and lifestyle publication for people living with food allergies and sensitivities.

EASY EATS

easyeats.com

An all-digital food and lifestyle magazine that challenges the traditional approach of what it means to be gluten free, by looking at life through a positive lens.

GLUTEN-FREE LIVING

glutenfreeliving.com

This magazine provides practical information about the gluten-free diet.

LIVING WITHOUT

livingwithout.com

A magazine for people with food allergies and sensitivities.

ORGANIZATIONS

AMERICAN CELIAC DISEASE ALLIANCE (ACDA)

2504 Duxbury Place
Alexandria, VA 22308
703-622-3331
americanceliac.org
A national organization devoted to advocating on behalf of the entire celiac community—patients, physicians, researchers, food manufacturers, and other service providers. The site offers the latest on the status of the long-anticipated gluten-free labeling legislation.

CELIAC DISEASE FOUNDATION (CDF)

20350 Ventura Blvd., Suite 240
Woodland Hills, CA 91364
818-716-1513
celiac.org
Dedicated to celiac awareness, education, advocacy, and research.

CELIAC SPRUE ASSOCIATION/USA INC.

PO Box 31700
Omaha, NE 68131-0700
877-272-4272
csaceliacs.org
The largest nonprofit celiac support group in America, with chapters and resource units across the country and members worldwide.

GLUTEN INTOLERANCE GROUP

31214 124th Avenue SE
Auburn, WA 98092-3667
253-833-6655
www.gluten.net
Oversees the Gluten-Free Certification Program (gfco.org) to assure food integrity and safety of gluten-free packaged products for consumers. The site provides a guide to more than 6,000 products, companies, and manufacturers that have met the group's strict standards confirmed by field inspections. Also runs the Gluten-Free Restaurant Awareness Program (glutenfreerestaurants.org), which helps restaurants establish gluten-free menus and provides a list of certified restaurants for consumers.

MEDICAL CENTERS

The following centers specialize in the expert diagnosis and treatment of people with celiac disease and other forms of gluten sensitivity. Many are involved in ongoing research and clinical trials.

CELIAC CENTER AT BETH ISRAEL DEACONESS MEDICAL CENTER

Harvard Medical School
330 Brookline Avenue
Boston, MA 02215
617-667-7000
celiacnow.org

CELIAC DISEASE CENTER AT COLUMBIA UNIVERSITY

Harkness Pavilion
180 Fort Washington Avenue, Suite 936
New York, NY 10032
212-342-4529
celiacdiseasecenter.org

CELIAC DISEASE CLINIC AT MAYO CLINIC

200 1st Street SW
Rochester, MN 55905
507-538-3270
mayoclinic.com/health /celiac-disease/DS00319

CENTER FOR CELIAC RESEARCH & TREATMENT

Yawkey Center for Outpatient Care
55 Fruit Street, Suite 6B
Boston, MA 02114
617-726-8705
celiaccenter.org

UNIVERSITY OF CHICAGO CELIAC DISEASE CENTER

5841 South Maryland Avenue, Mail Code 4069
Chicago, IL 60637
773-702-7593
cureceliacdisease.org

WILLIAM K. WARREN MEDICAL RESEARCH CENTER FOR CELIAC DISEASE

University of California, San Diego
9500 Gilman Drive, MC0623D
La Jolla, CA 92093-0623
858-822-1022
celiaccenter.ucsd.edu

INDEX

Underscored page references indicate boxed text. **Boldface** references indicate photographs.

VISIT SOUTHBEACHDIET.COM

For more health and weight loss tools, great recipes, customized meal plans, and support from registered dietitians and a vibrant community of South Beach Diet followers, visit SouthBeachDiet.com.